Sleep Disorders Management in Primary Care

Sleep Disorders Management in Primary Care

Guest Editor
Izolde Bouloukaki

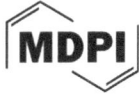

Basel • Beijing • Wuhan • Barcelona • Belgrade • Novi Sad • Cluj • Manchester

Guest Editor
Izolde Bouloukaki
Department of Social
Medicine
University of Crete
Heraklion
Greece

Editorial Office
MDPI AG
Grosspeteranlage 5
4052 Basel, Switzerland

This is a reprint of the Special Issue, published open access by the journal *Healthcare* (ISSN 2227-9032), freely accessible at: www.mdpi.com/journal/healthcare/special_issues/primary_care_sleep_medicine.

For citation purposes, cite each article independently as indicated on the article page online and as indicated below:

Lastname, A.A.; Lastname, B.B. Article Title. *Journal Name* **Year**, *Volume Number*, Page Range.

ISBN 978-3-7258-4438-8 (Hbk)
ISBN 978-3-7258-4437-1 (PDF)
https://doi.org/10.3390/books978-3-7258-4437-1

© 2025 by the authors. Articles in this book are Open Access and distributed under the Creative Commons Attribution (CC BY) license. The book as a whole is distributed by MDPI under the terms and conditions of the Creative Commons Attribution-NonCommercial-NoDerivs (CC BY-NC-ND) license (https://creativecommons.org/licenses/by-nc-nd/4.0/).

Contents

About the Editor vii

Izolde Bouloukaki, Theofilos Vouis, Antonios Velidakis, Violeta Moniaki, Eleni Mavroudi, George Stathakis, et al.
Polysomnography Differences Between Sleepy and Non-Sleepy Obstructive Sleep Apnea (OSA) Patients
Reprinted from: *Healthcare* **2025**, *13*, 478, https://doi.org/10.3390/healthcare13050478 1

Dimosthenis Lykouras, Eirini Zarkadi, Electra Koulousousa, Olga Lagiou, Dimitrios Komninos, Argyris Tzouvelekis and Kyriakos Karkoulias
Factors Affecting CPAP Adherence in an OSA Population during the First Two Years of the COVID-19 Pandemic
Reprinted from: *Healthcare* **2024**, *12*, 1772, https://doi.org/10.3390/healthcare12171772 14

Christina Alexopoulou, Maria Fountoulaki, Antigone Papavasileiou and Eumorfia Kondili
Sleep Habits, Academic Performance and Health Behaviors of Adolescents in Southern Greece
Reprinted from: *Healthcare* **2024**, *12*, 775, https://doi.org/10.3390/healthcare12070775 23

Kostas Archontogeorgis, Nicholas-Tiberio Economou, Panagiotis Bargiotas, Evangelia Nena, Athanasios Voulgaris, Konstantina Chadia, et al.
Sleepiness and Vitamin D Levels in Patients with Obstructive Sleep Apnea
Reprinted from: *Healthcare* **2024**, *12*, 698, https://doi.org/10.3390/healthcare12060698 36

Izolde Bouloukaki, Ioanna Tsiligianni, Giorgos Stathakis, Michail Fanaridis, Athina Koloi, Ekaterini Bakiri, et al.
Sleep Quality and Fatigue during Exam Periods in University Students: Prevalence and Associated Factors
Reprinted from: *Healthcare* **2023**, *11*, 2389, https://doi.org/10.3390/healthcare11172389 45

Ioanna Grigoriou, Paschalia Skalisti, Ioanna Papagiouvanni, Anastasia Michailidou, Konstantinos Charalampidis, Serafeim-Chrysovalantis Kotoulas, et al.
Smoking-Induced Disturbed Sleep. A Distinct Sleep-Related Disorder Pattern?
Reprinted from: *Healthcare* **2023**, *11*, 205, https://doi.org/10.3390/healthcare11020205 56

Abdullah N. Al-Rasheedi, Ashokkumar Thirunavukkarasu, Abdulhakeem Almutairi, Sultan Alruwaili, Hatem Alotaibi, Wasan Alzaid, et al.
Knowledge and Attitude towards Obstructive Sleep Apnea among Primary Care Physicians in Northern Regions of Saudi Arabia: A Multicenter Study
Reprinted from: *Healthcare* **2022**, *10*, 2369, https://doi.org/10.3390/healthcare10122369 70

Yi-Chieh Lee, Chun-Ting Lu, Wen-Nuan Cheng and Hsueh-Yu Li
The Impact of Mouth-Taping in Mouth-Breathers with Mild Obstructive Sleep Apnea: A Preliminary Study
Reprinted from: *Healthcare* **2022**, *10*, 1755, https://doi.org/10.3390/healthcare10091755 80

Athanasia Pataka, Seraphim Kotoulas, Asterios Tzinas, Nectaria Kasnaki, Evdokia Sourla, Evangelos Chatzopoulos, et al.
Sleep Disorders and Mental Stress of Healthcare Workers during the Two First Waves of COVID-19 Pandemic: Separate Analysis for Primary Care
Reprinted from: *Healthcare* **2022**, *10*, 1395, https://doi.org/10.3390/healthcare10081395 88

Panagiota K. Ntenta, Georgios D. Vavougios, Sotirios G. Zarogiannis and Konstantinos I. Gourgoulianis
Obstructive Sleep Apnea Syndrome Comorbidity Phenotypes in Primary Health Care Patients in Northern Greece
Reprinted from: *Healthcare* **2022**, *10*, 338, https://doi.org/10.3390/healthcare10020338 . . . . . . **105**

Maria Basta, Christina Belogianni, Mary Yannakoulia, Ioannis Zaganas, Symeon Panagiotakis, Panagiotis Simos and Alexandros N. Vgontzas
Poor Diet, Long Sleep, and Lack of Physical Activity Are Associated with Inflammation among Non-Demented Community-Dwelling Elderly
Reprinted from: *Healthcare* **2022**, *10*, 143, https://doi.org/10.3390/healthcare10010143 . . . . . . **115**

About the Editor

Izolde Bouloukaki

Dr. Izolde Bouloukaki serves as an Assistant Professor of Primary Care and Public Health at the Department of Social Medicine, School of Medicine, University of Crete, Greece, under the supervision of prof. I. Tsiligianni. She previously (till March 2023) served as a consultant in Family Medicine, employed in the Greek NHS, since 2012. She also, since 2003, serves as an attending physician in the Sleep Disorders Center, at the Department of Thoracic Medicine, in the University of Crete, at Heraklion, Crete, Greece, under the supervision of prof. S. Schiza. Dr. Bouloukaki received her Medical Degree in 2002 from the University of Crete. Her primary specialty is Family Medicine, which she completed in 2012. She earned a PhD degree in respiratory medicine (smoking cessation) in 2010 from the University of Crete. She specialized in Sleep Medicine, receiving a certification of Somnologist Expert in Sleep Medicine from the ESRS in 2014. Her primary scientific interests include epidemiology in primary care, pathophysiology, cardiovascular and metabolic consequences of sleep breathing disorders, IPF, COPD, asthma and smoking cessation. She has 115 publications in peer-reviewed journals, chapters in books and numerous invited lectures and abstracts in national and international congresses.

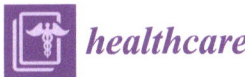

Article

Polysomnography Differences Between Sleepy and Non-Sleepy Obstructive Sleep Apnea (OSA) Patients

Izolde Bouloukaki *, Theofilos Vouis, Antonios Velidakis, Violeta Moniaki, Eleni Mavroudi, George Stathakis, Michail Fanaridis and Sophia Schiza

Department of Sleep Disorders Center, Department of Respiratory Medicine, Medical School, University of Crete, 71500 Heraklion, Greece; theofvouis@gmail.com (T.V.); vmoniaki@yahoo.gr (V.M.); elenima23@hotmail.com (E.M.); stathakisgg@gmail.com (G.S.); schizas@uoc.gr (S.S.)
* Correspondence: izolthi@gmail.com; Tel.: +30-2810-394933

Abstract: Background/Objectives: Factors underlying excessive daytime sleepiness (EDS) in obstructive sleep apnea (OSA) are not fully understood. We investigated whether polysomnography (PSG) parameters differed between non-sleepy and sleepy (based on the Epworth Sleepiness Scale (ESS)) OSA patients with the same disease severity, which may play a role in the presence of EDS. **Methods:** A total of 1307 patients, without cardiovascular, metabolic, respiratory, or inflammatory comorbidities, diagnosed with OSA (apnea–hypopnea index (AHI) $\geq$ 5 per hour of sleep) with type 1 PSG were included. Based on the AHI, patients were classified into mild- (AHI 5–14.9, n = 236), moderate- (AHI 15–29.9, n = 367), and severe-OSA (AHI $\geq$ 30, n = 704) groups. These groups were further divided into two subgroups based on the ESS, the most convenient and widely used tool to assess excessive daytime sleepiness: sleepy (ESS > 10) and non-sleepy (ESS $\leq$ 10). PSG data were compared between groups, and multivariable logistic regression was used to identify differences after adjustment for confounders. **Results:** For the entire population, male sex, younger age, obesity, depression, increased wakefulness after sleep onset (WASO), the arousal index, shorter sleep latency, and all indices of OSA severity (AHI, oxygen desaturation index, mean and lowest resting room air pulse oximetry (SpO_2), and sleep time with oxygen saturation < 90% (TST90)) were significantly associated with EDS. The arousal index consistently showed a strong association with EDS across all OSA severity groups. Moderate-OSA sleepy patients were younger, with shorter sleep latency and increased indices of OSA severity, excluding the AHI. Severe-OSA sleepy patients were younger, males, and obese; had depression, decreased slow-wave sleep (SWS) and sleep latency, and increased WASO; and presented an increase in all indices of OSA severity. **Conclusions:** Our results suggest that male sex, younger age, obesity, the presence of depression, WASO, lower sleep efficiency, the arousal index, and all indices of OSA severity may account for the presence or absence of EDS in OSA patients and could be useful for exploring the underlying pathophysiological mechanisms for precision medicine.

Keywords: obstructive sleep apnea; excessive daytime sleepiness; sleep architecture; indices of OSA severity; polysomnography; sleepy phenotype

1. Introduction

Obstructive sleep apnea (OSA) is a multifactorial disease characterized by recurrent episodes of upper-airway obstruction during sleep, leading to apnea or hypopnea (complete or partial cessation of airflow for 10 s or more during sleep), ultimately resulting in intermittent hypoxia (periodic alternating exposures to hypoxia and normoxia), disrupted sleep architecture (the structured organization of the various sleep stages), and intrathoracic pressure swings [1]. The presence of OSA poses a significant challenge for physicians and healthcare systems globally due to its increasing prevalence, ranging from 9% to 38% [2], and associated mental and medical comorbidities [3,4]. Conventionally, the assessment of OSA severity is based on the apnea–hypopnea index (AHI), the combined average number of apnea and hypopnea events that occur per hour of sleep [5]. To meet the diagnostic criteria for OSA, a person must have either more than 15 respiratory events per hour or more than 5 events per hour along with typical symptoms of OSA, such as snoring, fatigue, excessive daytime sleepiness (EDS), or comorbid conditions like hypertension, coronary artery disease, or stroke [1,6,7]. However, nowadays, diagnostic polysomnography (PSG), a multi-parameter type of sleep study used to diagnose sleep disorders, contains a plethora of information that can be used for a more comprehensive analysis of OSA, moving beyond the basic frequency-based measures like the AHI. This encompasses parameters such as ventilatory, hypoxic, and arousal burden; ventilatory patterns; and Pulse Wave Amplitude Drops (sudden drops in pulse wave amplitude that reflect peripheral vasoconstriction resulting from sympathetic activation) [8].

OSA is considered a heterogeneous disease, characterized by diverse symptoms, anthropometric features, polysomnographic findings, long-term outcomes, and comorbidities [9]. The symptoms of OSA can vary widely, and they may not necessarily reflect the severity of the disease [10]. The presence of EDS is common among patients with OSA, affecting 40.5–58% at initial diagnosis, and is recognized as a primary symptom of the syndrome [11]. If it is present, it can result in diminished quality of life and increased societal burden, which may impact healthcare utilization and costs. More specifically, patients with OSA and EDS are more prone to reporting lower mental well-being, impaired cognitive abilities, decreased productivity, and increased rates of work and car accidents [11–14].

The factors underlying EDS in OSA are not fully understood. Existing research suggests a possible relationship between polysomnographic measures (sleep architecture and OSA severity parameters) and EDS in these patients, but findings have been inconsistent. More specifically, several studies have revealed a lack of strong or consistent association among the indices of OSA severity, such as the AHI, and subjective EDS [15–18]. The presence of EDS has been also attributed to chronic intermittent hypoxia and sleep fragmentation [19]. OSA patients with EDS often exhibit alterations in macrostructural characteristics, including increased sleep efficiency, reduced sleep latency, a greater proportion of NREM, stage N1 sleep, and a decline in slow-wave sleep (SWS), as well as alterations in the microarchitecture, including an elevated arousal index, compared with those without EDS [18,20–22]. However, research findings on these associations have yielded mixed results [16,23,24]. The variability in findings may be attributed to discrepancies in the definition and measurement of EDS across studies or to methodological variations in the evaluation of sleep quality and architecture, which are susceptible to experimental and technical influences.

Given the serious public health implications of EDS and its medicolegal aspects [25], understanding the determinant of this OSA phenotype is an area of important future research. Such insights may be gained by investigating the association between the sleepy phenotype, OSA severity indices, and sleep architecture parameters. Exploring the sleepy phenotype within groups with different OSA severity could also yield valuable findings. Therefore, the aim of our study was to investigate whether PSG parameters differed between non-sleepy and sleepy OSA patients with the same OSA disease severity at the time of diagnosis, in a large cohort of newly diagnosed OSA patients, without comorbidities and before treatment initiation. We hypothesized that identifying the PSG characteristics of the patients with sleepiness is an essential step in elucidating the link between OSA pathophysiology and the EDS experienced by these patients.

2. Materials and Methods

2.1. Design and Sample

A cross-sectional study of individuals visiting the University of Crete's Sleep Disorders Center (Department of Respiratory Medicine, School of Medicine) in Greece for assessment of suspected OSA was conducted over an eight-year period (2015–2023). The inclusion criteria were (1) above 18 years of age, (2) with OSA diagnosis according to standard criteria (AHI $\geq$ 5 on PSG), and (3) treatment-naïve OSA.

Participants were excluded if they refused participation; had central sleep apnea syndrome, restrictive ventilatory syndrome, or any cardiovascular (coronary disease, atrial fibrillation, Cerebro-Vascular Accident/Transient Ischemic Attack, and/or heart failure), metabolic (except for hyperlipidemia), respiratory, or inflammatory comorbidities; had a personal or family history of mental illness, intake of benzodiazepines or similar sleep-inducing drugs, drug or alcohol abuse, or severe cognitive impairment; or had a history of narcolepsy or restless legs syndrome. Ethical approval (number 7370/04-06-2014) was granted by the University Hospital Ethics Committee, and all participants provided written informed consent.

Out of the 2884 adults who were assessed for suspected OSA, 2619 of them (91%) received a confirmed diagnosis of OSA. Following the exclusion of patients with specific comorbidities and missing data, our final sample comprised 1307 patients (Figure 1).

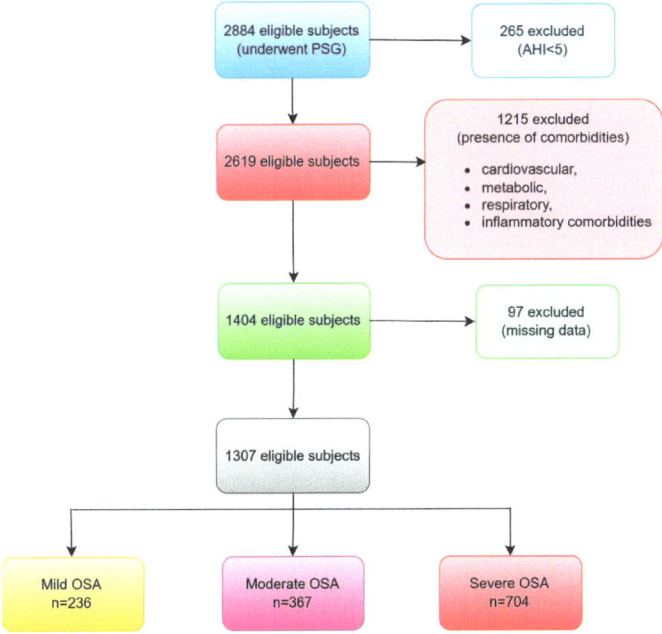

Figure 1. The flowchart of patients finally included. PSG: polysomnography; AHI: apnea–hypopnea index; OSA: obstructive sleep apnea.

2.2. Data Collection

A comprehensive evaluation was performed on all patients, including age, anthropometric data (body mass index (BMI) and circumferences of neck, waist, and hip), sleep-related symptoms, relevant medical history (including comorbidities), and histories of smoking, alcohol consumption, and substance abuse. Furthermore, attended overnight polysomnography (PSG) studies were performed. Participants' subjective daytime sleepiness levels were determined with the Epworth Sleepiness Scale (ESS).

Epworth Sleepiness Scale

The ESS is presently the most frequently employed self-reported measure of daytime sleepiness in clinical practice. This self-administered assessment consists of a concise eight-question questionnaire. The tool measures how likely someone is to fall asleep in eight typical situations. A score under 10 is within the normal range. Subjective daytime sleepiness increases proportionally with scores ranging from 10 to 24. An ESS score exceeding 10 points (ESS $\geq$ 11) suggests excessive daytime sleepiness (EDS) [26].

2.3. Polysomnography

Each patient received a single-night, full diagnostic PSG study using the Alice 5 Diagnostics System (Respironics, Murrysville, PA, USA), adhering to standard protocols and including the monitoring of the electroencephalogram (EEG; using 3 electroencephalogram derivations: frontal, central, and occipital), electro-oculogram, electromyogram, flow (by oronasal thermistor and nasal air pressure transducer), thoracic and abdominal respiratory effort (by respiratory inductance plethysmography), pulse oximetry (SpO_2), and body position. A microphone positioned on the anterior neck documented instances of snoring. Apnea and hypopnea were defined according to the American Academy of Sleep Medicine's standard criteria including the hypopnea rule, which requires $\geq$3% desaturation or EEG-based arousal [27]. The analysis included the following parameters: total sleep time (TST), sleep efficiency [SE (%), percentage of total time in bed actually spent in sleep], wakefulness after sleep onset (WASO, the amount of wake periods after sleep onset), arousal index (AI), apnea–hypopnea index (AHI), oxygen desaturation index (ODI), resting room air pulse oximetry (SpO_2), and sleep time with oxygen saturation < 90% (TST90). The AHI, computed as the hourly frequency of apnea and hypopnea events during sleep, served as the diagnostic criterion for OSA and its severity assessment. The severity of OSA was categorized according to the AHI: mild (5 to <15 events/h), moderate (15 to <30 events/h), and severe ($\geq$30 events/h). Only participants with an AHI of at least 5 events per hour were included in our study.

2.4. Statistical Analysis

For continuous variables, means and standard deviations (mean $\pm$ SD) are reported if they are normally distributed; otherwise, medians and interquartile ranges (25th–75th percentile) are given. The qualitative variables are represented by absolute numbers and percentages. Normally distributed variables were analyzed with ANOVA to determine differences among mild-, moderate-, and severe-OSA patient groups. Significant ANOVA results were followed by pairwise comparisons using the Tukey–Kramer post hoc test. For non-normally distributed variables, the Kruskal–Wallis test was used for comparing the three groups. Following a significant Kruskal–Wallis test, Dunn's pairwise comparisons were performed for the three group pairs, adjusting for multiple testing with the Bonferroni correction. Chi-square analysis was used to compare the three groups on categorical variables. Each of the three OSA severity groups was examined for association with prevalent EDS. A logistic regression analysis was conducted to determine the variables associated with EDS, controlling for age, gender, obesity indicators (BMI, waist-to-hip ratio, and neck circumference), smoking status, and comorbidities. An assessment of multicollinearity among predictors was conducted by using tolerance and the variance inflation factor (VIF) to maintain acceptable levels of collinearity. Age was categorized into groups of 18–59 and ≥ 60 years; the BMI was categorized as obese (BMI ≥ 30 kg/m^2) and non-obese (BMI < 30 kg/m^2); and EDS was categorized as sleepy (ESS >10) and non-sleepy (ESS ≤ 10). Statistical significance was established for *p*-values less than 0.05. Data analysis was conducted by using SPSS version 25 (SPSS Inc., Chicago, IL, USA).

3. Results

3.1. Patient Characteristics

The descriptive characteristics of the study population and the distribution of covariates are shown in Table 1. Overall, participants were predominantly males (79%), middle-aged (50 ± 14 years), and obese (BMI of 33 ± 7 kg/m^2). The majority of the participants (89%) had a spouse and had a higher level of education (68%). Individuals in the severe-OSA group were older and more obese, were more frequently males, and had higher prevalence of hypertension and hyperlipidemia compared with mild- and moderate-OSA patients.

Table 1. Clinical characteristics of patients according to OSA severity.

	Total Population N = 1307	Total Population According to AHI			*p*-Value Across All
		Mild-OSA Patients (AHI 5 to <15/h) N = 236	Moderate-OSA Patients (AHI 15 to <30/h) N = 367	Severe-OSA Patients (AHI $\geq$ 30/h) N = 704	
Demographics					
Sex, males (%)	1027 (79%)	172 (73%)	270 (74%)	585 (83%) **, #	<0.001
Age, years	50 ± 14	44 ± 13.0	51 ± 14 *	52 ± 14 **	<0.001
Age $\geq$ 60 years (%)	345 (27%)	27 (12%)	104 (28%) *	214 (30%) **	<0.001
BMI (kg/m^2)	33 ± 7	29 ± 5	31 ± 6*	35 ± 7 **, #	<0.001
BMI $\geq$ 30, n (%)	822 (63%)	87 (37%)	187 (51%) *	548 (78%) #, **	<0.001
NC (cm)	42 ± 5	39 ± 4	41 ± 4 *	43 ± 5 **, #	<0.001
WC (cm)	111 ± 16	101 ± 12	107 ± 12 *	117 ± 16 **, #	<0.001
HC (cm)	112 ± 15	105 ± 12	109 ± 12 *	117 ± 15 **, #	<0.001
Waist-to-hip ratio	0.99 ± 0.07	0.96 ± 0.08	0.99 ± 0.06 *	1.00 ± 0.07 **, #	<0.001
Education Level					
Primary level	61 (5%)	7 (3%)	19 (5%)	35 (5%)	
Secondary level	356 (27%)	52 (22%)	93 (25%)	211 (30%)	
Higher level	890 (68%)	177 (75%)	255 (69%)	458 (65%)	0.072
Married/with partner (%)	1160 (89%)	186 (78%)	328 (89%)	647 (92%)	<0.001
Smoking status					
Never, n (%)	501 (38%)	90 (38%)	152 (41%)	259 (37%)	
Current/former, n (%)	806 (62%)	146 (62%)	215 (59%)	445 (63%)	0.461
Daytime sleepiness					
ESS	10 ± 5	8 ± 5	9 ± 5	11 ± 6 **, #	<0.001
ESS > 10 (%)	644 (49%)	88 (38%)	165 (46%) *	391 (57%) **, #	<0.001
Comorbidities (%)					
Arterial hypertension	435 (33%)	29 (12%)	122 (33%) *	284 (40%) **, #	<0.001
Hyperlipidemia	469 (36%)	62 (26%)	136 (37%) *	271 (39%) **	0.003
Depression (on medications)	119 (9%)	18 (8%)	32 (9%)	69 (10%)	0.585

Data are presented as N (%) for categorical variables and mean values ± SDs or medians (25th–75th percentiles) for continuous variables. AHI: apnea–hypopnea index; BMI: body mass index; ESS: Epworth Sleepiness Scale; HC: hip circumference; NC: neck circumference; OSA: obstructive sleep apnea; WC: waist circumference. * $p < 0.05$, mild-OSA vs. moderate-OSA groups; ** $p < 0.05$, mild- vs. severe-OSA groups; # $p < 0.05$, moderate- vs. severe-OSA groups.

3.2. General Characteristics of the EDS Phenotype

Almost half of the population presented EDS, with significant differences between the three OSA severity groups (Table 1). The severe-OSA group exhibited the highest EDS (57 vs. 46 vs. 38%, $p < 0.001$). In the whole population, the sleepy phenotype was on average more often found in those who were males (82 vs. 75%, $p = 0.011$), younger than 60 years (77 vs. 70%, $p = 0.011$), and obese (67 vs. 59%, $p = 0.006$) compared with the non-sleepy phenotype. In the moderate-OSA group, the sleepy phenotype was more often found in those younger than 60 years (78 vs. 67%, $p = 0.02$), and in the severe-OSA group, the sleepy phenotype was more often found in those who were male (85 vs. 79%, $p = 0.042$) and younger than 60 years (73 vs. 65%, $p = 0.038$).

3.3. The Effect of PSG Parameters on EDS

Overall, the participants had moderate-to-severe OSA, with a median AHI of 31 (19, 61) events/hour. All patients and the patients in the three OSA severity groups were further divided into two categories based on their level of daytime sleepiness (Supplementary Table S1, Table 2, Figure 2): those who experienced EDS (ESS > 10) and those who did not (ESS $\leq$ 10). In all patients, SWS sleep (7 vs. 8% TST, $p = 0.02$) and sleep latency were lower (35 vs. 41, $p < 0.001$), whereas the arousal index (47 vs. 41, $p < 0.001$), WASO (110 vs. 103, $p = 0.004$), and NREM sleep (91 vs. 89, $p = 0.03$) were higher. The indices of OSA severity (AHI, ODI, mean and lowest SpO_2, and TST90, all $p < 0.001$) were worse in sleepy OSA patients compared with non-sleepy ones. Mild-OSA sleepy patients exhibited higher WASO (92 vs. 88, $p = 0.03$) compared with non-sleepy patients. Decreased sleep latency (32 vs. 39, $p = 0.03$) was noted in moderate-OSA sleepy patients. Statistically significant differences were observed in the mean (93 vs. 94%, $p = 0.005$) and lowest SpO_2 (84 vs. 84%, $p = 0.01$) and in TST90 (26 vs. 19, $p = 0.001$); however, these differences lacked clinical significance. In the severe-OSA sleepy subgroup, SWS sleep (7 vs. 8% TST, $p = 0.001$) and sleep latency were lower (38 vs. 45, $p < 0.001$), whereas the arousal index (54 vs. 50, $p = 0.001$) was higher. Additionally, the indices of OSA severity (AHI, ODI, mean and lowest SpO_2, and TST90, all $p < 0.001$) were worse in severe-OSA sleepy patients.

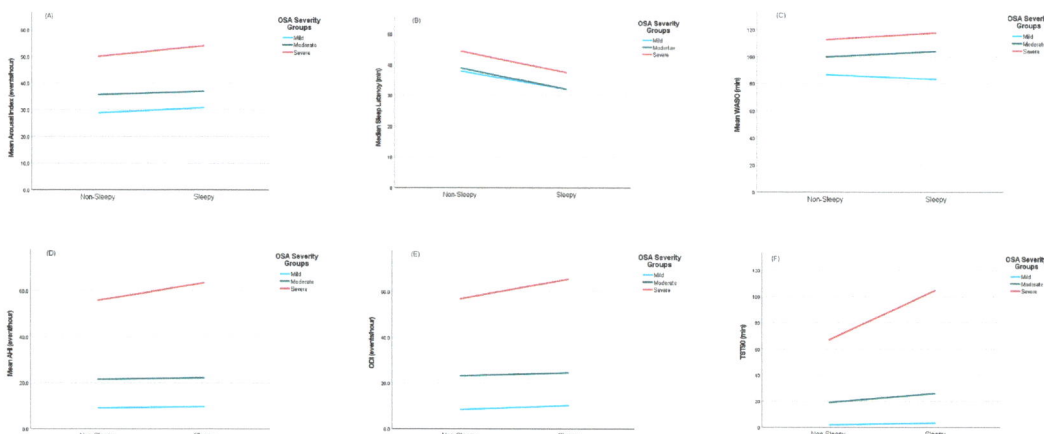

Figure 2. Comparison of arousal index (**A**), sleep latency (**B**), WASO (**C**), AHI (**D**), ODI (**E**), and TST90 (**F**) between sleepy and non-sleepy groups within OSA severity groups.

Table 2. Comparison of study subgroups with or without EDS within OSA severity groups.

	Mild OSA			Moderate OSA			Severe OSA		
	ESS ≤ 10	ESS > 10	p-Value	ESS ≤ 10	ESS > 10	p-Value	ESS ≤ 10	ESS > 10	p-Value
TST (min)	292 ± 49	296 ± 48	0.66	275 ± 56	281 ± 52	0.28	262 ± 61	261 ± 54	0.86
Sleep efficiency (%)	70 ± 10	72 ± 10	0.35	66 ± 12	67 ± 11	0.33	62 ± 13	63 ± 11	0.42
NREM (%TST)	89 ± 8	89 ± 4	0.94	88 ± 7	90 ± 7	0.86	91 ± 6	90 ± 3	0.86
SWS (%TST)	8 ± 4	8 ± 3	0.70	8 ± 3	8 ± 4	0.93	8 ± 4	7 ± 3	0.001 *
REM (%TST)	11 ± 4	12 ± 4	0.62	10 ± 4	11 ± 4	0.24	10 ± 8	9 ± 4	0.51
Arousal index	30 ± 9	31 ± 7	0.65	37 ± 8	37 ± 7	0.54	50 ± 14	54 ± 13	0.001 *
Sleep latency (min)	38 (26, 58)	32 (21, 53)	0.24	39 (25, 61)	32 (22, 52)	0.03 *	45 (29, 75)	38 (24, 59)	<0.001 *
WASO (min)	88 ± 33	92 ± 33	0.03 *	106 ± 38	107 ± 38	0.63	118 ± 39	122 ± 40	0.19
AHI	9 ± 3	10 ± 3	0.06	21 ± 4	22 ± 4	0.13	55 ± 20	63 ± 23	<0.001 *
AHI REM	12 ± 7	13 ± 7	0.52	29 ± 13	30 ± 12	0.40	59 ± 23	64 ± 23	0.01 *
ODI	8 ± 3	10 ± 9	0.11	24 ± 9	24 ± 6	0.52	57 ± 22	65 ± 24	<0.001 *
Mean SpO$_2$ (%)	95 ± 1	95 ± 1	0.23	94 ± 2	93 ± 1	0.005 *	91 ± 2	90 ± 3	<0.001 *
Lowest SpO$_2$ (%)	88 ± 3	88 ± 4	0.39	84 ± 3	83 ± 4	0.01 *	78 ± 7	74 ± 8	<0.001 *
TST90 (min)	2 (0, 7)	4 (1, 9)	0.12	19 (10, 33)	26 (14, 43)	0.001 *	67 (38, 108)	105 (59, 171)	<0.001 *
TST90 (%)	0.8 (0, 2.3)	1.3 (0.3, 1.3)	0.11	7.2 (3.6, 12.0)	9.4 (4.7, 15.6)	0.001 *	25.9 (13.8, 46.0)	42.7 (21.8, 71.4)	<0.001 *

AHI: apnea–hypopnea index; AI: arousal index; ESS: Epworth Sleepiness Scale; ODI: oxygen desaturation index; OSA: obstructive sleep apnea; SE: sleep efficiency; SpO$_2$: resting room air pulse oximetry; TST: total sleep time; TST90: sleep time with oxygen saturation < 90%; WASO, wakefulness after sleep onset. * p-Value < 0.05.

Table 3 summarizes the results of a multiple stepwise logistic regression analysis exploring the association between EDS and various independent factors, considering the entire patient population and the OSA severity classifications separately. After adjustments for age, gender, BMI, smoking status, and comorbidities, we found that for the entire population, male sex, younger age (<60 years), obesity (BMI ≥ 30kg/m^2), the presence of depression, WASO, lower sleep efficiency, the arousal index, and all indices of OSA severity were significantly associated with the presence of EDS. An arousal index exceeding 30 was the most significant predictor, demonstrating a two-fold increased likelihood of developing EDS.

Table 3. Multiple stepwise logistic regression analysis of relationship between EDS and various independent variables in OSA severity groups.

	All OSA Patients		Mild-OSA Patients		Moderate-OSA Patients		Severe-OSA Patients	
	OR (95%CI)	p-Value	OR (95%CI)	p-Value	OR (95%CI)	p-Value	OR (95%CI)	p-Value
Males vs. females	1.499 (1.129–1.991)	0.005 *	0.751 (0.393–1.436)	0.386	1.399 (0.821–2.386)	0.217	1.797 (1.160–2.784)	0.009 *
Age ≤ 60	1.418 (1.080–1.864)	0.012 *	0.433 (0.149–1.254)	0.123	1.802 (1.079–3.012)	0.025 *	1.359 (1.053–1.938)	0.041 *
BMI ≥ 30	1.351 (1.069–1.707)	0.012 *	0.887 (0485–1.624)	0.699	0.931 (0.588–1.474)	0.759	1.025 (1.002–1.049)	0.035 *
Depression	1.688 (1.128–2.527)	0.011 *	1.033 (0.367–2.905)	0.952	1.692 (0.785–3.648)	0.180	1.829 (1.051–3.184)	0.033 *
Sleep efficiency (%)	1.003 (0.993–1.013)	0.582	1.028 (0.996–1.060)	0.090	1.015 (0.994–1.037)	0.161	1.015 (0.999–1.031)	0.063
WASO	1.004 (1.001–1.007)	0.015 *	0.997 (0.989–1.006)	0.543	1.003 (0.996–1.009)	0.418	1.002 (0.998–1.007)	0.049 *
Sleep latency	0.995 (0.991-.998)	0.003 *	1.000 (0.990–1.009)	0.969	0.993 (0.986–1.000)	0.038 *	0.989 (0.983–0.944)	<0.001 *
NREM (%TST)	1.000 (0.999–1.002)	0.633	1.011 (0.969–1.055)	0.601	0.966 (0.963–1.031)	0.841	1.000 (0.999–1.002)	0.633
SWS (%TST)	0.960 (0.928–0.993)	0.018 *	0.964 (0.870–1.069)	0.487	1.050 (0.953–1.156)	0.325	0.922 (0.874–0.972)	0.003 *
REM (%TST)	0.995 (0.973–1.018)	0.658	1.005 (0.942–1.071)	0.889	1.080 (0.976–1.195)	0.139	0.986 (0.954–1.020)	0.418
Arousal index	1.026 (1.017–1.035)	<0.001 *	1.043 (1.003–1.085)	0.036 *	1.026 (1.007–1.055)	0.038 *	1.020 (1.008–1.033)	0.002 *
Arousal index ≥ 30	2.398 (1.702–3.380)	<0.001 *	2.412 (1.373–4.239)	0.002 *	2.229 (1.236–4.020)	0.008 *	2.001 (0.326–12.267)	0.033 *
AHI	1.014 (1.009–1.018)	<0.001 *	1.098 (0.987–1.222)	0.086	1.065 (0.997–1.138)	0.062	1.016 (1.007–1.024)	<0.001 *
AHI REM	1.011 (1.006–1.015)	<0.001 *	1.008 (0.968–1.049)	0.699	1.013 (0.994–1.033)	0.190	1.008 (1.001–1.016)	0.032 *
ODI	1.014 (1.010–1.019)	<0.001 *	1.050 (0.971–1.136)	0.221	1.046 (1.011–1.082)	0.009 *	1.016 (1.008–1.024)	<0.001 *

Table 3. Cont.

	All OSA Patients		Mild-OSA Patients		Moderate-OSA Patients		Severe-OSA Patients	
	OR (95%CI)	p-Value	OR (95%CI)	p-Value	OR (95%CI)	p-Value	OR (95%CI)	p-Value
Mean SaO$_2$	0.817 (0.775–0.861)	<0.001 *	0.828 (0.632–1.085)	0.171	0.712 (0.602–0.842)	<0.001 *	0.794 (0.726–0.870)	<0.001 *
Lowest SaO$_2$	0.936 (0.920–0.953)	<0.001 *	0.948 (0.844–1.065)	0.368	0.890 (0.831–0.954)	0.001 *	0.926 (0.899–0.952)	<0.001 *
TST90 (%)	1.019 (1.014–1.024)	<0.001 *	1.051 (0.960–1.150)	0.278	1.022 (1.004–1.040)	0.016 *	1.018 (1.012–1.024)	<0.001 *

All models were adjusted for the participants' age, sex, obesity, smoking status, and comorbidities. * p-Value < 0.05.

It is also noteworthy that the arousal index consistently showed a strong correlation with EDS across all OSA severity groups; this was particularly true for the mild-OSA group, in which it was the only significant predictor. Male gender, obesity, and the presence of depression, along with WASO and lower SWS, remained significant predictors of EDS only in the severe-OSA group. Patients with moderate-to-severe OSA who were younger and exhibited shorter sleep latencies were more likely to experience EDS. While the AHI significantly predicted EDS only in severe-OSA cases, the ODI, the mean and lowest SpO2, and TST90 were predictive of EDS in both moderate- and severe-OSA groups.

4. Discussion

This study explores differences in PSG characteristics between sleepy and non-sleepy patients in a large cohort of treatment-naïve patients with different levels of OSA severity. Our findings indicate the presence of distinct sleepy phenotypes, varying according to the severity of OSA. More specifically, the mild-OSA sleepy patient was characterized by a higher arousal index, whereas the moderate-OSA sleepy patient was younger, with shorter sleep latency and increased indices of OSA severity, excluding the AHI in addition to an increased arousal index. Patients in the severe-OSA sleepy group tended to be younger, males, obese, and diagnosed with depression (on medication). Those patients also exhibited decreased SWS and sleep latency, increased WASO, an arousal index, and an increase in all indices of OSA severity.

One major finding of our study is that an increased arousal index ($\geq$30) was associated with a 2.4 greater likelihood of subjective EDS regardless of OSA severity. This finding is in accordance with previous studies [18,20,22,28–30]; however, other studies [16,30–32] have failed to establish a statistically significant association between the arousal index and sleepiness in OSA. Evidence suggests that recurrent cortical arousals indicate physiological stress and impair the restorative function of sleep, resulting in daytime sleepiness and cognitive impairment [33]. Although they present as promising predictors of EDS, EEG-based arousals are scored less reliably compared with respiratory events and are influenced by sleep stages [34,35]. Additionally, their association with sympathetic activation is unclear [36], suggesting the need for alternative methods of measuring arousal during sleep. The addition of "arousal intensity" to arousal frequency has been recommended as a potential way to improve their predictive value [37]. Notably, a recent study explored markers of arousal intensity, in addition to the arousal index [30]. The authors suggested that while the number of arousals may be similar between sleepy and not sleepy patients, sleepy phenotypes might experience more disruptive or severe arousals accompanied by sympathetic nervous system activation, potentially resulting in heightened daytime sleepiness [30]. Additionally, it has been shown that cortical arousals with a duration greater than 15 s exhibit a more robust association with ESS scores than shorter cortical arousals (3–15 s) [38]. In light of these findings, we consider that arousal events during sleep deserve increased attention in polysomnographic scoring, as they reliably reflect daytime sleepiness and sleep quality. However, additional research is essential to gaining a more comprehensive understanding of this association.

We also explored other markers of sleep architecture, and we found that in moderate-to-severe-OSA patients, the sleepy phenotype, compared with the not sleepy phenotype, had shorter sleep latency, spent more time awake after sleep onset and had less SWS in severe OSA, in accordance with previous studies [20,22,39]. New research using innovative methods to assess sleep architecture reinforces the association between EDS and reduced SWS [40]. In this study, OSA patients with severe objective EDS, identified by the Multiple Sleep Latency Test, exhibited lower N3 sleep continuity and duration [40]. Our findings, however, contradict earlier research in OSA patients that did not link EDS to alterations in sleep architecture [16,23,30,31].

Another important finding of our study is that the EDS in our cohort was associated with more severe hypoxemia, as indicated by increased ODI and TST90, as well as lower mean and lowest SpO_2, in moderate-to-severe-OSA patients. These findings are in line with prior research [6,16,17,29–31], which consistently found significantly worse hypoxemia in OSA patients with EDS. While several mechanisms have been proposed for how hypoxemia induces sleepiness in OSA, including inflammation, oxidative injury, neuronal damage, and cell loss in wake-promoting regions of the brain [41–43], the exact mechanisms that lead to EDS in OSA are still unclear. Importantly, our study found that the association between OSA severity as traditionally measured by the AHI and EDS was only evident in patients with severe OSA. This is not unexpected, given that the relationship between the AHI and EDS is uncertain and even poor [3,15–18,20,22]. In this context, models utilizing hypoxemia metrics as predictors of EDS could be considered preferable to those relying on the AHI. The OSA-specific hypoxic burden, measuring the frequency, depth, and duration of desaturation during respiratory events, could show promise due to its significant associations with various negative health outcomes [44].

While most research has focused on moderate and severe OSA, this study delves deeper by exploring predictors of EDS separately for each severity level, including mild OSA. Our study shows a high rate of EDS among patients with mild OSA, aligning with results from previous studies [45–47]. The EDS experienced by patients with mild OSA may be a result of an increased arousal index, as observed in our study. This suggests that these patients could represent a unique subgroup within the OSA population, and the arousal index might be a better marker for their sleepiness than traditional OSA severity measures. However, it is important to consider that there may be additional unmeasured factors contributing to EDS in these patients, such as habitual sleep duration and medications other than benzodiazepines that could influence EDS.

Demographic characteristics that may be associated with EDS in OSA patients have also been described in our study. Younger age has been associated with EDS, particularly in moderate- and severe-OSA patients [11], and this is consistent with previous studies [20,48]. However, the influence of aging on the self-reported daytime sleepiness in OSA [49] should be taken into account, particularly when the ESS, one of the most common screening instruments for assessing sleepiness, is used [26]. The ESS evaluates sleepiness by questioning the tendency to fall asleep in eight common everyday scenarios [26], where older individuals may not engage in all of them [50]. Consequently, lower ESS score and EDS prevalence are expected in this age group. Our findings also indicate a higher prevalence of EDS in males, especially in the group with severe OSA. It appears that the ESS is more likely to identify sleepiness in men than in women [13,51]. This might be because women answer questions about sleepiness differently and might not experience the typical symptoms of OSA [52,53]. The higher BMI in severe-OSA sleepy patients noted in our study has also been independently associated with sleepiness in OSA patients in previous studies [22,54].

Our study expands upon existing knowledge of OSA by identifying factors that predict EDS in clinical populations with OSA. Examining the PSG factors contributing to the sleepiness phenotype is a critical step in understanding the association between OSA's pathophysiology and EDS experienced by patients. The identification of these distinctive PSG findings can facilitate clinicians in providing a more precise assessment of EDS in these patients, thus promoting effective individualized management and mitigating potential health complications.

One strength of this study is the large, well-characterized sample of treatment naïve patients with OSA, with detailed characterization of PSG parameters. We also excluded patients with major comorbidities and other sleep disorders that could influence sleep architecture, and we explored how the observed relationships between the sleepiness phenotypes may differ based on clinical and PSG characteristics. Furthermore, we had data on depression available; therefore, we found that this variable might influence our sleepiness phenotype. There are also limitations. The patients with OSA were recruited from a sleep center and do not necessarily represent patients with OSA found in the general population. Moreover, as males were overrepresented in our population, our findings may not be generalizable to females. Another limitation is that the ESS was used for EDS evaluation, which is less reliable than an objective assessment of sleepiness, such as the Multiple Sleep Latency Test, and may underestimate sleepiness severity in older subjects [50]. An objective assessment of sleepiness is highly warranted in future studies to validate these results. Further research is also needed to establish causal relationships between PSG parameters and EDS; investigate these differences in more diverse populations, with a particular focus on including a greater number of female participants; and explore additional contributing factors, such as habitual sleep time and medications for EDS in OSA patients.

5. Conclusions

Our results suggest that male sex, younger age, obesity, the presence of depression, parameters of sleep architecture, and indices of OSA severity may account for the presence or absence of EDS in OSA patients. Despite identifying distinct sleepy phenotypes based on OSA severity, the arousal index consistently showed a strong correlation with EDS across all OSA severity groups. The next important step is to explore the role and mechanisms of these factors in causing sleepiness and find valid sleepiness measures that can accurately predict health risks in OSA patients.

Supplementary Materials: The following supporting information can be downloaded at: https://www.mdpi.com/article/10.3390/healthcare13050478/s1, Supplementary Table S1: Comparison of PSG characteristics in total population based on their level of daytime sleepiness.

Author Contributions: Conceptualization, I.B. and S.S.; methodology, I.B., T.V., A.V., E.M. and V.M.; formal analysis, I.B., G.S. and M.F.; writing—original draft preparation, I.B., G.S. and S.S.; writing—review and editing, I.B., G.S. and M.F.; Supervision, S.S. All authors have read and agreed to the published version of the manuscript.

Funding: This research received no external funding.

Institutional Review Board Statement: This study adhered to the guidelines specified in the Declaration of Helsinki and received approval from the University Hospital Ethics Committee (Protocol number 7370/04-06-2014).

Informed Consent Statement: Informed consent was obtained from all subjects involved in the study.

Data Availability Statement: The data presented in this study are available upon request from the corresponding author. The data are not publicly available due to privacy restrictions.

Conflicts of Interest: The authors declare no conflicts of interest.

References

1. Kapur, V.K.; Auckley, D.H.; Chowdhuri, S.; Kuhlmann, D.C.; Mehra, R.; Ramar, K.; Harrod, C.G. Clinical practice guideline for diagnostic testing for adult obstructive sleep apnea: An American Academy of Sleep Medicine clinical practice guideline. *J. Clin. Sleep Med.* 2017, *13*, 479–504. [CrossRef]
2. Senaratna, C.V.; Perret, J.L.; Lodge, C.J.; Lowe, A.J.; Campbell, B.E.; Matheson, M.C.; Hamilton, G.S.; Dharmage, S.C. Prevalence of obstructive sleep apnea in the general population: A systematic review. *Sleep Med. Rev.* 2017, *34*, 70–81. [CrossRef] [PubMed]
3. Randerath, W.; Bassetti, C.L.; Bonsignore, M.R.; Farre, R.; Ferini-Strambi, L.; Grote, L.; Hedner, J.; Kohler, M.; Martinez-Garcia, M.A.; Mihaicuta, S.; et al. Challenges and perspectives in obstructive sleep apnoea: Report by an ad hoc working group of the Sleep Disordered Breathing Group of the European Respiratory Society and the European Sleep Research Society. *Eur. Respir. J.* 2018, *52*, 1702616. [CrossRef] [PubMed]
4. Heinzer, R.; Vat, S.; Marques-Vidal, P.; Marti-Soler, H.; Andries, D.; Tobback, N.; Mooser, V.; Preisig, M.; Malhotra, A.; Waeber, G.; et al. Prevalence of sleep-disordered breathing in the general population: The HypnoLaus study. *Lancet Respir. Med.* 2015, *3*, 310–318. [CrossRef]
5. Gabryelska, A.; Łukasik, Z.M.; Makowska, J.S.; Białasiewicz, P. Obstructive Sleep Apnea: From Intermittent Hypoxia to Cardiovascular Complications via Blood Platelets. *Front. Neurol.* 2018, *9*, 635. [CrossRef] [PubMed]
6. American Academy of Sleep Medicine. Obstructive sleep apnea, adult. In *International Classification of Sleep Disorders*, 3rd ed.; American Academy of Sleep Medicine: Darien, IL, USA, 2014; pp. 53–62.
7. Sateia, M.J. International classification of sleep disorders-third edition: Highlights and modifications. *Chest* 2014, *146*, 1387–1394. [CrossRef] [PubMed]
8. Azarbarzin, A.; Labarca, G.; Kwon, Y.; Wellman, A. Physiologic Consequences of Upper Airway Obstruction in Sleep Apnea. *Chest* 2024, *166*, 1209–1217. [CrossRef]
9. Randerath, W.; de Lange, J.; Hedner, J.; Ho, J.P.T.F.; Marklund, M.; Schiza, S.; Steier, J.; Verbraecken, J. Current and novel treatment options for obstructive sleep apnoea. *ERJ Open Res.* 2022, *8*, 00126–2022. [CrossRef]
10. Bixler, E.O.; Vgontzas, A.N.; Lin, H.M.; Calhoun, S.L.; Vela-Bueno, A.; Kales, A. Excessive daytime sleepiness in a general population sample: The role of sleep apnea, age, obesity, diabetes, and depression. *J. Clin. Endocrinol. Metab.* 2005, *90*, 4510–4515. [CrossRef] [PubMed]
11. Bjorvatn, B.; Lehmann, S.; Gulati, S.; Aurlien, H.; Pallesen, S.; Saxvig, I.W. Prevalence of excessive sleepiness is higher whereas insomnia is lower with greater severity of obstructive sleep apnea. *Sleep Breath.* 2015, *19*, 1387–1393. [CrossRef] [PubMed]
12. Baldwin, C.M.; Griffith, K.A.; Nieto, F.J.; O'Connor, G.T.; Walsleben, J.A.; Redline, S. The association of sleep-disordered breathing and sleep symptoms with quality of life in the sleep heart health study. *Sleep* 2001, *24*, 96–105. [CrossRef] [PubMed]
13. Baldwin, C.M.; Kapur, V.K.; Holberg, C.J.; Rosen, C.; Nieto, F.J. Associations between gender and measures of daytime somnolence in the Sleep Heart Health Study. *Sleep* 2004, *27*, 305–311. [CrossRef] [PubMed]
14. Stansbury, R.C.; Strollo, P.J. Clinical manifestations of sleep apnea. *J. Thorac. Dis.* 2015, *7*, E298–E310. [PubMed]
15. Garbarino, S.; Scoditti, E.; Lanteri, P.; Conte, L.; Magnavita, N.; Toraldo, D.M. Obstructive Sleep Apnea With or Without Excessive Daytime Sleepiness: Clinical and Experimental Data-Driven Phenotyping. *Front. Neurol.* 2018, *9*, 505. [CrossRef] [PubMed]
16. Jacobsen, J.H.; Shi, L.; Mokhlesi, B. Factors associated with excessive daytime sleepiness in patients with severe obstructive sleep apnea. *Sleep Breath.* 2013, *17*, 629–635. [CrossRef] [PubMed]
17. Ulander, M.; Hedner, J.; Stillberg, G.; Sunnergren, O.; Grote, L. Correlates of excessive daytime sleepiness in obstructive sleep apnea:results from the nationwide SESAR cohort including patients. *J. Sleep Res.* 2022, *31*, e13690. [CrossRef]
18. Prasad, B.; Steffen, A.D.; Van Dongen, H.P.A.; Pack, F.M.; Strakovsky, I.; Staley, B.; Dinges, D.F.; Maislin, G.; Pack, A.I.; Weaver, T.E. Determinants of sleepiness in obstructive sleep apnea. *Sleep* 2018, *41*, zsx199. [CrossRef]
19. Lal, C.; Weaver, T.E.; Bae, C.J.; Strohl, K.P. Excessive Daytime Sleepiness in Obstructive Sleep Apnea. Mechanisms and Clinical Management. *Ann. Am. Thorac. Soc.* 2021, *18*, 757–768. [CrossRef] [PubMed]
20. Oksenberg, A.; Arons, E.; Nasser, K.; Shneor, O.; Radwan, H.; Silverberg, D.S. Severe obstructive sleep apnea: Sleepy versus nonsleepy patients. *Laryngoscope* 2010, *120*, 643–648. [CrossRef] [PubMed]
21. Shao, C.; Qi, H.; Lang, R.; Yu, B.; Tang, Y.; Zhang, L.; Wang, X.; Wang, L. Clinical features and contributing factors of excessive daytime sleepiness in Chinese obstructive sleep apnea patients: The role of comorbid symptoms and polysomnographic variables. *Can. Respir. J.* 2019, *2019*, 5476372. [CrossRef] [PubMed]
22. Sun, Y.; Ning, Y.; Huang, L.; Lei, F.; Li, Z.; Zhou, G.; Tang, X. Polysomnographic characteristics of daytime sleepiness in obstructive sleep apnea syndrome. *Sleep Breath.* 2012, *16*, 375–381. [CrossRef] [PubMed]
23. Rey de Castro, J.; Rosales-Mayor, E. Clinical and polysomnographic differences between OSAH patients with/without excessive daytime sleepiness. *Sleep Breath.* 2013, *17*, 1079–1086. [CrossRef] [PubMed]
24. Chen, R.; Xiong, K.P.; Lian, Y.X.; Huang, J.Y.; Zhao, M.Y.; Li, J.X.; Liu, C.F. Daytime sleepiness and its determining factors in Chinese obstructive sleep apnea patients. *Sleep Breath.* 2011, *15*, 129–135. [CrossRef]

25. Bonsignore, M.R.; Randerath, W.; Riha, R.; Smyth, D.; Gratziou, C.; Gonçalves, M.; McNicholas, W.T. New rules on driver licensing for patients with obstructive sleep apnea: European Union Directive 2014/85/EU. *J. Sleep Res.* **2016**, *25*, 3–4. [CrossRef] [PubMed]
26. Johns, M.W. A new method for measuring daytime sleepiness: The Epworth sleepiness scale. *Sleep* **1991**, *14*, 540–545. [CrossRef]
27. Berry, R.B.; Brooks, R.; Gamaldo, C.E.; Harding, S.M.; Lloyd, R.M.; Quan, S.F.; Troester, M.T.; Vaughn, B.V. *The AASM Manual for the Scoring of Sleep and Associated Events: Rules, Terminology and Technical Specifications, Version 2.3*; American Academy of Sleep Medicine: Darien, IL, USA, 2016.
28. Goncalves, M.A.; Paiva, T.; Ramos, E.; Guilleminault, C. Obstructive sleep apnea syndrome, sleepiness, and quality of life. *Chest* **2004**, *125*, 2091–2096. [CrossRef] [PubMed]
29. Archontogeorgis, K.; Economou, N.T.; Bargiotas, P.; Nena, E.; Voulgaris, A.; Chadia, K.; Trakada, G.; Romigi, A.; Steiropoulos, P. Sleepiness and Vitamin D Levels in Patients with Obstructive Sleep Apnea. *Healthcare* **2024**, *12*, 698. [CrossRef]
30. Thorarinsdottir, E.H.; Pack, A.I.; Gislason, T.; Kuna, S.T.; Penzel, T.; Yun Li, Q.; Cistulli, P.A.; Magalang, U.J.; McArdle, N.; Singh, B.; et al. Polysomnographic characteristics of excessive daytime sleepiness phenotypes in obstructive sleep apnea: Results from the international sleep apnea global interdisciplinary consortium. *Sleep* **2024**, *47*, zsae035. [CrossRef] [PubMed]
31. Kapur, V.K.; Baldwin, C.M.; Resnick, H.E.; Gottlieb, D.J.; Nieto, F.J. Sleepiness in patients with moderate to severe sleep-disordered breathing. *Sleep* **2005**, *28*, 472–477. [CrossRef]
32. Mediano, O.; Barcelo, A.; de la Pena, M.; Gozal, D.; Agusti, A.; Barbe, F. Daytime sleepiness and polysomnographic variables in sleep apnoea patients. *Rev. Port. Pneumol.* **2007**, *13*, 896–898. [CrossRef] [PubMed]
33. Gottlieb, D.J.; Punjabi, N.M. Diagnosis and management of obstructive sleep apnea: A review. *JAMA* **2020**, *323*, 1389–1400. [CrossRef] [PubMed]
34. Whitney, C.W.; Gottlieb, D.J.; Redline, S.; Norman, R.G.; Dodge, R.R.; Shahar, E.; Surovec, S.; Nieto, F.J. Reliability of scoring respiratory disturbance indices and sleep staging. *Sleep* **1998**, *21*, 749–757. [CrossRef] [PubMed]
35. Dingli, K.; Fietze, I.; Assimakopoulos, T.; Quispe-Bravo, S.; Witt, C.; Douglas, N.J. Arousability in sleep apnoea/hypopnoea syndrome patients. *Eur. Respir. J.* **2002**, *20*, 733–740. [CrossRef] [PubMed]
36. Mansukhani, M.P.; Wang, S.; Somers, V.K. Chemoreflex physiology and implications for sleep apnoea: Insights from studies in humans. *Exp. Physiol.* **2015**, *100*, 130–135. [CrossRef] [PubMed]
37. Azarbarzin, A.; Ostrowski, M.; Hanly, P.; Younes, M. Relationship between arousal intensity and heart rate response to arousal. *Sleep* **2014**, *37*, 645–653. [CrossRef] [PubMed]
38. Schwartz, D.J.; Moxley, P. On the potential clinical relevance of the length of arousals from sleep in patients with obstructive sleep apnea. *J. Clin. Sleep Med.* **2006**, *15*, 175–180.
39. Li, N.; Wang, J.; Wang, D.; Wang, Q.; Han, F.; Jyothi, K.; Chen, R. Correlation of sleep microstructure with daytime sleepiness and cognitive function in young and middle-aged adults with obstructive sleep apnea syndrome. *Eur. Arch. Otorhinolaryngol.* **2019**, *276*, 3525–3532. [CrossRef] [PubMed]
40. Chen, X.; Leppänen, T.; Kainulainen, S.; Howarth, T.P.; Oksenberg, A.; Töyräs, J.; Terrill, P.I.; Korkalainen, H. Sleep stage continuity is associated with objective daytime sleepiness in patients with suspected obstructive sleep apnea. *J. Clin. Sleep Med.* **2024**, *20*, 1595–1606. [CrossRef] [PubMed]
41. Veasey, S.C.; Davis, C.W.; Fenik, P.; Zhan, G.; Hsu, Y.J.; Pratico, D.; Gow, A. Long-term intermittent hypoxia in mice: Protracted hypersomnolence with oxidative injury to sleep-wake brain regions. *Sleep* **2004**, *27*, 194–201. [CrossRef]
42. Zhu, Y.; Fenik, P.; Zhan, G.; Xin, R.; Veasey, S.C. Degeneration in arousal neurons in chronic sleep disruption modeling sleep apnea. *Front. Neurol.* **2015**, *6*, 109. [CrossRef] [PubMed]
43. Zhu, Y.; Fenik, P.; Zhan, G.; Mazza, E.; Kelz, M.; Aston-Jones, G.; Veasey, S.C. Selective loss of catecholaminergic wake active neurons in a murine sleep apnea model. *J. Neurosci.* **2007**, *27*, 10060–10071. [CrossRef] [PubMed]
44. Martinez-Garcia, M.A.; Sánchez-de-la-Torre, M.; White, D.P.; Azarbarzin, A. Hypoxic Burden in Obstructive Sleep Apnea: Present and Future. *Arch. Bronconeumol.* **2023**, *59*, 36–43. [CrossRef] [PubMed]
45. Landzberg, D.; Bagai, K. Prevalence of objective excessive daytime sleepiness in a cohort of patients with mild obstructive sleep apnea. *Sleep Breath.* **2022**, *26*, 1471–1477. [CrossRef] [PubMed]
46. Omobomi, O.; Batool-Anwar, S.; Quan, S.F. Clinical and Polysomnographic Correlates of Subjective Sleepiness in Mild Obstructive Sleep Apnea. *Sleep Vigil.* **2019**, *3*, 131–138. [CrossRef] [PubMed]
47. Lee, S.A.; Paek, J.H.; Han, S.H. Sleep hygiene and its association with daytime sleepiness, depressive symptoms, and quality of life in patients with mild obstructive sleep apnea. *J. Neurol. Sci.* **2015**, *359*, 445–449. [CrossRef]
48. Roure, N.; Gomez, S.; Mediano, O.; Duran, J.; de la Peña, M.; Capote, F.; Teran, J.; Masa, J.F.; Alonso, M.L.; Corral, J.; et al. Daytime sleepiness and polysomnography in obstructive sleep apnea patients. *Sleep Med.* **2008**, *9*, 727–731. [CrossRef] [PubMed]
49. Ramos, A.R.; Figueredo, P.; Shafazand, S.; Chediak, A.D.; Abreu, A.R.; Dib, S.I.; Torre, C.; Wallace, D.M. Obstructive sleep apnea phenotypes and markers of vascular disease: A review. *Front. Neurol.* **2017**, *8*, 659. [CrossRef] [PubMed]

50. Onen, F.; Moreau, T.; Gooneratne, N.S.; Petit, C.; Falissard, B.; Onen, S.H. Limits of the Epworth sleepiness scale in older adults. *Sleep Breath.* **2013**, *17*, 343–350. [CrossRef] [PubMed]
51. Drakatos, P.; Ghiassi, R.; Jarrold, I.; Harris, J.; Abidi, A.; Douiri, A.; Hart, N.; Kosky, C.; Williams, A.J.; Partridge, M.R.; et al. The use of an online pictorial Epworth Sleepiness Scale in the assessment of age and gender specific differences in excessive daytime sleepiness. *J. Thorac. Dis.* **2015**, *7*, 897–902. [PubMed]
52. Lin, C.M.; Davidson, T.M.; Ancoli-Israel, S. Gender differences in obstructive sleep apnea and treatment implications. *Sleep Med. Rev.* **2008**, *12*, 481–496. [CrossRef] [PubMed]
53. Valipour, A.; Lothaller, H.; Rauscher, H.; Zwick, H.; Burghuber, O.C.; Lavie, P. Genderrelated differences in symptoms of patients with suspected breathing disorders in sleep: A clinical population study using the sleep disorders questionnaire. *Sleep* **2007**, *30*, 312–319. [CrossRef]
54. Ng, W.L.; Orellana, L.; Shaw, J.E.; Wong, E.; Peeters, A. The relationship between weight change and daytime sleepiness: The Sleep Heart Health Study. *Sleep Med.* **2017**, *36*, 109–118. [CrossRef] [PubMed]

Disclaimer/Publisher's Note: The statements, opinions and data contained in all publications are solely those of the individual author(s) and contributor(s) and not of MDPI and/or the editor(s). MDPI and/or the editor(s) disclaim responsibility for any injury to people or property resulting from any ideas, methods, instructions or products referred to in the content.

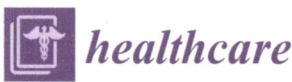
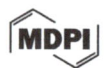

Article

Factors Affecting CPAP Adherence in an OSA Population during the First Two Years of the COVID-19 Pandemic

Dimosthenis Lykouras [†], Eirini Zarkadi [†], Electra Koulousousa, Olga Lagiou, Dimitrios Komninos, Argyris Tzouvelekis and Kyriakos Karkoulias *

Department of Respiratory Medicine, University Hospital of Patras, 26500 Patras, Greece; lykouras@upatras.gr (D.L.); edzarka@gmail.com (E.Z.); komninos312@gmail.com (D.K.); argyris.tzouvelekis@gmail.com (A.T.)
* Correspondence: karkoulias@upatras.gr
[†] These authors contributed equally to this work.

Abstract: Background: Obstructive sleep apnea (OSA) is a common disorder associated with major cardiovascular and neurocognitive sequelae. Continuous positive airway pressure (CPAP) is the standard treatment for OSA. The aim of this study was to investigate the prevalence and associations of long-term CPAP adherence in newly diagnosed OSA patients. **Methods:** We enrolled patients who were diagnosed with OSA during the COVID-19 pandemic. Adherence was defined as CPAP use ≥4 h per night on ≥70% of nights over 30 consecutive days. Patient demographics were retrieved from medical records, and CPAP adherence at 6 months and 1 year after initiation was monitored. **Results:** Overall, 107 patients were included in the analysis. A number of 73 (68%) and 63 (59%) patients were adherent to CPAP treatment at 6 months and 12 months accordingly. Among the factors examined and analyzed (age, gender, BMI, Apnea–Hypopnea Index (AHI)), no significant correlation was found. Further analysis revealed the potential role of comorbidities. CPAP compliance at 6 months was shown to be associated with better CPAP adherence at 12 months. **Conclusions:** CPAP adherence at 6 months is correlated to long-term adherence to treatment. Therefore, early close follow-up is important. Further prospective studies are needed to identify other potential predictors.

Keywords: CPAP; OSA; CPAP adherence; telemedicine

1. Introduction

Modern society and technological advances render our lifestyle incompatible with good sleep [1]. Obstructive sleep apnea (OSA) is a common sleep disorder that affects up to 23% of middle-aged women and 50% of middle-aged men [2]. It is characterized by repeated collapses of the upper airway, causing interrupted sleep, lower oxygen levels, and increased sympathetic activity, leading to high blood pressure. OSA may also result in cognitive issues and daytime sleepiness, which can significantly affect quality of life [3].

Continuous positive airway pressure (CPAP) is widely recognized as the primary treatment option for OSA. Despite ongoing debates about its impact on cardiovascular outcomes, CPAP is proven to reduce daytime sleepiness and enhance mood and quality of life [4]. A patient with OSA may need to use CPAP for at least 4 h a night to experience a reduction in daytime symptoms, especially sleepiness and neurocognitive function, and reduce the risk of developing cardiovascular and metabolic comorbidities. An overall CPAP use of >4 h per night on most nights during a week (>70% of nights) marks optimal CPAP adherence in most studies [5]. However, its efficacy can be hampered by poor adherence to the therapy [6].

Facing difficulties with CPAP therapy is a frequent issue seen in clinical settings. Research indicates that adherence to CPAP therapy usually ranges from 30 to 60%. In cases of mild OSA, where the symptoms are typically less severe and thus easier to manage, adherence to CPAP therapy may potentially be even lower [7].

A myriad of both medical and non-medical factors may contribute to configuring CPAP adherence and numerous studies have attempted to investigate the determinants. Several demographic variables, such as age, gender, and body mass index (BMI), are reported to have an effect on compliance. The severity of OSA, as indicated by a high Apnea–Hypopnea Index (AHI) and excessive daytime sleepiness, has been associated with better adherence to CPAP therapy. The presence of comorbidities, as well as socioeconomic factors, such as economic, educational, and civil status, have also been shown to interfere with treatment compliance. Moreover, device-related factors, which can include physical discomfort while using the device, financial and insurance reimbursement issues, and the associated psychological stress [8], have also been highlighted. Finally, early compliance is pointed out as a positive predictive factor, while interventions such as the use of telemedicine may favorably influence long-term adherence [9].

Therefore, a comprehensive and individualized approach is required to optimize patient care and mitigate the risk of treatment failure [10]. However, even though the issue has been extensively addressed, several studies have yielded conflicting results, and there is still no consensus on which specific factors are associated with CPAP adherence.

Adding to the above, since the onset of the COVID-19 pandemic in 2020, the world has rapidly transformed. This transformation has particularly affected patients with sleep-disordered breathing conditions, especially OSA, who face potentially more severe COVID-19 outcomes due to the shared risk factors and comorbidities of both diseases. Initially, continuous positive airway pressure (CPAP) therapy, the primary option for moderate to severe OSA, was marked as a high-risk aerosol-generating procedure causing fear of potential COVID-19 transmission. To address these issues, several scientific societies have issued recommendations on screening, diagnosing, and treating sleep-disordered breathing during the pandemic. The pandemic caused a decrease in patient visits in clinics across Europe, Greece included. Most centers have had to restrict themselves to phone-based follow-ups and handling high-priority cases [11].

The aim of this study was to investigate the prevalence of long-term CPAP adherence in newly diagnosed OSA patients and identify specific factors that are linked to improved adherence. The study time frame was during the first 2 years of the COVID-19 pandemic.

2. Materials and Methods

2.1. Subjects

This is a retrospective observational study of patients referred to the sleep laboratory of the Department of Respiratory Medicine, University Hospital of Patras, Greece. All patients recruited for the study underwent night polysomnography (NPSG) between January 2020 and December 2022, during the initial phase of the COVID-19 pandemic. Only adult patients who were diagnosed for the first time with OSA and started CPAP treatment were included in the study analysis. Old CPAP users and patients who did not start CPAP treatment for any reason (declined, reimbursement issues, patient preference) were excluded from the analysis. Patients with overt cardiovascular disease and patients with a diagnosis of active cancer at the time of data collection after the phone contact were not included.

The diagnosis of OSA is made when a patient undergoing a diagnostic sleep study has an AHI of 5 or more. Patients were classified by AHI into mild (AHI $\geq$ 5 and <15), moderate ($\geq$15 and <30), and severe (AHI $\geq$ 30) OSA. CPAP adherence was defined as at least 4 h/night use on 70% of nights. Patients who had a diagnosis other than OSA, such as insomnia and obesity hypoventilation syndrome, were excluded from the study. We also excluded patients with increased AHI who were prescribed non-invasive ventilation (NIV) for other indications.

It should be noted that the recruitment period was during the initial phase of the COVID-19 pandemic; a time during which mandatory sleep laboratory closures led to limited access for patients to some of our services. Patients initially undergo a sleep study in the laboratory, and then a titration study follows. After CPAP initiation at home, they return to an outpatient clinic, or they receive a follow-up phone call at 1 month to check initial compliance and treatment efficacy. Afterwards, regular visits happen every 6 months, when a prescription for reimbursement is needed as well. Restrictive measures during the pandemic reduced subsequently in-person visits.

The medical records of included patients were accessed, and data regarding demographics (age, gender, profession, marital status, body mass index (BMI)), sleep questionnaires (Epworth Sleepiness Score (ESS), Athens Insomnia Scale (AIS)), and sleep study parameters (Apnea–Hypopnea Index (AHI)) were collected. We did not explore other sleep study parameters, such as the oxygen desaturation index (ODI) or the average desaturation percentage. Sleep studies were scored according to current American Academy of Sleep Medicine (AASM) diagnostic criteria [12]. We also collected medical information regarding chronic concomitant diseases, including diabetes, hypertension and heart failure, chronic obstructive pulmonary disease, and depression. Patients should have been on treatment for at least 3 months to be regarded as suffering from the respective diseases. The CPAP start date was noted as the initial checkpoint for the study.

2.2. Data Collection

CPAP usage information was collected through the AirView platform for patients using ResMed CPAP machines. More specifically, patients were checked for adherence to their treatment at 6 months and 12 months after CPAP initiation. Additional information was obtained by a phone call. Patients who were using other CPAP machines were only interviewed by phone call.

The investigators managed to identify CPAP patients and then gathered information regarding CPAP usage and adherence to treatment according to the study protocol from existing information. Afterwards, study participants were contacted via telephone, and structured interviews were performed containing questions on side effects, co-morbidities, lifestyle, and other factors that could possibly have impaired adherence. It should be noted that telephone interviews may be linked to patient reporting bias. We combined these data with information from electronic patient records and other medical records available at our site.

Adherence was defined as adequate use of CPAP for ≥ 4 h on at least >70% of nights during the last month prior to study checkpoints (before 6 months and before 12 months). Patients were grouped accordingly to adherent and non-adherent.

2.3. Statistical Analysis

Statistical analysis was performed using IBM SPSS version 28 (IBM, Armonk, NY, USA), and $p < 0.05$ was statistically significant. All results are presented as mean values and standard deviations (SD) unless stated otherwise. Comparisons between the two groups of patients (compliant at 1 year and non-compliant at 1 year) were made using chi-square for binary variables, t-test for normally distributed variables, and Wilcoxon rank test for not normally distributed variables. We performed bivariate analysis to investigate the potential correlations between participants' characteristics and their adherence to CPAP treatment at 6 months and 12 months after starting their CPAP treatment.

2.4. Ethical Considerations

The study has been approved by the Institutional ethical committee and review board (approval code 143/2024). The study was performed according to the Declaration of Helsinki. All participants had provided verbal consent to participate in the study via telephone call or had already provided consent for the online data management platform. The verbal consent was documented by the interviewing physician.

3. Results

The overall number of patients who underwent a night study during the studied period was 240. A total of 134 patients were eligible for entry in the study, as they were diagnosed with OSA and started CPAP during the years 2020–2022. As this is a retrospective analysis, the dataset was reduced to 107 patients on CPAP because of corrupt contact information (21 subjects had either given a number that was not receiving or patients were not responding) and unwillingness to participate in the study (6 subjects).

Baseline characteristics of the OSA patients started on CPAP are shown in Table 1. They were divided into two groups according to their adherence to CPAP treatment 1 year after CPAP titration and CPAP initiation. The mean age for the non-adherent and adherent group at 1 year were 53.4 (10.2) and 56.2 (11.0) years, respectively. Both genders were represented, but the number of men was slightly higher, without any impact on data interpretation. The mean BMI (33.7 versus 36.7), AHI (46.8 versus 51.0), and ESS (11.4 versus 10.3) were not significantly different between the groups. Thus, the groups were matched, and any outcome variation was not due to baseline predisposition. A key point in our analysis was the fact that patients both near the site and far away showed similar adherence to CPAP treatment (20 patients near the site city and 23 patients in remote areas in the non-adherent group) (34 near the site city and 30 in the remote area adherent group).

Table 1. Baseline characteristics of study subjects.

	CPAP Non-Adherent at 1 Year (n = 43)	CPAP Adherent at 1 Year (n = 64)	All Patients (n = 107)	*p*-Value
Age (years)	53.4 (10.2)	56.2 (11.0)	55.2 (10.7)	0.434
Gender (M/F)	35/8 (81.3%/18.7%)	51/13 (79.6%/20.4%)	86/21 (80.3%/19.7%)	0.516
Height (cm)	174.3 (8.1)	173.6 (10.0)	173.9 (9.2)	0.270
Weight (kg)	102.1 (19.3)	109.8 (21.0)	106.7 (20.6)	0.988
BMI (kg/m^2)	33.7 (7.0)	36.7 (8.1)	35.5 (7.8)	0.238
AHI (events/h)	46.8 (24.4)	51.0 (27.4)	49.3 (26.2)	0.215
Epworth Sleepiness Scale (ESS) score	11.4 (4.9)	10.3 (5.1)	10.7 (5.0)	0.920
Athens Insomnia Scale (AIS) score	7.8 (4.4)	7.2 (3.9)	7.4 (4.1)	0.406
Residence (site city/remote)	20/23 (46.5%/53.5%)	34/30 (53.1%/46.9%)	54/53 (50.4%/50.6%)	0.318
Diabetes	7 (16.2%)	15 (23.4%)	22 (20.5%)	0.467
Hypertension	24 (55.8%)	30 (46.8%)	54 (50.4%)	0.432
Heart failure	14 (32.5%)	18 (28.1%)	32 (29.9%)	0.670
COPD	9 (20.9%)	15 (23.4%)	24 (22.4%)	0.817
Depression	6 (13.9%)	18 (28.1%)	24 (22.4%)	0.102

Values are presented as mean (SD) unless stated otherwise.

A total number of 73 patients were using CPAP treatment at 6 months after treatment initiation, with an adherence level of 68.2%. The percentage of adherence fell 1 year after treatment initiation and was as high as 59.8%, as demonstrated in Table 1.

We attempted to analyze factors that may result in this important reduction in treatment compliance. Age, gender, weight, height, BMI, Apnea–Hypopnea Index (AHI) at diagnosis, and residence of patients (in the city of the site or in remote areas) were tested in the analysis. None of these factors were shown to be associated with worse adherence to CPAP treatment.

A percentage of 23% of those who discontinued CPAP usage reported that difficulties with its use (noise, mask interface issues, leakages) had urged them to do so. Another 10% of non-compliant patients had stopped their treatment due to financial issues and lack of insurance, thus reflecting an important aspect to be considered, especially in long-term treatments.

We also attempted to explore the role that comorbidities may play in adherence to treatment. Therefore, we tested the effect of diabetes, hypertension, heart failure, COPD, and depression on CPAP adherence at the end of the first year of treatment. However, none of these variables demonstrated statistical significance.

We performed bivariate analysis to further investigate the potential correlations between the patients' characteristics and their adherence to CPAP treatment at 6 months and 1 year after treatment initiation (Table 2). The analysis revealed some statistically significant correlations that could enable the prediction of CPAP adherence based on the baseline characteristics in our study population. Older age was a predictor in both groups ($p = 0.049$ at 6 months and $p = 0.029$ at 1 year), and increased BMI was a determinant of better adherence at 1 year of CPAP use ($p = 0.020$). As for the comorbidities, a significant correlation was found for CPAP users with depression ($p = 0.037$), who were more likely to have better compliance at 1 year of treatment.

Table 2. CPAP online management and CPAP usage at 6-month correlation to overall CPAP adherence at 1 year.

	CPAP Non-Adherent at 1 Year (n = 43)	CPAP Adherent at 1 Year (n = 64)	p-Value
CPAP online management (yes/no)	16/27 (37.2%/62.8%)	30/34 (46.8%/53.2%)	0.215
CPAP adherence at 6 months (yes/no)	11/32 (25.6%/74.6%)	62/2 (96.8%/3.2%)	<0.001

Further multivariate analysis of our data was performed to elucidate the most important factors affecting CPAP adherence at 1 year after treatment initiation. The results showed that patients with optimal adherence at 6 months had a higher likelihood of continuing their treatment ($p < 0.001$). Patients on treatment for depression ($p = 0.033$) were showing better compliance, and patients using telemedicine tools for device monitoring had a tendency ($p = 0.072$) to have improved compliance with their CPAP treatment.

Our study shows that patients showing good compliance at 6 months may also have good CPAP compliance at 1 year (Table 2). Online management tools were not directly associated with improvements in compliance, yet a trend towards improvement was recorded in our data, as patients who did not use available telemedicine tools tended to be non-adherent 1 year after CPAP treatment initiation.

4. Discussion

CPAP is the treatment of choice for OSA and is seen as the benchmark. Research shows that CPAP treatment can reduce the risk of cardiovascular disease in patients with moderate to severe OSA, improving their quality of life and daytime sleepiness. CPAP adherence is important for treatment outcomes, but adherence rates have been reported to vary between 30 and 60% in different previous studies.

In our study, we found that 68% of the patients were using CPAP 6 months after treatment initiation. This finding is in line with the 6-month adherence rate of 63.9% and 70.3% reported in previous studies in the field [13,14]. Those patients were using their treatment according to guidelines for CPAP use, that is, at least 4 h every night and at least >70% of nights every month.

A recent study investigating long-term adherence to CPAP treatment in mild OSA showed that only 25.7% of patients continued using their machine 1 year after starting it. Further analysis showed that older patients with lower BMI and the presence of a bed partner had a better chance of remaining on the treatment [15]. A large study, in a population in Asia that recruited OSA patients with mild up to severe disease, revealed that a total of 78.5% of CPAP users remained adhering to their treatment 1 year after treatment had started. They also concluded that trial treatment of 1 month was improving overall treatment adherence [16]. Our results from our single-site population revealed quite a high percentage of adherence to CPAP treatment in the patients, which is comparable to studies recruiting patients at all stages of disease severity.

CPAP therapy can be intrusive for patients, and low adherence can be a major problem. One of the first studies in the field of CPAP adherence was published back in 1993 [17].

CPAP was available in clinical practice for less than 10 years at that time. In this study, memory chips were used to accurately track adherence data. They analyzed key metrics, including mean nightly usage time, the number of nights the therapy was used, and side effects. Their findings suggested that using the therapy for at least 4 h on 70% of nights was a reliable indicator of treatment compliance. In another study investigating CPAP adherence patterns, the authors discovered two groups of CPAP users among their participants. The "intermittent" users tended to skip 1–7 nights per week and used the therapy for fewer hours each night. On the other hand, the "consistent" users applied their devices on 90% of nights or more and typically used them for longer periods [18].

Our study shows that adherence to CPAP at 6 months after treatment initiation is predictive of CPAP adherence at 1 year. This finding is in accordance with previous studies showing that if CPAP adherence is achieved early, CPAP compliance can last [19]. In the SAVE (Sleep Apnea Cardiovascular Endpoints) study, only compliance at 1 month and the presence of side effects of CPAP therapy were independent predictors of its use at 12 months. Similarly, previous studies have reported that CPAP usage patterns within the first week are predictive of long-term use [20].

The examination of other factors that could be correlated to optimal CPAP adherence at 1 year, such as sex, age, increased BMI or worse AHI, did not reveal any significant results. However, a further bivariate logistic regression analysis showed that CPAP users who were older and had a higher BMI were more likely to comply with treatment at 1 year. A retrospective observational study of 1339 OSA patients found no association between CPAP adherence and demographic or polysomnographic variables, which is in accordance with our negative results. The association between AHI and CPAP adherence was not confirmed in a study of 188 patients with moderate to severe OSA [21].

Hypersomnolence, as indicated by high ESS, has been proposed as a predictor of compliance. In our analysis, we found no significant correlation. In agreement with our results, a previous study also predicted no association with ESS, which can also be justified by the fact reported by some authors that ESS score is poorly correlated with OSA severity [22].

Moreover, several studies have suggested that rural residence might be a potential barrier for OSA patients to diagnosis and care. An important prospective cohort study of 242 uncomplicated patients with OSA, urban versus rural residence, was not associated with CPAP use or adherence [23]. Correspondingly, we found no significant difference between patients coming from the city and those from remote areas.

Another issue to be addressed is comorbidities in patients under CPAP treatment for OSA. Diseases, including diabetes, hypertension, COPD and depression, are highly prevalent in the OSA population, and we intended to determine their role in adherence to CPAP treatment. Interestingly, patients under treatment for depression were more likely to be compliant with CPAP treatment one year after starting it. However, a large-scale study of a similar population in Greece did not demonstrate a potential role of any comorbidity in adherence to treatment.

An important finding of our study is that patients who demonstrated good compliance at 6 months may also have good CPAP compliance at 1 year. Therefore, close monitoring during the first months of CPAP usage is of paramount importance for long-term compliance. Future studies may consider shorter monitoring periods of 3 months in the initial phases of CPAP treatment to further clarify this issue.

The online management tool that was used by some of our patients, ResMed Airview, was also not found to improve compliance in our analysis. Indeed, previous studies have reported comparable findings. A multinational study indicated that telemonitoring did not improve 1-month and 3-month CPAP adherence compared with usual care, while in a cohort of 120 patients with OSA, the usage of telemedicine during the critical habituation phase for CPAP did not alter daily CPAP use or treatment adherence at 3 and 12 months [24]. In contrast, a recent meta-analysis of 11 studies with 1358 revealed that telemedicine interventions may improve CPAP adherence in patients with OSA compared to no intervention [25]. However, although the efficacy of telemonitoring systems has been inconsistent, most trials have shown that such tools could prove more cost-effective and source-saving. Meanwhile, especially in a setting simulating the COVID-19 pandemic, with reduced footfall in healthcare facilities, telemonitoring could prove of significant value. Moreover, in our region in Greece, we treat patients from remote areas of the islands, and telemedicine is of great value in this setting as well.

A large prospective study from Greece that investigated the impact of the COVID-19 pandemic on the CPAP adherence of patients already on CPAP concluded that it did not actually affect device usage. Moreover, the use of telemedicine was important to overcome barriers caused by lockdowns in order to facilitate regular follow-ups and increase CPAP treatment adherence [11].

The treatment rejection rate at 1 year in our study is acceptable. The reasons for treatment discontinuation included difficulties with CPAP daily use, such as noise, mask interface issues, and leakages. Another important aspect of CPAP discontinuation is the relatively high cost of obtaining a CPAP machine either privately or through insurance coverage. A substantial minority (10%) of patients non-compliant with CPAP prematurely discontinued treatment due to financial issues and lack of insurance.

Our study was designed to demonstrate CPAP adherence among patients during the years of the pandemic. At that time, several lockdowns in Greece appreciably affected sleep laboratory services and sleep clinics. Nevertheless, regular follow-up visits and phone consultations may have resulted in quite high CPAP adherence in our cohort. Furthermore, several studies have reported ameliorated CPAP adherence during the COVID-19 pandemic. In a cohort of 7485 patients with OSA, the investigators reported a 3.9% increase in adherence from a mean value of 386 min per night pre-COVID-19 to 401 min per night during lockdown [26]. Another study also observed that improved CPAP adherence in severe OSA patients during the COVID-19 lockdown was more pronounced in women and younger and pre-lockdown CPAP adherers [27].

Our study has some limitations. Firstly, this is a retrospective study; therefore, missing information may have reduced our initial sample size. Secondly, phone interviews may have intrinsic defects with regard to the accuracy of information derived from patients. Thirdly, the retrospective design did not allow us to have correlations with other comorbidities that could affect adherence levels, such as hypertension and diabetes. The last remark is that our study is a single-site retrospective study that may have selection bias caused by the availability of some technologies or geographic distribution.

5. Conclusions

Effective CPAP treatment can be affected by several factors. Patients who were adherent to CPAP treatment at 6 months were more likely to continue using their device and on a long-term basis, thus, showing sustained adherence at 1 year and subsequently a lower drop-out rate. Other factors, including OSA severity, BMI, or sleepiness severity, were not significantly correlated with long-term CPAP adherence. Further prospective studies may be needed to clarify other potential predictors of treatment compliance.

Author Contributions: D.L.: conception, data collection, data analysis, and manuscript preparation, E.Z.: data collection and manuscript preparation, E.K.: data collection and manuscript preparation, O.L.: data analysis and manuscript preparation, D.K.: data collection, A.T.: conception and manuscript preparation, K.K.: conception and manuscript preparation. All authors have read and agreed to the published version of the manuscript.

Funding: This research received no external funding.

Institutional Review Board Statement: The study has been approved by the Institutional ethical committee and review board (approval code 143/2024, approved on 14 March 2024). The study was performed according to the Declaration of Helsinki.

Informed Consent Statement: All participants provided verbal consent to participate in the study via telephone call or had already provided consent for the online data management platform. Written informed consent for publication has been waived due to already existing and/or documented verbal consent.

Data Availability Statement: Data are contained within the article.

Conflicts of Interest: The authors declare no conflicts of interest.

References

1. Bendaoud, I.; Sosso, F.A.E. Socioeconomic Position and Excessive Daytime Sleepiness: A Systematic Review of Social Epidemiological Studies. *Clocks Sleep* **2022**, *4*, 240–259. [CrossRef]
2. Heinzer, R.; Vat, S.; Marques-Vidal, P.; Marti-Soler, H.; Andries, D.; Tobback, N.; Mooser, V.; Preisig, M.; Malhotra, A.; Waeber, G.; et al. Prevalence of sleep-disordered breathing in the general population: The HypnoLaus study. *Lancet Respir. Med.* **2015**, *3*, 310–318. [CrossRef]
3. McEvoy, R.; Antic, N.; Heeley, E.; Luo, Y.; Ou, Q.; Zhang, X.; Mediano, O.; Chen, R.; Drager, L.F.; Liu, Z.; et al. CPAP for Prevention of Cardiovascular Events in Obstructive Sleep Apnea. *N. Engl. J. Med.* **2016**, *375*, 919–931. [CrossRef] [PubMed]
4. Abuzaid, A.; Al Ashry, H.; Elbadawi, A.; Ld, H.; Saad, M.; Elgendy, I.Y.; Elgendy, A.; Mahmoud, A.N.; Mentias, A.; Barakat, A.; et al. Meta-Analysis of Cardiovascular Outcomes With Continuous Positive Airway Pressure Therapy in Patients With Obstructive Sleep Apnea. *Am. J. Cardiol.* **2017**, *120*, 693–699. [CrossRef] [PubMed]
5. Engleman, H.; Martin, S.; Douglas, N. Compliance with CPAP therapy in patients with the sleep apnoea/hypopnoea syndrome. *Thorax* **1994**, *49*, 263–266. [CrossRef] [PubMed]
6. Weaver, T.; Grunstein, R. Adherence to continuous positive airway pressure therapy: The challenge to effective treatment. *Proc. Am. Thorac. Soc.* **2008**, *5*, 173–178. [CrossRef]
7. Lin, H.; Prasad, A.; Pan, C.; Rowley, J.A. Factors associated with noncompliance to treatment with positive airway pressure. *Arch. Otolaryngol.-Head Neck Surg.* **2007**, *133*, 69–72. [CrossRef] [PubMed]
8. Hussain, S.; Irfan, M.; Waheed, Z.; Alam, N.; Mansoor, S.; Islam, M. Compliance with continuous positive airway pressure (CPAP) therapy for obstructive sleep apnea among privately paying patients—A cross sectional study. *BMC Pulm. Med.* **2014**, *14*, 188. [CrossRef]
9. Tsuyumu, M.; Tsurumoto, T.; Iimura, J.; Nakajima, T.; Kojima, H. Ten-year adherence to continuous positive airway pressure treatment in patients with moderate-to-severe obstructive sleep apnea. *Sleep Breath.* **2020**, *24*, 1565–1571. [CrossRef]
10. Sawyer, A.; Gooneratne, N.; Marcus, C.; Ofer, D.; Richards, K.C.; Weaver, T.E. A systematic review of CPAP adherence across age groups: Clinical and empiric insights for developing CPAP adherence interventions. *Sleep Med. Rev.* **2011**, *15*, 343–356. [CrossRef]
11. Bouloukaki, I.; Pataka, A.; Mauroudi, E.; Moniaki, V.; Fanaridis, M.; Schiza, S.E. Impact of the COVID-19 pandemic on positive airway pressure adherence and patients' perspectives in Greece: The role of telemedicine. *J. Clin. Sleep Med.* **2023**, *19*, 1743–1751. [CrossRef]
12. Berry, R.; Budhiraja, R.; Gottlieb, D.; Gozal, D.; Iber, C.; Kapur, V.K.; Marcus, C.L.; Mehra, R.; Parthasarathy, S.; Quan, S.F.; et al. Rules for scoring respiratory events in sleep: Update of the 2007 AASM Manual for the Scoring of Sleep and Associated Events. Deliberations of the Sleep Apnea Definitions Task Force of the American Academy of Sleep Medicine. *J. Clin. Sleep Med.* **2012**, *8*, 597–619. [CrossRef]
13. Basoglu, O.; Midilli, M.; Midilli, R.; Bilgen, C. Adherence to continuous positive airway pressure therapy in obstructive sleep apnea syndrome: Effect of visual education. *Sleep Breath.* **2012**, *16*, 1193–1200. [CrossRef] [PubMed]
14. Riachy, M.; Najem, S.; Iskandar, M.; Choucair, J.; Ibrahim, I.; Juvelikian, G. Factors predicting CPAP adherence in obstructive sleep apnea syndrome. *Sleep Breath.* **2017**, *21*, 295–302. [CrossRef] [PubMed]
15. Qiao, M.; Xie, Y.; Wolff, A.; Kwon, J. Long term adherence to continuous positive Airway pressure in mild obstructive sleep apnea. *BMC Pulm. Med.* **2023**, *23*, 320. [CrossRef] [PubMed]
16. Tan, B.; Tan, A.; Chan, Y.H.; Mok, Y.; Wong, H.S.; Hsu, P.P. Adherence to Continuous Positive Airway Pressure therapy in Singaporean patients with Obstructive Sleep Apnea. *Am. J. Otolaryngol.* **2018**, *39*, 501–506. [CrossRef]
17. Kribbs, N.; Pack, A.; Kline, L.; Smith, P.L.; Schwartz, A.R.; Schubert, N.M.; Redline, S.; Henry, J.N.; Getsy, J.E.; Dinges, D.F. Objective measurement of patterns of nasal CPAP use by patients with obstructive sleep apnea. *Am. Rev. Respir. Dis.* **1993**, *147*, 887–895. [CrossRef] [PubMed]
18. Weaver, T.; Kribbs, N.; Pack, A.; Kline, L.R.; Chugh, D.K.; Maislin, G.; Smith, P.L.; Schwartz, A.R.; Schubert, N.M.; Gillen, K.A.; et al. Night-to-night variability in CPAP use over the first three months of treatment. *Sleep* **1997**, *20*, 278–283. [CrossRef]
19. Nadal, N.; De Batlle, J.; Barbé, F.; Marsal, J.R.; Sánchez-De-La-Torre, A.; Tarraubella, N.; Lavega, M.; Sánchez-De-La-Torre, M. Predictors of CPAP compliance in different clinical settings: Primary care versus sleep unit. *Sleep Breath.* **2018**, *22*, 157–163. [CrossRef]
20. Van Ryswyk, E.; Anderson, C.S.; Antic, N.A.; Barbe, F.; Bittencourt, L.; Freed, R.; Heeley, E.; Liu, Z.; Loffler, K.A.; Lorenzi-Filho, G.; et al. Predictors of long-term adherence to continuous positive airway pressure in patients with obstructive sleep apnea and cardiovascular disease. *Sleep* **2019**, *42*, zsz152. [CrossRef]

21. Chiu, H.; Chen, P.; Chuang, L.; Chen, N.; Tu, Y.; Hsieh, Y.; Wang, Y.; Guilleminault, C. Diagnostic accuracy of the Berlin questionnaire, STOP-BANG, STOP, and Epworth sleepiness scale in detecting obstructive sleep apnea: A bivariate meta-analysis. *Sleep Med. Rev.* **2017**, *36*, 57–70. [CrossRef] [PubMed]
22. Balakrishnan, K.; James, K.; Weaver, E.M. Predicting CPAP Use and Treatment Outcomes Using Composite Indices of Sleep Apnea Severity. *J. Clin. Sleep Med.* **2016**, *12*, 849–854. [CrossRef]
23. Corrigan, J.; Tsai, W.; Ip-Buting, A.; Ng, C.; Ogah, I.; Peller, P.; Sharpe, H.; Laratta, C.; Pendharkar, S.R. Treatment outcomes among rural and urban patients with obstructive sleep apnea: A prospective cohort study. *J. Clin. Sleep Med.* **2022**, *18*, 1013–1020. [CrossRef] [PubMed]
24. Turino, C.; de Batlle, J.; Woehrle, H.; Mayoral, A.; Castro-Grattoni, A.L.; Gómez, S.; Dalmases, M.; Sánchez-De-La-Torre, M.; Barbé, F. Management of continuous positive airway pressure treatment compliance using telemonitoring in obstructive sleep apnoea. *Eur. Respir. J.* **2017**, *49*, 1601128. [CrossRef] [PubMed]
25. Hu, Y.; Su, Y.; Hu, S.; Ma, J.; Zhang, Z.; Fang, F.; Guan, J. Effects of telemedicine interventions in improving continuous positive airway pressure adherence in patients with obstructive sleep apnoea: A meta-analysis of randomised controlled trials. *Sleep Breath.* **2021**, *25*, 1761–1771. [CrossRef]
26. Attias, D.; Pepin, J.; Pathak, A. Impact of COVID-19 lockdown on adherence to continuous positive airway pressure by obstructive sleep apnoea patients. *Eur. Respir. J.* **2020**, *56*, 2001607. [CrossRef]
27. Demirovic, S.; Lusic Kalcina, L.; Pavlinac Dodig, I.; Pecotic, R.; Valic, M.; Ivkovic, N.; Dogas, Z. The COVID-19 Lockdown and CPAP Adherence: The More Vulnerable Ones Less Likely to Improve Adherence? *Nat. Sci. Sleep* **2021**, *13*, 1097–1108. [CrossRef]

Disclaimer/Publisher's Note: The statements, opinions and data contained in all publications are solely those of the individual author(s) and contributor(s) and not of MDPI and/or the editor(s). MDPI and/or the editor(s) disclaim responsibility for any injury to people or property resulting from any ideas, methods, instructions or products referred to in the content.

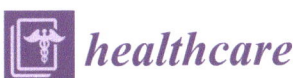

Article

Sleep Habits, Academic Performance and Health Behaviors of Adolescents in Southern Greece

Christina Alexopoulou [1,*], Maria Fountoulaki [2], Antigone Papavasileiou [3] and Eumorfia Kondili [1]

- [1] Department of Intensive Care and Sleep Laboratory, University Hospital of Heraklion, 71110 Heraklion, Greece; kondylie@uoc.gr
- [2] Attikon University Hospital, 12462 Athens, Greece; mafountoulaki@gmail.com
- [3] Pediatric Neurology, IASO Children Hospital Athens, 15123 Marousi, Greece; theon@otenet.gr
- * Correspondence: calexopoulou@pagni.gr

Abstract: Adolescents often experience insufficient sleep and have unhealthy sleep habits. Our aim was to investigate the sleep patterns of secondary education students in Heraklion, Crete, Greece and their association with school performance and health habits. We conducted a community-based cross-sectional study with 831 students aged 13–19 years who completed an online self-reported questionnaire related to sleep and health habits. The data are mostly numerical or categorical, and an analysis was performed using t-tests, chi-square tests and multiple logistic regression. During weekdays, the students slept for an average of 7 ± 1.1 h, which is significantly lower than the 7.8 ± 1.5 h average on weekends ($p < 0.001$). Nearly 79% reported difficulty waking up and having insufficient sleep time, while 73.8% felt sleepy at school at least once a week. Having sufficient sleep time ≥ 8 h) was positively correlated with better academic performance (OR: 1.48, CI: 1.06–2.07, $p = 0.022$) and frequent physical exercise (never/rarely: 13.5%, adequate: 21.2%, often: 65.3%; $p = 0.002$). Conversely, there was a negative correlation between adequate sleep and both smoking (OR: 0.29, CI: 0.13–0.63) and alcohol consumption (OR: 0.51, CI: 0.36–0.71, $p = 0.001$). In conclusion, this study shows that students in Heraklion, Crete frequently experience sleep deprivation, which is associated with compromised academic performance, reduced physical activity and an increased likelihood of engaging in unhealthy behaviors like smoking and alcohol consumption.

Keywords: sleep; sleep hygiene; adolescents; sleep habits; sleep deprivation; academic performance; health behavior

1. Introduction

Sleep behavior among adolescents is a major health concern worldwide [1]. When discussing adolescent sleep behavior, it is important to consider various key points such as the onset of sleep time, sleep patterns and duration and how they correlate with gender, the day of the week, parental sleep behaviors and other social factors. Studies have shown that the quality of sleep can be negatively affected depending on these factors [2,3].

Various studies have reported that the timing of sleep onset differs according to age, particularly in adolescents. Specifically, older adolescents tend to fall asleep later on both school nights and weekends [1,2,4–6]. However, they tend to sleep longer on weekends than on school nights. School demands often disrupt adolescents' sleep–wake cycles, leading to inconsistent sleep patterns. They often become deprived of sleep during the week and make up for it by sleeping more during the weekends. However, more research is required to determine the appropriate sleep duration for young patients aged 13–19. Previous reports have suggested that adolescents need approximately 9 h of sleep per night on average [6,7]. Nevertheless, this differs significantly from the actual time they spend sleeping, which decreases with each passing decade in some areas of the world. The teenage population in the US and Sweden tends to have a shorter sleep duration in later decades compared to past decades, although the average sleep requirement for all adolescents is considered to be 9 h [1,2,4–6]. North American, European, Chinese and Australian studies have revealed that older adolescents (15–16 years) have a borderline sleep onset time (in order to achieve the full 9 h sleep they need), while Icelandic adolescents of all ages go to sleep later than others (borderline to insufficient) [1]. According to Gariepi et al. [2], the sleep recommendation times were, on average, lower on school days than on non-school days with great variation among countries, especially on school days and between genders.

Additionally, the onset of puberty varies considerably in an individualized fashion, and some adolescents are still prepubertal when they enter middle school. It should be noted that the sleep needs in the prepubertal pediatric population are not yet known [8].

Differences in sleep duration between boys and girls have been described, with some studies pointing out that boys sleep less and others concluding that they sleep more than girls [4–6,9].

The quality of sleep has been linked to academic performance and social jet lag [8,10]. Sleep deprivation, characterized by insomnia and daytime sleepiness, can have negative effects on adolescents' school performance as well as their somatic and psychosocial health [8]. Sleep behavior is a prime example of how external factors like parental bedtime setting, cognitive behavioral therapy for insomnia (CBT-I) and a practice of good 'sleep hygiene' can modify children's and adolescents' physiological and developmental needs, leading to important outcomes for cognition, emotion regulation, motivation and mental health [11–14]. Environmental factors can vary between countries and regions, highlighting the need for further studies on sleep behaviors in different populations.

To the authors' knowledge, there is no study in the literature examining sleep habits, academic performances and health behaviors and the correlation between them in adolescents in Greece, so we conducted this study to assess both the duration and quality of sleep, examining factors such as bedtime, wake-up time, variations between school days and weekends and experiences of difficulties in waking up or daytime sleepiness. Additionally, we sought to investigate any correlation between sleep patterns and various aspects such as academic performance and health behaviors, including smoking, the consumption of coffee and alcohol intake as well as the use of electronic devices.

2. Materials and Methods

2.1. Participants and Methods

This was a cross-sectional, community-based study with a self-reported questionnaire. The participants were school students during their sixth years of secondary education, separated into two groups corresponding to the first part of 3 years of Gymnasium and the second part of 3 years of Lyceum each, in accordance with the Greek educational system. This study was conducted in 2018 among students aged between 13 and 19 years in Crete, Southern Greece before the emergence of the COVID-19 pandemic. This study was approved by the Ethics Committee of the University Hospital of Heraklion, Crete, Greece. One of the teachers in each class was responsible for informing the parents and students about the study and obtaining parental consent. All parents consented and all students who were recruited participated in the study.

As part of the study, 831 students aged between 13 and 19 were asked to anonymously complete an online 28-question questionnaire. The questions covered their everyday habits, including sleep duration and bedtime, sleepiness in class, difficulties in waking up, sleep hygiene and habits before bed, such as the use of electronic devices. Additionally, the students were asked to record their coffee and alcohol intake, exercise routines and school performances. They were also asked about their parents' sleep habits because it seems that there is a correlation. The questionnaire was accessible through http://j.mp/sleep1718 accessed on 15 January 2018 (Table 1).

Table 1. Questionnaire (translated to English).

	Sleep in Adolescent Students	
	A1. Sex	
Female		Male
	A2. Class	
1st Gymnasium	2nd Gymnasium	3rd Gymnasium
1st Lyceum	2nd Lyceum	3rd Lyceum
	A3. Year of birth	
1999	2000	2001
2002	2003	2004
2005		
A4. Your grades (without gymnastics) on the first quartermaster this year. If you haven't received your grades yet please select your estimation. (max 20)		
18.1–20	16.1–18	13.1–16
9.5–13	>9.5	
	A5. Do you exercise?	
Never	Sometimes	On a regular often basis
	A6. Do you smoke?	
Not at all	Sometimes	Almost every day
	A7. Do you drink any alcohol?	
Not at all	Sometimes	Almost every day

		Sleep Duration at Home			
	B1. How many hours do you sleep the nights before school?				
4 h or less	about 4.5 h	about 5 h	about 5.5 h	about 6 h	about 6.5 h
about 7 h	about 7.5 h	about 8 h	about 8.5 h	about 9 h	about 9.5 h
>9 h					
	B2. The same days how many hours do your parents sleep?				
4 h or less	about 4.5 h	about 5 h	about 5.5 h	about 6 h	about 6.5 h
about 7 h	about 7.5 h	about 8 h	about 8.5 h	about 9 h	about 9.5 h
>9 h					
B3. During Friday Saturday and holiday eves, when you don't have to go to school the next morning, how many hours do you sleep?					
4 h or less	about 4.5 h	about 5 h	about 5.5 h	about 6 h	about 6.5 h
about 7 h	about 7.5 h	about 8 h	about 8.5 h	about 9 h	about 9.5 h
>9 h					
	B4. The same days how many hours do your parents sleep?				
4 h or less	about 4.5 h	about 5 h	about 5.5 h	about 6 h	about 6.5 h
about 7 h	about 7.5 h	about 8 h	about 8.5 h	about 9 h	about 9.5 h
>9 h					
	B5. During holiday season how many hours do you sleep?				
4 h or less	about 4.5 h	about 5 h	about 5.5 h	about 6 h	about 6.5 h
about 7 h	about 7.5 h	about 8 h	about 8.5 h	about 9 h	about 9.5 h
>9 h					
	B6. The same days how many hours do your parents sleep?				
4 h or less	about 4.5 h	about 5 h	about 5.5 h	about 6 h	about 6.5 h
about 7 h	about 7.5 h	about 8 h	about 8.5 h	about 9 h	about 9.5 h
>9 h					

	About bed time at home	
	C1. At what time do you sleep the nights before school?	
Around 8:30 p.m. or earlier	Around 09:00 p.m.	Around 09:30 p.m.
Around 10:00 p.m.	Around 10:30 p.m.	Around 11:00 p.m.
Around 11:30 p.m.	Around midnight	Around 12:30 a.m.
Around 1:00 a.m	Around 01: 30 a.m.	Later than 01:30 a.m.
	C2. The same days at what time do your parents sleep?	
Around 8:30 p.m. or earlier	Around 09:00 p.m.	Around 09:30 p.m.
Around 10:00 p.m.	Around 10:30 p.m.	Around 11:00 p.m.
Around 11:30 p.m.	Around midnight	Around 12:30 a.m.
Around 1:00 a.m.	Around 01:30 a.m.	Later than 01:30 a.m.

Table 1. Cont.

C3. During Friday Saturday and holiday eves, when you don't have to go to school the next morning, at what time do you sleep?		
Around 8:30 pm or earlier	Around 09:00 p.m.	Around 09:30 p.m.
Around 10:00 p.m	Around 10:30 p.m.	Around 11:00 p.m.
Around 11:30 p.m.	Around midnight	Around 12:30 a.m.
Around 1:00 a.m.	Around 01:30 a.m.	Later than 01:30 a.m.
C4. At the same days at what time do your parents sleep?		
Around 8:30 p.m. or earlier	Around 09:00 p.m.	Around 09:30 p.m.
Around 10:00 p.m.	Around 10:30 p.m.	Around 11:00 p.m.
Around 11:30 p.m.	Around midnight	Around 12:30 a.m.
Around 1:00 a.m.	Around 01:30 a.m.	Later than 01:30 a.m.
C5. During holiday season at what time do you sleep?		
Around 8:30 pm or earlier	Around 09:00 p.m.	Around 09:30 p.m.
Around 10:00 p.m.	Around 10:30 p.m.	Around 11:00 p.m.
Around 11:30 p.m.	Around midnight	Around 12:30 a.m.
Around 1:00 a.m.	Around 01:30 a.m.	Later than 01:30 a.m.
C6. At the same days at what time do your parents sleep?		
Around 8:30 p.m. or earlier	Around 09:00 p.m.	Around 09:30 p.m.
Around 10:00 p.m.	Around 10:30 p.m.	Around 11:00 p.m.
Around 11:30 p.m.	Around midnight	Around 12:30 a.m.
Around 1:00 a.m.	Around 01:30 a.m.	Later than 01:30 a.m.
Everyday sleep and wake		
D1. Do you have any difficulties to wake up in the morning during school days?		
Never or rarely	Sometimes	Almost always
D2. How do you go to school usually?		
On foot		By car or bus
D3. What time do you usually leave from home to go to school?		
....		
D4. During the daytime at school do your feel sleepy?		
Never or rarely	1–2 days/week	>2 days/week
D5. Do your parents believe that you need more sleep during schooldays and do they advise you to sleep more or earlier?		
Never or rarely	Sometimes	Almost always
Not only during school days but everyday		
D6. During schooldays do you take a nap?		
Never or rarely	1–2 naps per week	>2 naps per week
D7. During the school year your everyday afterschool activities (sports, extra lessons etc.) stop at:		
7:00 p.m. 8:00 p.m. 9:00 p.m. 10:00 p.m. Later than 10:00 p.m.		
D8. During the school year what is the latest thing you do before sleep?		
Watch TV Use PC or smartphone Read a book Listen Music Play without electronic means Homework		
Else:...		
D9. During school year do you take any caffeine products or energy drinks or substances in order to stay awake?		
Never or rarely	Sometimes	Almost everyday

2.2. Statistical Analysis

Categorical variables were expressed as frequencies and percentages. Continuous variables were presented as mean ± standard deviation (SD) or median and 25–75% interquartile range (25–75 IQR), as appropriate. Categorical variables are compared using the Fisher exact test, and continuous variables were compared using the Kruskal–Wallis, Friedman and Wilcoxon or Mann–Whitney tests, as appropriate. Spearman's rho was used to evaluate correlations between continuous and categorical variables, as appropriate. To investigate if sleep habits and other variables were independently associated with poor academic performance, a multiple logistic regression model (with odds ratios [ORs] and two-sided 95% confidence intervals [CIs]) was performed. A p-value of < 0.05 was considered statistically significant. Pairwise comparisons were performed using the

Kruskal–Wallis test followed by Bonferroni's correction for multiple comparisons. The adjusted significance level was set at 0.001. Statistical analyses were performed using an IBM SPSS Statistics 24.0 statistical package.

3. Results

A total of 831 students completed the questionnaires. The age and gender distributions at Gymnasium and Lyceum and class levels are listed in Table 2. Most of the participants (70.2%) were Lyceum students. There were no significant age and gender differences within the education and class levels ($p > 0.05$).

Table 2. Participants' characteristics. Distributions based on gender, class and educational level.

		Sex								
		Boys (n = 421)			Girls (n = 410)			Total (n = 831)		
		n	% #	% *	N	% #	% *	n	% *	p
Age (years)	13	57	48.7	13.5	60	51.3	14.6	117	14.1	0.434
	14	44	50.0	10.5	44	50.0	10.7	88	10.6	
	15	21	44.7	5.0	26	55.3	6.3	47	5.7	
	16	130	57.0	30.9	98	43.0	23.9	228	27.4	
	17	96	49.7	22.8	97	50.3	23.7	193	23.2	
	18	70	46.4	16.6	81	53.6	19.8	151	18.2	
	19	3	42.9	0.7	4	57.1	1.0	7	0.8	
Educational Level	Gymnasium	120	48.4	28.5	128	51.6	31.2	248	29.8	0.392
	Lyceum	301	51.6	71.5	282	48.4	68.8	583	70.2	
Class	Gymnasium 1st	56	48.7	13.3	59	51.3	14.4	115	13.8	0.316
	Gymnasium 2nd	44	50.6	10.5	43	49.4	10.5	87	10.5	
	Gymnasium 3rd	20	43.5	4.8	26	56.5	6.3	46	5.5	
	Lyceum 1st	135	57.0	32.1	102	43.0	24.9	237	28.5	
	Lyceum 2nd	93	48.2	22.1	100	51.8	24.4	193	23.2	
	Lyceum 3rd	73	47.7	17.3	80	52.3	19.5	153	18.4	

#: percentage per gender for the same class; *: percentage of the total students in the same class.

3.1. Sleep Habits

We observed that, regardless of the level of education, the students slept for a significantly shorter duration on weekdays (median 7.0 h, with an interquartile range (IQR) of 6–7 h) compared to weekends (median 8.0 h, IQR 7–9 h, $p < 0.001$), as shown in Figure 1. A similar pattern was observed in the sleep durations of the students' parents, with shorter sleep durations on weekdays (median 7.0 h, IQR 6–8 h) compared to weekends (median 8.0 h, IQR 7–8 h), as shown in Table 3. The distributions of students and students' parents at six different hours of sleep duration (4–9 h) are presented in Figure 2. The sleep durations in the six different classes during weekdays and weekends are presented in Figure 3 and Table 4. Overall, a significant decrease in sleep duration with an increase in educational year was observed. The sleep duration decreased from 8 (IQR 7–8) hours in the first Gymnasium class to 7 (6–7) hours in the third Lyceum class, indicating a decline in sleep duration with the progression of educational level ($p < 0.001$). Pairwise comparisons of sleep during weekdays and weekends between the six classes are detailed in Tables S1 and S2.

Table 3. Sleep durations on weekdays and weekends for students and students' parents.

Sleep Duration (Hours) (Median, IQR 25–75)	Weekdays	Weekends	p-Value
Students	7 (6–8)	8 (7–9)	<0.001
Students' Parents	7 (6–8)	8 (7–8)	<0.001

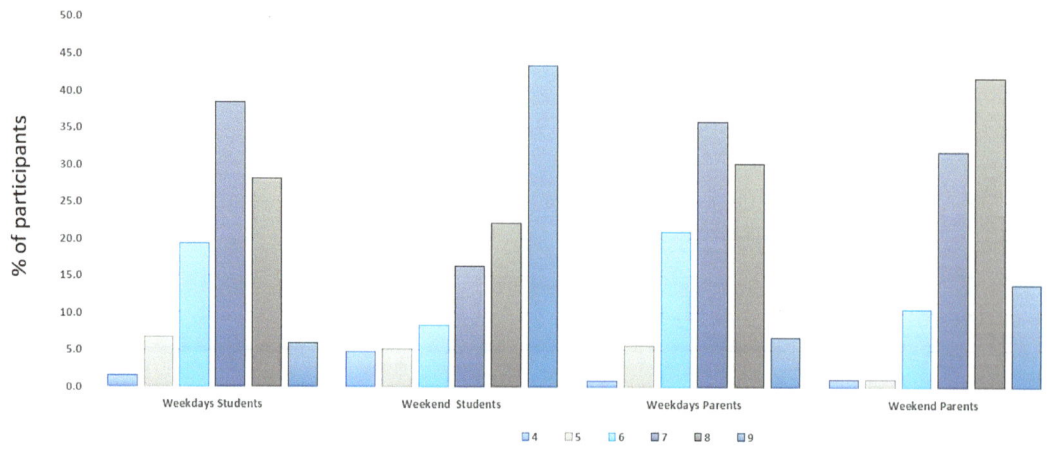

Figure 1. Percentages of students and students' parents at 5 different ranges of sleep duration during weekdays and weekends.

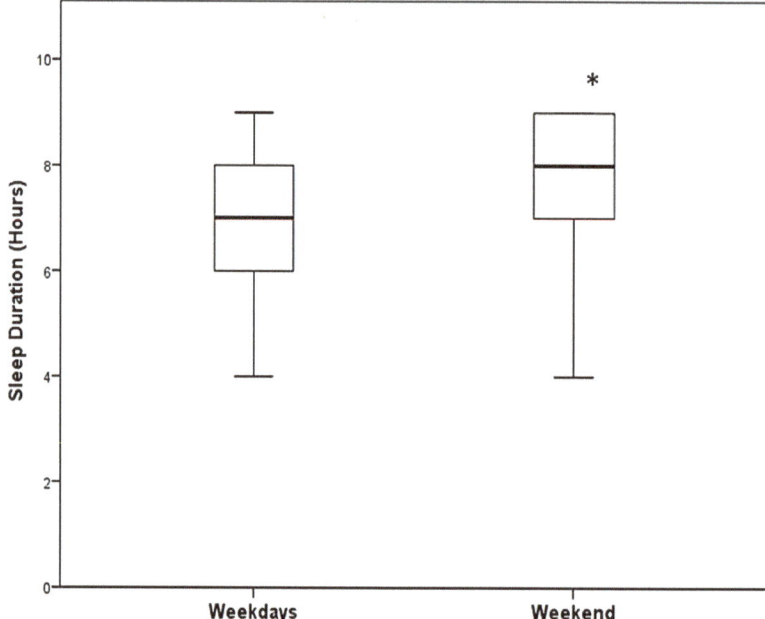

Figure 2. Box and whisker plots representing a comparison of sleep duration on weekdays and weekends for students./ The lower and upper edges of the box represent the 25th and 75th percentiles, respectively. The lines within the box show the median values. The whiskers depict the adjacent values. (*) denotes a statistically significant difference between the values; $p < 0.05$.

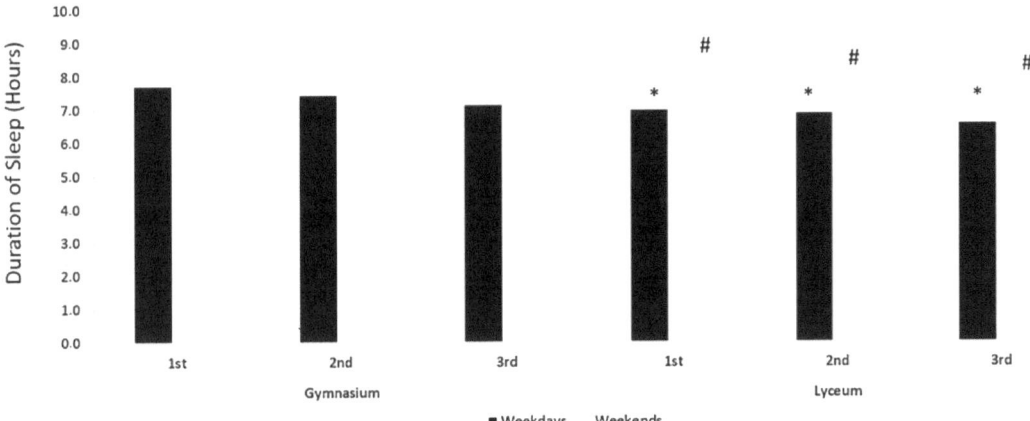

Figure 3. Sleep duration during weekdays (black columns) and weekend days (light grey columns) for each school class. Pairwise comparisons performed using Kruskal–Wallis test, followed by Bonferroni's correction for multiple comparisons. * represents significant difference from Gymnasium 1st class for weekdays, $p < 0.0001$, while # represents significant difference from Gymnasium 1st class for weekends.

Table 4. Sleep durations based on class on weekdays and weekends.

Sleep Duration (Hours), Median (IQR 25–75)	Class					
	Gymnasium 1st	Gymnasium 2nd	Gymnasium 3rd	Lyceum 1st	Lyceum 2nd	Lyceum 3rd
Weekdays	8 (7–8)	8 (7–8)	7 (7–8)	7 (6–8)	7 (6–7)	7 (6–7)
Weekends	8 (7–9)	8 (7–9)	8 (7–9)	9 (7–9)	8 (7–9)	8 (7–9)

A significant bedtime delay was observed on weekdays as the students progressed to higher educational levels. The bedtime was reported to be 22:30 for the first class of Gymnasium, 23:30 for the third class of Gymnasium and 00:10 for the third class of Lyceum, ($p < 0.001$). Bedtime delays during weekends followed a similar pattern across different educational levels, with bedtimes shifting later as the educational levels increased, being 23:54 in the first Gymnasium class and 1.06 in the third Lyceum class. Weekends showed a consistent trend of delayed bedtimes compared to weekdays across all educational levels ($p < 0.001$).

Of the 831 students surveyed, 193 (23.2%) reported adhering to the recommended sleep durations for their ages (equal to or exceeding 8 h). A total of 250 students (19.7%) disclosed having at least one nap per week, whereas 86 students (10.3%) admitted to having more than two nap days per week. No statistically significant differences in nap patterns were observed between the male and female students.

Regarding pre-sleep habits involving electronic devices, a substantial portion of the surveyed students—529 individuals (63.7%)—acknowledged using electronic devices before bedtime. We found a difference between genders in regard to using electronic devices before sleep, with a significantly higher rate observed among boys compared to girls; 69.6% of boys reported using electronic devices before sleep compared to 57.6% of girls ($p < 0.001$).

3.2. Health Habits

The students' health habits, encompassing behaviors related to smoking, alcohol consumption and physical activity, were examined and are presented in Table 5. Among the surveyed students, 25 individuals (3.0%) admitted to frequent smoking, while 56 students

(6.7%) reported occasional smoking. We found a significant gender disparity in smoking frequency: 5.0% of boys acknowledged frequent smoking, and 8.3% disclosed occasional smoking. In comparison, only 1.0% of girls reported frequent smoking, and 5.1% admitted to occasional smoking ($p < 0.001$).

Table 5. Health habits (smoking, drinking and exercise) of boys and girls.

| | | Sex | | | | | | | | | |
| | | Boy | | | Girl | | | Total | | | |
		N	%[1]	%[2]	N	%[1]	%[2]	N	%[1]	%[2]	p-Value
Smoking	Never/Rarely	365	48.7	86.7	385	51.3	93.9	750	100.0	90.3	<0.001
	Sometimes	35	62.5	8.3	21	37.5	5.1	56	100.0	6.7	
	Often	21	84.0	5.0	4	16.0	1.0	25	100.0	3.0	
	Total (per gender)	421			410						
Drinking alcohol	Never/Rarely	202	45.7	48.0	240	54.3	58.5	442	100.0	53.2	<0.001
	Sometimes	207	55.5	49.2	166	44.5	40.5	373	100.0	44.9	
	Often	12	75.0	2.9	4	25.0	1.0	16	100.0	1.9	
	Total (per gender)	421			410						
Exercise	Never/Rarely	73	47.4	17.3	81	52.6	19.8	154	100.0	18.5	0.046
	Sometimes	102	45.1	24.2	124	54.9	30.2	226	100.0	27.2	
	Often	246	54.5	58.4	205	45.5	50.0	451	100.0	54.3	
	Total (per gender)	421			410						
Coffee or caffeine	Never/Rarely	253	51.5	60.1	238	48.5	58.0	491	100.0	59.1	0.821
	Sometimes	112	49.8	26.6	113	50.2	27.6	225	100.0	27.1	
	Often	56	48.7	13.3	59	51.3	14.4	115	100.0	13.8	
	Total (per gender)	421			410						

[1]: Percentage of total number of participants at each frequency condition (Never/Rarely, Sometimes and Often);
[2]: percentage of total number of participants within same gender at each frequency condition; $p < 0.001$ represents statistically significant difference.

For alcohol consumption, occasional drinking "drinking alcohol sometimes" was reported by 373 participants (44%), with a significantly higher prevalence among boys (207, 49.2%) compared to girls (166, 40.5%) ($p < 0.001$). A relatively uniform prevalence of coffee and caffeine consumption was found between boys and girls. The consumption of coffee and caffeine-containing products was reported among 115 students (13.8%), and no significant difference was found among both genders. A majority of students (54.3%) reported exercising often, with boys exercising at a higher proportion (58.4%) than girls (50.0%) ($p = 0.046$). Health habits per age are presented in Supplementary Table S3. The percentage of students who reported never or rarely smoking decreased significantly with age, starting at 97% at the age of 13 and reaching 81.5% and 42.9% at 18 and 19, respectively. A similar pattern was observed for drinking alcohol (89.7% at the age of 13 and 34.2% and 27.8% at the ages of 18 and 19, respectively) and consuming coffee and caffeine products (77.8% at the age of 13 and 33.8% and 28.6% at the ages of 18 and 19, respectively).

Regarding physical activity, we found an increase in the proportion of students who reported never or rarely engaging in physical activity with age, from 8.5% at the age of 13 to 33.4% and 57.1% at the ages of 18 and 19, respectively. Furthermore, there was a significant decrease in the proportion of students who reported engaging in physical activity often as they became older, from 76.9% at the age of 13 to 26.5% and 28.6% at the ages of 18 and 19, respectively.

3.3. Sleep Quality

The evaluation of sleep quality centered on difficulties in waking up and experiencing daytime sleepiness. Among the surveyed students, a substantial majority, comprising 656 individuals (78.9%), reported difficulties when waking up. Within this group, 292 students (35.1%) encountered these difficulties often. A total of 304 students (36.6%) admitted to feeling sleepy at school for one to two days per week, while 309 students (37.2%) reported feeling the same for over two days per week. Significantly more boys than girls were found to never or rarely feel sleepy at school (29.7% vs. 22.7%, $p < 0.05$).

A significant positive correlation emerged between sufficient sleep duration, defined as a sleep duration of ≥ 8 h, and academic performance (18.1 vs. < 18.0), as indicated by the school grades (OR: 1.48 CI 1.06–2.07, $p = 0.022$) after adjusting gender and educational level (Lyceum/Gymnasium) (Table S4). Additionally, sufficient sleep duration exhibited a positive association with the frequency of engaging in physical exercise, with higher rates observed among those who exercised often (65.3%) compared to those who exercised sometimes (21.2%) or rarely (13.5%) ($p = 0.002$). Conversely, sufficient sleep demonstrated a negative correlation with both smoking (OR: 0.29, CI 0.13–0.63) and alcohol consumption (OR: 0.51, CI 0.36–0.71) ($p = 0.001$).

4. Discussion

The results of this cross-sectional study reveal that a significant proportion of adolescents in Crete, Greece fail to attain good sleep health. Specifically, this study shows that most adolescents are unable to achieve adequate sleep duration, appropriate timing and sustained alertness during waking hours. Furthermore, this study identifies a correlation between insufficient sleep time, lower academic performance and an increased prevalence of unhealthy habits. The current study found that the total sleep time was lower than that considered appropriate for each age group. According to the literature, less than 8 h of sleep is not appropriate for optimal health for individuals aged between 13 and 18 [7,10]. Sleep duration decreased from 8 (IQR 7–8) hours in the first Gymnasium class to 7 (6–7) hours in the third Lyceum class, indicating a decline in sleep duration with the progression of educational level ($p < 0.001$). Sleep duration was increased during weekends but still not sufficient. Previous studies reported inconsistent findings regarding gender-based disparities in sleep quality among adolescents, including daytime sleepiness, difficulty initiating sleep and sleep onset latency [1,11,15–19]. However, the present study did not find significant differences in sleep quality indices between genders, with the exception of boys reporting lower levels of daytime sleepiness compared to girls. Regardless of their education level (Gymnasium or Lyceum), we found that students have shorter sleep durations on weekdays than on weekends. The same pattern was also observed in the students' parents. Furthermore, with the progression of the academic level, there was a noticeable reduction in sleep duration on both weekdays and weekends. This finding aligns with the consensus statement of the American Academy of Sleep Medicine in 2016 (7) indicating a sleep phase delay as children move through secondary school years. Notably, adolescents in Lyceum tend to sleep less than 8 h per night, which is significantly less than the recommended time for their age [7]. During the transition from Gymnasium to Lyceum, students are exposed to various environmental demands, such as school demands and socialization, which may affect their sleep quantity. This period is particularly risky as students are expected to balance their educational and extracurricular activities, leading to inadequate sleep. Insufficient sleep during this critical period may have negative impacts on students' mental and physical health, academic performance and overall well-being [20].

A considerable proportion of students reported taking at least one nap per week. Remarkably, there was no apparent disparity in napping patterns between genders. However, it is difficult to interpret the significance of this finding, as napping needs have been linked to factors such as insufficient sleep at night or ethnic, socio-cultural and racial differences [8]. Nevertheless, this finding emphasizes the need for further research studies in specific geographical regions. Although young individuals are unlikely to require different sleep durations across different continents, they may have diverse sleep patterns that are influenced by environmental factors such as warm climates or socio-cultural norms.

Using electronic devices before sleep was reported by the majority of the students, with a significantly higher rate in boys than girls. This finding holds significant importance as such behavior has been linked to delayed sleep onset. Prior research has consistently demonstrated that the use of electronic devices before bedtime has detrimental effects on sleep quality, including delayed onset, reduced duration and disrupted sleep patterns [21–23].

According to this study's results, a considerable number of participants experienced poor sleep quality, as evidenced by difficulties waking up and feeling sleepy during the day. This finding is significant since inadequate sleep during adolescence has been linked to cognitive dysfunction, learning challenges, poor emotional well-being and metabolic disorders that can lead to obesity [24–31].

The present study has revealed a positive correlation between sleep duration and physical exercise frequency. Specifically, children who reported experiencing good sleep quality were found to engage in physical exercise significantly more frequently than their peers who exercised seldomly or not at all. This finding is in accordance with the study by Nixon et al. [32], who reported that adolescents with poor sleep quality might engage in less physical activity. Both studies suggest that the quality and quantity of sleep are important factors in determining physical activity levels and overall health in children and emphasize the importance of quality sleep and its impact on children's physical well-being.

In the current study, we found that good sleep is linked with lower rates of smoking and alcohol consumption. This finding is consistent with previous studies that have shown a connection between poor sleep and risky behaviors in adolescents [33–36]. A national sample of US adolescents revealed that those with late bedtimes had an increased likelihood of using cigarettes, alcohol and drugs. They were also more prone to violent behaviors and emotional distress [37]. Furthermore, the impact of sleep quality on cognitive function has been highlighted in healthy adolescents and those with neurodevelopmental and psychiatric conditions [38]. Previous studies have demonstrated that sleep quality is critically involved in learning and memory [11].

A significant finding of this study is that sufficient sleep duration, defined as at least eight hours of sleep daily, was positively related to academic performance, as assessed by school grades. This finding is in accordance with previous studies reporting that adequate sleep quality is associated with higher academic performance [39]. The association between good sleep quality and high academic performance has been extensively investigated, and multiple possible factors have been proposed [40]. Sleep is crucial for cognitive functions like attention, memory and decision making. Adequate sleep can enhance these functions, enabling adolescents to concentrate better in class, retain information effectively and perform well in academic tasks. Moreover, good sleep quality is essential for memory consolidation and enhancing learning. Sufficient sleep may promote memory and recall information processes, leading to increased learning capacity and, ultimately, high academic performance [41,42].

Addressing and improving sleep hygiene, promoting consistent sleep schedules, creating a conducive sleep environment and raising awareness about the importance of adequate sleep among adolescents and their parents can significantly mitigate these effects and potentially improve academic outcomes.

Limitations

The limitation of this study is the reliance upon retrospective data to measure sleep instead of employing sleep diaries, which is regarded as the most reliable method for subjectively assessing sleep. Sleep diaries are easy to use, transportable and cost-effective. They measure sleep proactively, thereby eliminating any bias attributed to the tendency to recollect recent experiences [43].

The questionnaire used was made on the Google platform for the needs of this study and was not a validated scale that already existed in the literature. The aim was to cover all of the aspects of interest without using many different scales, which would eliminate the answering rates among school students due to long answering times. It is of great interest that the participation rate among the students was almost 100%. All health-associated behaviors were self-reported, and the data on alcohol and smoking were crude. As a measure of academic achievement, we only used the school grades at the moment of participation in the study, which may not reflect the overall academic performance of a student. This study was conducted on Crete, which is the biggest island in Greece, but it is a specific region and the generalization of the results is limited. Further studies are needed to better evaluate the sleep habits and health-related behaviors among adolescents as well as the effects of specific interventions in order to improve their sleep and well-being.

5. Conclusions

In conclusion, this cross-sectional study showed that most Greek adolescents residing on Crete experience poor sleep quality and sleep deprivation. As the adolescents grew older, their sleep duration tended to decrease, and no distinctions were observed between genders in this regard within this sample. More importantly, this research highlighted a positive correlation between good sleep habits and both academic achievement and the avoidance of early risky behaviors among these adolescents. These findings have implications for academic and healthcare professionals working with adolescents in Greece and beyond. Promoting good sleep hygiene may be an effective strategy for improving academic performance and reducing risky behaviors in this population. Further research is warranted to gain a more comprehensive understanding of the factors that influence sleep behaviors in adolescents.

Supplementary Materials: The following supporting information can be downloaded at https://www.mdpi.com/article/10.3390/healthcare12070775/s1, Supplementary S1: Table S1: Sleeping hours of students during working days at 6 different classes, post hoc analysis, $p < 0.001$: significant difference. Table S2: Sleeping hours of students during working days at 6 different classes, post hoc analysis, $p < 0.001$: significant difference. Table S3: Health habits based on age. Table S4. Adjusted ORs with 95% CIs of sleeping ≥ 8 h per day based on students' grades.

Author Contributions: Conceptualization, C.A.; methodology, C.A.; data curation, C.A., M.F., A.P. and E.K.; writing—original draft, C.A., M.F., A.P. and E.K.; writing—review and editing, C.A., M.F., A.P. and E.K. All authors have read and agreed to the published version of the manuscript.

Funding: This research received no external funding.

Institutional Review Board Statement: This study was approved by the Ethics Committee of the University Hospital of Heraklion, Crete, Greece (20244 on 29 September 2022). One of the teachers in each class was responsible for informing the parents and students about the study and obtaining parental consent.

Informed Consent Statement: Informed consent was obtained from all subjects involved in the study.

Data Availability Statement: Data are contained within the article.

Acknowledgments: We thank Antonios Margaritis and Periklis Georgiadis (Peiramatiko Lyceum of Heraklion, Greece) for their contributions.

Conflicts of Interest: The authors declare no conflicts of interest.

References

1. Gradisar, M.; Gardner, G.; Dohnt, H. Recent worldwide sleep patterns and problems during adolescence: A review and meta-analysis of age, region, and sleep. *Sleep Med.* **2011**, *12*, 110.e8. [CrossRef] [PubMed]
2. Gariepy, G.; Danna, S.; Gobina, I.; Rasmussen, M.; de Matos, M.G.; Tynjälä, J.; Janssen, I.; Kalman, M.; Villeruša, A.; Husarova, D.; et al. How Are Adolescents Sleeping? Adolescent Sleep Patterns and Sociodemographic Differences in 24 European and North American Countries. *J. Adolesc. Health* **2020**, *66* (Suppl. S6), S81–S88. [CrossRef] [PubMed]
3. Jeon, E.; Kim, N. Correspondence between Parents' and Adolescents' Sleep Duration. *Int. J. Environ. Res. Public Health* **2022**, *19*, 1034. [CrossRef] [PubMed]

4. Keyes, K.M.; Maslowsky, J.; Hamilton, A.; Schulenberg, J. The Great Sleep Recession: Changes in Sleep Duration Among US Adolescents, 1991–2012. *Pediatrics* **2015**, *135*, 460.e8. [CrossRef] [PubMed]
5. Norell-Clarke, A.; Hagquist, C. Changes in sleep habits between 1985 and 2013 among children and adolescents in Sweden. *Scand. J. Public Health* **2017**, *45*, 869.e77. [CrossRef] [PubMed]
6. Patte, K.A.; Qian, W.; Leatherdale, S.T. Sleep duration trends and trajectories among youth in the COMPASS study. *Sleep Health* **2017**, *3*, 309.e16. [CrossRef] [PubMed]
7. Paruthi, S.; Brooks, L.J.; D'Ambrosio, C.; Hall, W.A.; Kotagal, S.; Lloyd, R.M.; Malow, B.A.; Maski, K.; Nichols, C.; Quan, S.F.; et al. Recommended Amount of Sleep for Pediatric Populations: A Consensus Statement of the American Academy of Sleep Medicine. *Sleep Med.* **2016**, *12*, 785–786. [CrossRef] [PubMed]
8. Meltzer, L.J.; Williamson, A.A.; Mindell, J.A. Pediatric sleep health: It matters, and so does how we define it. *Sleep Med. Rev.* **2021**, *57*, 101425. [CrossRef] [PubMed]
9. Díaz-Morales, J.F.; Escribano, C. Social jetlag, academic achievement and cognitive performance: Understanding gender/sex differences. *Chrono-Int.* **2015**, *32*, 822.e31. [CrossRef] [PubMed]
10. Carskadon, M.A.; Orav, E.J.; Dement, W.C. Evolution of sleep and daytime sleepiness in adolescents. In *Sleep/Wake Disorders: Natural History, Epidemiology, and Long-Term Evolution*; Guilleminault, C., Lugaresi, E., Eds.; Raven Press: New York, NY, USA, 1983; pp. 201–216.
11. Tarokh, L.; Saletin, J.M.; Carskadon, M.A. Sleep in adolescence: Physiology, cognition and mental health. *Neurosci. Biobehav. Rev.* **2016**, *70*, 182–188. [CrossRef]
12. Carskadon, M.A. *The Encyclopedia of Sleep*; Kushida, C., Ed.; Academic Press: Cambridge, MA, USA, 2013; pp. 86–87.
13. de Bruin, E.J.; Oort, F.J.; Bögels, S.M.; Meijer, A.M. Efficacy of Internet and Group-Administered Cognitive Behavioral Therapy for Insomnia in Adolescents: A Pilot Study. *Behav. Sleep Med.* **2014**, *12*, 235–254. [CrossRef] [PubMed]
14. Bootzin, R.R.; Stevens, S.J. Adolescents, substance abuse, and the treatment of insomnia and daytime sleepiness. *Clin. Psychol. Rev.* **2005**, *25*, 629–644. [CrossRef] [PubMed]
15. Shochat, T.; Cohen-Zion, M.; Tzischinsky, O. Functional consequences of inadequate sleep in adolescents: A systematic review. *Sleep Med. Rev.* **2014**, *18*, 75.e87. [CrossRef] [PubMed]
16. Lytle, L.A.; Pasch, K.E.; Farbakhsh, K. The Relationship Between Sleep and Weight in a Sample of Adolescents. *Obesity* **2011**, *19*, 324–331. [CrossRef] [PubMed]
17. Williams, J.A.; Zimmerman, F.J.; Bell, J.F. Norms and Trends of Sleep Time Among US Children and Adolescents. *JAMA Pediatr.* **2013**, *167*, 55–60. [CrossRef]
18. Mitchell, J.A.; Rodriguez, D.; Schmitz, K.H.; Audrain-McGovern, J. Sleep Duration and Adolescent Obesity. *Pediatrics* **2013**, *131*, e1428. [CrossRef] [PubMed]
19. Kocevska, D.; Lysen, T.S.; Dotinga, A.; Koopman-Verhoeff, M.E.; Luijk, M.P.C.M.; Antypa, N.; Biermasz, N.R.; Blokstra, A.; Brug, J.; Burk, W.J.; et al. Sleep characteristics across the lifespan in 1.1 million people from the Netherlands, United Kingdom and United States: A systematic review and meta-analysis. *Nat. Hum. Behav.* **2020**, *5*, 113–122. [CrossRef] [PubMed]
20. Mitchell, J.A.; Morales, K.H.; Williamson, A.A.; Huffnagle, N.; Ludwick, A.; Grant, S.F.; Dinges, D.F.; Zemel, B.A. Changes in Sleep Duration and Timing During the Middle-to-High School Transition. *J. Adolesc. Health* **2020**, *67*, 829–836. [CrossRef] [PubMed]
21. Hale, L.; Guan, S. Screen time and sleep among school-aged children and adolescents: A systematic literature review. *Sleep Med. Rev.* **2014**, *21*, 50–58. [CrossRef] [PubMed]
22. Gradisar, M.; Wolfson, A.R.; Harvey, A.G.; Hale, L.; Rosenberg, R.; Czeisler, C.A. The sleep and technology use of Americans: Findings from the National Sleep Foundation's 2011 Sleep in America poll. *J. Clin. Sleep Med.* **2013**, *9*, 1291–1299. [CrossRef] [PubMed]
23. Hysing, M.; Pallesen, S.; Stormark, K.M.; Jakobsen, R.; Lundervold, A.J.; Sivertsen, B. Sleep and use of electronic devices in adolescence: Results from a large population-based study. *BMJ Open* **2015**, *5*, e006748. [CrossRef] [PubMed]
24. Tragomalou, A.; Moschonis, G.; Manios, Y.; Kassari, P.; Ioakimidis, I.; Diou, C.; Stefanopoulos, L.; Lekka, E.; Maglaveras, N.; Delopoulos, A.; et al. Novel e-Health Applications for the Management of Cardiometabolic Risk Factors in Children and Adolescents in Greece. *Nutrients* **2020**, *12*, 1380. [CrossRef] [PubMed]
25. Miller, M.A.; Kruisbrink, M.; Wallace, J.; Ji, C.; Cappuccio, F.P. Sleep duration and incidence of obesity in infants, children, and adolescents: A systematic review and meta-analysis of prospective studies. *Sleep* **2018**, *41*, 169–181. [CrossRef] [PubMed]
26. Cappuccio, F.P.; Taggart, F.M.; Kandala, N.-B.; Currie, A.; Peile, E.; Stranges, S.; Miller, M.A. Meta-Analysis of Short Sleep Duration and Obesity in Children and Adults. *Sleep* **2008**, *31*, 619–626. [CrossRef] [PubMed]
27. Czeisler, C.A.; Shanahan, T.L. Problems Associated with Use of Mobile Devices in the Sleep Environment—Streaming Instead of Dreaming. *JAMA Pediatr.* **2016**, *170*, 1146–1147. [CrossRef] [PubMed]
28. Dewald, J.F.; Meijer, A.M.; Oort, F.J.; Kerkhof, G.A.; Bögels, S.M. The influence of sleep quality, sleep duration and sleepiness on school performance in children and adolescents: A meta-analytic review. *Sleep Med. Rev.* **2010**, *14*, 179–189. [CrossRef] [PubMed]
29. Gruber, M.J.; Gelman, B.D.; Ranganath, C. States of Curiosity Modulate Hippocampus-Dependent Learning via the Dopaminergic Circuit. *Neuron* **2014**, *84*, 486–496. [CrossRef] [PubMed]
30. Bagley, E.J.; Kelly, R.J.; Buckhalt, J.A.; El-Sheikh, M. What keeps low-SES children from sleeping well: The role of presleep worries and sleep environment. *Sleep Med.* **2015**, *16*, 496–502. [CrossRef] [PubMed]

31. Gregory, A.M.; Sadeh, A. Sleep, emotional and behavioral difficulties in children and adolescents. *Sleep Med. Rev.* **2012**, *16*, 129–136. [CrossRef] [PubMed]
32. Nixon, G.M.; Thompson, J.M.D.; Han, D.Y.; Becroft, D.M.; Clark, P.M.; Robinson, E.; Waldie, K.E.; Wild, C.J.; Black, P.N.; Mitchell, E.A. Short Sleep Duration in Middle Childhood: Risk Factors and Consequences. *Sleep* **2008**, *31*, 71–78. [CrossRef] [PubMed]
33. Wong, N.T.; Zimmerman, M.A.; Parker, E.A. A Typology of Youth Participation and Empowerment for Child and Adolescent Health Promotion. *Am. J. Community Psychol.* **2010**, *46*, 100–114. [CrossRef]
34. Vazsonyi, A.T.; Jiskrova, G.K.; Ksinan, A.J.; Blatný, M. An empirical test of self-control theory in Roma adolescents. *J. Crim. Justice* **2016**, *44*, 66–76. [CrossRef]
35. Lundahl, A.; Kidwell, K.M.; Van Dyk, T.R.; Nelson, T.D. A Meta-Analysis of the Effect of Experimental Sleep Restriction on Youth's Attention and Hyperactivity. *Dev. Neuropsychol.* **2015**, *40*, 104–121. [CrossRef] [PubMed]
36. Sheikh, M.; Kelly, R.J. Sleep in children: Links with marital conflict and child development. In *Sleep and Development: Familial and Socio-Cultural Considerations*; El-Sheikh, M., Ed.; Oxford University Press: Oxford, UK, 2011; pp. 3–28. [CrossRef]
37. McGlinchey, E.L.; Harvey, A.G. Risk Behaviors and Negative Health Outcomes for Adolescents with Late Bedtimes. *J. Youth Adolesc.* **2015**, *44*, 478–488. [CrossRef] [PubMed]
38. Kotagal, S. Sleep in Neurodevelopmental and Neurodegenerative Disorders. *Semin. Pediatr. Neurol.* **2015**, *22*, 126–129. [CrossRef] [PubMed]
39. Escribano, C.; Díaz-Morales, J.F. Sleep Habits And Chronotype Effects On Academic And Cognitive Performance in Spanish Adolescents: A Review. *Int. Online J. Educ. Sci.* **2016**, *8*. [CrossRef]
40. Boergers, J.; Gable, C.J.B.; Owens, J.A. Later School Start Time Is Associated with Improved Sleep and Daytime Functioning in Adolescents. *J. Dev. Behav. Pediatr.* **2014**, *35*, 11–17. [CrossRef] [PubMed]
41. Hysing, M.; Harvey, A.G.; Linton, S.J.; Askeland, K.G.; Sivertsen, B. Sleep and academic performance in later adolescence: Results from a large population-based study. *J. Sleep Res.* **2016**, *25*, 318–324. [CrossRef] [PubMed]
42. Hoedlmoser, K. Sleep and Memory in Children. *Curr. Sleep Med. Rep.* **2020**, *6*, 280–289. [CrossRef]
43. Short, M.A.; Arora, T.; Gradisar, M.; Taheri, S.; Carskadon, M.A. How Many Sleep Diary Entries Are Needed to Reliably Estimate Adolescent Sleep? *Sleep* **2017**, *40*, zsx006. [CrossRef] [PubMed]

Disclaimer/Publisher's Note: The statements, opinions and data contained in all publications are solely those of the individual author(s) and contributor(s) and not of MDPI and/or the editor(s). MDPI and/or the editor(s) disclaim responsibility for any injury to people or property resulting from any ideas, methods, instructions or products referred to in the content.

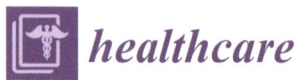 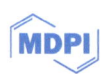

Article

Sleepiness and Vitamin D Levels in Patients with Obstructive Sleep Apnea

Kostas Archontogeorgis [1], Nicholas-Tiberio Economou [1], Panagiotis Bargiotas [2], Evangelia Nena [3], Athanasios Voulgaris [1], Konstantina Chadia [1], Georgia Trakada [4], Andrea Romigi [5,6] and Paschalis Steiropoulos [1,*]

[1] Department of Pneumonology, Medical School, Democritus University of Thrace, 68100 Alexandroupolis, Greece; k.archontogeorgis@yahoo.it (K.A.); nt_economou@yahoo.it (N.-T.E.); thanasisvoul@hotmail.com (A.V.); con_chadia@yahoo.gr (K.C.)
[2] Sleep-Wake Lab, Department of Neurology, Medical School, University of Cyprus, Nicosia 2408, Cyprus; bargiotas.panagiotis@ucy.ac.cy
[3] Laboratory of Hygiene and Environmental Protection, Medical School, Democritus University of Thrace, 68100 Alexandroupolis, Greece; evangelianena@yahoo.gr
[4] Division of Pulmonology, Department of Clinical Therapeutics, School of Medicine, National and Kapodistrian University of Athens, Alexandra Hospital, 11635 Athens, Greece; gtrakada@hotmail.com
[5] IRCCS Neuromed Istituto Neurologico Mediterraneo Pozzilli (IS), 86077 Pozzilli, Italy; andrea.romigi@gmail.com
[6] Faculty of Psychology, Uninettuno Telematic International University, 00186 Rome, Italy
* Correspondence: steiropoulos@yahoo.com

Abstract: Study Objectives: The aim of this cross-sectional study is to explore the association between serum 25-hydroxyvitamin D [25(OH)D] levels, a marker of Vitamin D status, and excessive daytime sleepiness (EDS), expressed as increased scores of the Epworth Sleepiness Scale (ESS), in a group of prospectively enrolled patients with obstructive sleep apnea (OSA). Methods: Newly diagnosed patients with OSA, divided into two groups, those with EDS (ESS > 10) and those without EDS (ESS < 10). All patients underwent night polysomnography. Measurement of serum 25(OH)D vitamin was performed using a radioimmunoassay. Results: In total, 217 patients with OSA (197 males and 20 females) were included. Patients with EDS had higher AHI ($p < 0.001$) values and lower mean serum 25(OH)D levels, compared with those of non-somnolent patients [17.4 (12.2–25.7) versus 21.1 (15.3–28.8) ng/mL, respectively, $p = 0.005$]. In patients with EDS, serum 25(OH)D levels correlated with average oxyhemoglobin saturation during sleep ($r = 0.194$, $p = 0.043$), and negatively with ESS score ($r = -0.285$, $p = 0.003$), AHI ($r = -0.197$, $p = 0.040$) and arousal index ($r = -0.256$, $p = 0.019$). Binary regression analysis identified Vit D serum levels ($\beta = -0.045$, OR: 0.956, 95% CI: 0.916–0.997, $p = 0.035$), total sleep time ($\beta = 0.011$, OR: 1.011, 95% CI: 1.002–1.021, $p = 0.016$) and AHI ($\beta = 0.022$, OR: 1.022, 95% CI: 1.003–1.043, $p = 0.026$) as independent predictors of EDS in patients with OSA. In patients with EDS, multiple regression analysis indicated that ESS score was negatively associated with Vit D serum levels ($\beta = -0.135$, $p = 0.014$) and minimum oxyhemoglobin saturation during sleep ($\beta = -0.137$, $p = 0.043$). Conclusions: In the present study, EDS in patients with OSA is associated with low levels of Vitamin D, while sleep hypoxia may play a role in this process.

Keywords: vitamin D; sleepiness; obstructive sleep apnea (OSA); sleep apnea; Epworth sleepiness scale (ESS)

1. Introduction

Obstructive sleep apnea (OSA) is characterized by intermittent cessation of breathing during sleep due to partial or complete upper airway obstruction [1]. By definition, these episodes are always accompanied by respiratory effort and result in oxyhemoglobin desaturation and sleep fragmentation [1]. Currently, OSA is the most frequent sleep-related breathing disorder, with an estimated prevalence between 10–17% for men and 3–9% for women in the Western countries [2]. OSA-related symptoms could be divided into nocturnal, such as loud snoring and a choking sensation during sleep, and diurnal, such as excessive daytime sleepiness (EDS), which among others is recognized as the most common and disabling daytime feature of OSA [3].

EDS is a frequently reported symptom of OSA and it may affect from 19% to 87.2% of patients diagnosed with OSA [4]. Although the prevalence of EDS in OSA exhibits significant variability in epidemiological studies, these evident differences in the prevalence data might be attributed to a complex interplay of several factors, including the methodologies employed for EDS measurement, sample sizes, age, gender, severity of OSA, ethnicity, the presence of comorbidities, and other unrecognized factors that could impact OSA manifestation [5]. EDS is characterized by the inability to remain alert and maintain wakefulness during the day, with sleep occurring unintentionally or at inappropriate times almost daily for at least three months [6]. Well-studied risk factors for this condition include increased BMI and neck circumference, older age, male gender and anatomical variations causing narrowing of the upper airway [7]. As the syndrome evolves, and while at the same time remains undiagnosed and untreated, EDS becomes debilitating resulting in impaired quality of life, reduced work performance and increased probability for traffic accidents [3].

Information regarding Vit D is now widely accessible not only in the scientific literature, but also across various platforms on the internet [8,9]. Vitamin D (Vit D) is a fat-soluble vitamin produced in the skin after exposure to solar radiation. Vit D exists in various forms and serum 25-hydroxyvitamin D [25(OH)D] is considered the marker of choice for the measurement of Vit D levels [8]. Interestingly, Vit D insufficiency (defined as Vit D levels < 20 ng/mL) and deficiency (defined as Vit D levels < 10 ng/mL) has an increased prevalence worldwide and is present in numerous pulmonary diseases, such as viral and bacterial respiratory infections, asthma, chronic obstructive pulmonary disease and cancer [10]. Recent data reported lower Vit D serum levels in patients with OSA compared with non-apneic individuals, while CPAP treatment showed beneficial effects on Vit D concentrations in this particular population of patients [11,12].

Data regarding the relationship between Vit D serum levels and EDS in OSA are still scarce. Hence, the aim of the present cross-sectional study is to compare Vit D serum levels in OSA patients with and without EDS and to explore potential associations between Vit D levels and the degree of excessive daytime sleepiness in these patients. In addition, secondary endpoints of the study are to examine possible correlations between Vit D levels and different anthropometric and sleep characteristics, focusing on the subgroup of patients with EDS.

2. Materials and Methods

2.1. Patients

Patients who underwent polysomnography in our Institution and were consecutively diagnosed with OSA were included in the study.

Patient recruitment took place between 1 April and 31 October 2017, in order to avoid significant variations in exposure to sunlight, which could affect Vit D levels. The following exclusion criteria were applied: Vit D supplementation, central sleep apnea syndrome, corticosteroid and/or diuretic therapy, conditions known to affect calcium, phosphorus and Vit D metabolism and absorption, heart failure, inflammatory diseases, cancer, liver or kidney disease, osteoporosis and patients with no OSA-related EDS [13].

Overall, 289 patients with OSA [250 males and 39 females with a median age 57 (48–65) years] were evaluated for inclusion in the present study. A detailed medical history regarding past medical conditions, known comorbidities, current medication use, focusing on Vit D supplements, and tobacco smoking was recorded. A clinical examination and the assessment of anthropometric characteristics (including height, weight, neck circumference, hip, and waist circumference as well as waist/hip circumference ratio and body mass index-BMI) were performed.

OSA was defined as AHI ≥ 15 events/hour of sleep or as AHI ≥ 5 events/hour of sleep accompanied by symptoms of disturbed sleep, such as excessive daytime sleepiness, gasping or choking during sleep, observed loud snoring or breathing interruption [3].

Sleepiness was evaluated using the validated Greek version of the Epworth Sleepiness Scale (ESS) [14], a self-administered questionnaire which includes eight questions referring to typical everyday situations. By attributing a score from 0 to 3, the patient rates the possibility of falling asleep in each situation. A score > 10 indicates EDS.

Pulmonary function testing, analysis of arterial blood gases and a 12-lead electrocardiogram were also performed in order for potential coexistent pulmonary and cardiovascular diseases to be excluded.

2.2. Polysomnography

An attended overnight polysomnography was performed from 22:00 to 06:00 h and variables were recorded on a computer system (Alice® 4, Philips Respironics, Murrysville, PA, USA). A standard montage of electroencephalogram, electro-occulogram, electromyogram and electrocardiogram signals was used for sleep staging. Pulse oximetry was registered and airflow was detected using combined oronasal thermistors for apneas and nasal pressure for hypopneas. Chest and abdominal motion were detected using inductive plethysmography. Sleep staging and respiratory events were scored manually according to standard criteria [15]. Apnea was defined as a ≥90% of reduction in airflow for at least 10 s [15]. Hypopnea was defined as a ≥30% reduction in airflow for at least 10 s in combination with oxyhemoglobin desaturation of at least 3% or an arousal registered by the electroencephalogram [15]. The apnea–hypopnea index (AHI) was calculated as the average number of apneas and hypopneas per hour of PSG-recorded sleep time [15].

2.3. Blood Samples and Measurements

Venous blood samples were collected from all participants the morning after polysomnography after at least 8 h of fasting. Samples were obtained from the antecubital vein and were left to coagulate and then centrifuged (3000 rpm for 10 min). Biochemical parameters regarding renal and liver function, as well as glucose, C-reactive protein (CRP) serum levels and lipid profile were measured using an automated analyzer. Serum concentrations of 25(OH)D were determined using a commercial radioimmunoassay kit and the manufacturer's specifications the same day as that of the blood sampling (DiaSorin, Stillwater, MN, USA).

2.4. Statistical Analysis

The sample size was determined by using the G*Power software version 3.1.9.7. It was evaluated that the minimum sample size to yield a statistical power of at least 0.8 with an alpha of 0.05 and a medium effect size (d = 0.35) was 102. All analyses were carried out using IBM Statistical Package for Social Sciences (SPSS Inc. Released 2008. SPSS Statistics for Windows, Version 17.0. Chicago, IL, USA: SPSS Inc.). The normality of distribution for continuous variables was tested with the Shapiro–Wilk test. All data are expressed as the median (25th–75th percentile). Comparison of percentages between groups was performed with the chi-squared test. In normally distributed variables, correlations were analyzed with Pearson's correlation coefficient, while comparisons between means were studied with the Student's *t*-test. In case of skewed distribution, the Spearman's correlation and non-parametric Mann–Whitney test was applied. Independent predictors of EDS between the two groups were identified using binary logistic regression analysis. In the EDS group, independent factors of EDS were further determined using multiple linear regression analysis. Reported *p*-values are two-tailed and significance was defined at $p < 0.05$.

2.5. Ethics Approval

All procedures were carried out in accordance with the Helsinki Declaration of Human Rights and patients gave their informed consent [16]. The study protocol was approved by the Institutional ethics committee of the University General Hospital of Alexandroupolis (approval date: 13 October 2014).

3. Results

In total, 217 patients with OSA (197 males and 20 females) participated in the present study. Included patients were middle-aged [age was 55 (46.5–62.5) years] and obese [BMI was 35.3 (31.4–38.3) kg/m^2], while median serum Vit D levels were of 19.4 (13.3–26.5) ng/mL. Females exhibited lower 25(OH)D serum levels compared with males [15.5 (9.7–20.6) versus 20.2 (13.4–26.7), respectively, $p = 0.048$)].

Participants were divided according to the presence or not of EDS into two groups: non-sleepy (ESS score $\leq$ 10), which included 108 patients (96 males and 12 females), and sleepy (ESS score > 10), which included 109 patients (101 males and 8 females). No differences were identified between the two groups in terms of gender, age, and BMI. Anthropometric and demographic characteristics of included patients are presented in Table 1.

Table 1. Comparison of anthropometric characteristics between OSA patients with and without EDS.

	OSA Patients without EDS n = 108	OSA Patients with EDS n = 109	p
Gender (male/female)	96/12	101/8	0.337
Age (years)	55.5 (46–64)	54 (47–62)	0.839
BMI (kg/m^2)	34.3 (30.7–37.7)	36 (32.1–38.9)	0.103
Neck circumference (cm)	44 (42–47)	45 (42–48)	0.502
Waist circumference (cm)	121 (113–129)	121 (112–130)	0.764
Hip circumference (cm)	116 (111–124)	116 (110–123)	0.937
WHR	1.03 (0.99–1.06)	1.03 (0.99–1.08)	0.406
Smoking (%)	24.1%	28.4%	0.465

BMI: body mass index; EDS: excessive daytime sleepiness; OSA: obstructive sleep apnea; WHR: waist-to-hip ratio.

In sleepy patients, the following findings were demonstrated: a longer total sleep time, higher sleep efficiency, higher values of arousal index, AHI and worse indices of hypoxia during sleep when compared with patients without EDS. Sleep characteristics of patients are presented in Table 2.

Table 2. Comparison of sleep characteristics between OSA patients with and without EDS.

	OSA Patients without EDS n = 108	OSA Patients with EDS n = 109	p
TST (min)	311 (263–339)	340 (311–360)	<0.001
N1 (%)	12.3 (5.5–18.7)	7.7 (4.4–15.3)	0.055
N2 (%)	70.1 (59.2–77.9)	72.2 (61.9–85.1)	0.046
N3 (%)	7.5 (1.8–15.2)	5.2 (0–13.6)	0.074
REM (%)	7.5 (1.4–12.9)	5.4 (1.3–10.5)	0.171
AHI (events/h)	33.9 (15–62.3)	54.9 (35.2–73)	<0.001
Aver SpO$_2$ (%)	92 (90–94)	91 (89–93)	0.002
Min SpO$_2$ (%)	77 (69–82)	73 (63–79)	0.008
T < 90% (%)	11.8 (3.2–38.3)	30.9 (12.8–59.6)	<0.001
Arousal index	27.5 (13.5–35.7)	35.2 (19.2–49.5)	0.034
Sleep efficiency (%)	83.7 (75.7–90)	88.6 (80.2–92.7)	0.004
ESS score	7 (5–9)	14 (12–17)	<0.001

AHI: apnea-hypopnea index, Aver SpO$_2$: average oxyhemoglobin saturation, EDS: excessive daytime sleepiness, ESS: Epworth sleepiness scale, Min SpO$_2$: minimum oxyhemoglobin saturation, N1: sleep stage 1, N2: sleep stage 2, N3: sleep stage 3, OSA: obstructive sleep apnea, REM: rapid eye movement, TST: total sleep time, T < 90%: time with oxyhemoglobin saturation < 90%.

Additionally, patients with EDS had a poorer lipidemic profile, as expressed by higher triglycerides levels and lower HDL-C, compared with patients without EDS. Moreover, sleepy patients with OSA had significantly lower serum 25(OH)D levels than those without EDS [21.1 (15.3–28.8) versus 17.4 (12.2–25.7) ng/mL, respectively; $p = 0.005$]. Results of blood examinations of patients are presented in Table 3 and results from pulmonary function testing are presented in Table 4.

Table 3. Comparison of laboratory results between OSA patients with and without EDS.

	OSA Patients without EDS n = 108	OSA Patients with EDS n = 109	p
Glucose (mg/dL)	103 (92–117)	114 (94.3–128.8)	0.078
Creatinine (mg/dL)	0.9 (0.8–1)	0.9 (0.8–1)	0.316
Cholesterol (mg/dL)	201 (176.8–234)	198 (176–234.8)	0.735
Triglycerides (mg/dL)	136.5 (98–181)	167 (112.5–211.8)	0.013
LDL-C (mg/dL)	125.9 (96.3–151.5)	118.2 (102–142.3)	0.899
HDL-C (mg/dL)	47 (42–57.3)	42 (37–52)	0.007
AST (U/L)	23 (19–27)	21.5 (18–27.8)	0.390
ALT (U/L)	25 (17–33)	24.5 (20–35)	0.604
CRP (mg/dL)	0.25 (0.1–0.79)	0.40 (0.20–0.66)	0.376
25(OH)D (ng/mL)	21.1 (15.3–28.8)	17.4 (12.2–25.7)	0.005

ALT: alanine aminotransferase, AST: aspartate aminotransferase, CRP: C—reactive protein, HDL-C: high-density lipoprotein cholesterol, LDL-C: low-density lipoprotein cholesterol.

Table 4. Comparison of pulmonary function testing results between OSA patients with and without EDS.

	OSA Patients without EDS n = 108	OSA Patients with EDS n = 109	p
FEV_1 (% predicted)	93.8 (81.9–103)	92.3 (75.9–106.8)	0.736
FVC (% predicted)	90.7 (78.1–99.3)	85.9 (73.8–97.8)	0.137
FEV_1/FVC (%)	86.5 (82–110.3)	83 (79–95)	0.323
pO_2 (mmHg)	79 (73–85.6)	78.5 (68.5–86)	0.344
pCO_2 (mmHg)	41 (38.9–44)	42 (39–45)	0.327

FEV_1: forced expiratory volume in 1st sec, FVC: forced vital capacity, pCO_2: carbon dioxide partial pressure, pO_2: oxygen partial pressure.

Further analysis in the group of sleepy patients showed that serum 25(OH)D levels were positively correlated with average oxyhemoglobin saturation during sleep (r = 0.194, $p = 0.043$) and negatively associated with the ESS score (r = −0.285, $p = 0.003$), AHI (r = −0.197, $p = 0.040$) and arousal index (r = −0.256, $p = 0.019$). Conversely, among non-sleepy OSA patients, Vit D serum levels were positively associated with average oxyhemoglobin saturation (r = 0.250, $p = 0.009$) and negatively associated with time with oxyhemoglobin saturation <90% (r = −0.214, $p = 0.028$) during sleep.

Age, sex, BMI, indices of oxygenation during sleep (average and minimum oxyhemoglobin saturation and time with oxyhemoglobin saturation <90%), total sleep time, sleep efficiency, AHI, arousal index and Vit D serum levels were included in a binary logistic regression analysis model in order to identify independent predictors of EDS. This analysis revealed that Vit D serum levels (β = −0.045, OR: 0.956, 95% CI: 0.916-0.997, $p = 0.035$), total sleep time (β = 0.011, OR: 1.011, 95% CI: 1.002–1.021, $p = 0.016$) and AHI (β = 0.022, OR: 1.022, 95% CI: 1.003–1.043, $p = 0.026$) emerged as independent predictors of EDS in patients with OSA.

In the group of OSA patients with EDS, correlations of ESS score with other indicators were determined using a multivariate linear regression analysis. In this analysis, ESS score was set as the outcome, whereas age, sex, BMI, indices of oxygenation during sleep (average and minimum oxyhemoglobin saturation and time with oxyhemoglobin saturation <90%), total sleep time, sleep efficiency, AHI, arousal index and Vit D serum levels were set as covariates (regression equation: y = 13.255 − 0.02a − 0.254b + 0.041c + 0.204d − 0.137e + 0.008f + 0.001g − 0.034h − 0.029j + 0.033k − 0.135m). Results indicated that the ESS score was negatively associated with Vit D serum levels ($\beta = -0.135$, $p = 0.014$) and minimum oxyhemoglobin saturation during sleep ($\beta = -0.137$, $p = 0.043$). In the group of OSA patients without EDS, a similar analysis showed that the ESS score was positively associated with sleep efficiency ($\beta = 0.138$, $p = 0.001$).

4. Discussion

The present study reported significantly lower levels of 25(OH)D in patients with OSA and EDS compared with patients with OSA and without EDS. Additionally, Vit D serum levels, AHI and total sleep time were identified as independent predictors of EDS. Finally, 25(OH)D levels were associated with indices of hypoxia during sleep and total sleep time.

Both decreased serum 25(OH)D levels and the severity of OSA were associated with EDS in the group of patients with OSA. The relationship between EDS and hypovitaminosis D has been a subject of interest in previous studies. In a previous study, an association was shown between Vit D status and excessive daytime sleepiness in patients with sleep disorders, of which OSA was the most prevalent [17]. Interestingly, only in Black patients with Vit D deficiency (defined as <20 ng/mL) were Vit D levels correlated with sleepiness ($r = 0.48$, $p < 0.05$), expressed as scores in ESS ≥ 10 [17]. In addition, multiple lines of evidence indicate that patients with OSA are more prone to Vit D deficiency than those without OSA [18,19], and that treatment with CPAP could increase Vit D levels either after short-term application and in male patients with OSA [20], and after long-term application in sleepy patients and those with severe OSA [21], or more specifically in male obese patients with OSA [12]. However, the association between Vit D and OSA remains controversial. In a recent study that included 133 patients suspected of having OSA, no difference was noted between hypertensive and normotensive subjects [22]. Polysomnography was conducted following the classification of subjects into hypertensive and normotensive groups. Therefore, not all individuals in the study were diagnosed with OSA. The inclusion of individuals without OSA in the study population may explain the discrepancy in these findings. In the same study, a negative association between the calcium concentration and arousal index and a correlation between AHI and Vit D concentration was observed. These findings indeed suggest a potential relationship between Vitamin D and OSA [22].

In the present study, differences between sleepy and non-sleepy patients with OSA in terms of polysomnographic parameters were noted. Specifically, OSA patients with EDS exhibited an increased AHI, total sleep time, arousal index and sleep efficiency, and presented worse hypoxia during sleep compared with those individuals without EDS. These results confirm previous reports on the association of EDS (assessed either by subjective or objective tools [23]) with anthropometric and polysomnographic characteristics in OSA patients, including a higher BMI, longer total sleep time, increased arousal index and decreased minimum oxyhemoglobin saturation during REM and NREM sleep [24].

Hypoxia may serve as an underlying mechanism explaining the association between hypovitaminosis D and EDS. Previous studies have reported a clear link between impaired oxygenation during sleep and EDS in individuals with OSA, suggesting a potential causal relationship between nocturnal hypoxia and EDS [23,24]. Concurrently, hypoxia and hypoxia-related factors, such as hypoxia-inducible factor-1α subunit (HIF-1α) and vascular endothelial growth factor (VEGF), are inversely correlated to serum 25(OH)D levels [25,26]. Indeed, in our study we confirmed previous reports that patients with OSA exhibit decreased 25(OH)D levels in comparison to healthy controls, and these diminished 25(OH)D levels are correlated with average oxyhemoglobin saturation and with the percentage of time with oxyhemoglobin saturation <90% during sleep [18]. Thus, the over-expression of inflammatory factors promoted by hypoxia during sleep may mediate the relationship between low Vit D levels and increased levels of EDS in OSA patients.

Moreover, several other pathogenetic mechanisms have been proposed in order to elucidate the link between Vit D and EDS. An underlining hypothesis suggests that low Vit D serum levels could lead to EDS through mechanisms involving the upregulation of inflammatory mediators and hypnogenic cytokines such as TNF-α, IL-1, IL-6 and prostagladin-2 [27,28]. The relationship between EDS and increased AHI has been proven in some, but not in all studies [29–31]. Excluding AHI, other factors, including metabolic and psychological conditions, are associated with an increased risk of EDS in OSA patients [32]. EDS has been frequently reported among diabetic patients without OSA and constitutes a risk factor for severe hypoglycemia [28,33]. Recently, reduced serum Vit D levels have been associated with increased insulin resistance in patients with OSA [34]. Similarly, in patients with OSA and EDS associations have been shown between insulin resistance and glucose deregulation [35,36]. Moreover, in a median follow-up of 8.1 years, lower serum Vit D concentrations were associated with increased risk of type 2 diabetes, with daytime sleepiness being the major contributor [37]. Thus, insulin resistance may mediate the emergence of EDS in patients with OSA and Vit D insufficiency.

Notably, studies exploring the association between EDS and Vit D serum levels in conditions other than OSA have reported conflicting results. In the study of Carlander et al. [38], serum 25(OH)D concentrations were decreased in patients with narcolepsy compared with healthy controls. Patients with narcolepsy were at increased risk of Vit D deficiency compared with non-narcoleptic subjects (72.5% versus 50.9%, respectively) [38]. Conversely, another study showed similar levels of 25(OH) D between patients with narcolepsy type 1 and healthy controls [39]. In patients with narcolepsy, no significant association was found between Vit D deficiency and disease duration or severity [39]. OSA and narcolepsy frequently coexist (about 25%) and this fact may explain the puzzling results regarding the association between Vit D and narcolepsy [40].

Certainly, our study has a number of limitations. Firstly, our data were obtained from middle-aged adults and no generalization of the results could be performed in older patients with OSA. Of note, regression analysis failed to demonstrate age as an influencing factor for EDS in our participants. Secondly, data regarding skin pigmentation, clothing and dietary habits were not recorded in the current study. Nevertheless, the study was conducted in a short time interval (6 months), and included Caucasian patients, living in the same area, with relatively similar sun exposure and dietary habits. Additionally, the number of included female patients was relatively small and thus the study results should be interpreted with caution. However, at regression analysis, gender was excluded as a cofounder regarding the relationship between Vit D deficiency and EDS. It should be noted that the index of females/males was the result of an increased male referral and did not result from a female exclusion process. Finally, EDS was evaluated using the ESS and not an objective method, such as the multiple sleep latency test. However, there is evidence suggesting that ESS can be a valid tool for the evaluation of EDS [41]. Potential mechanisms of EDS in OSA are still not entirely clear [42].

5. Conclusions

In conclusion, our results show that both AHI and Vit D serum levels predict EDS in a group of patients with OSA. Hypoxia during sleep may play an important role in this process. A possible bi-directional relationship between OSA and hypovitaminosis D could partially explain our findings. Further research is needed in order to better elucidate the interaction between serum Vit D levels and EDS in patients with OSA.

Author Contributions: K.A. and P.S. conception and design of the study; interpretation of data; statistical analysis; drafting of manuscript; critical revision of the manuscript for important intellectual content. N.-T.E., E.N., A.V., A.R., K.C., G.T. and P.B. analysis and interpretation of data; critical revision of the manuscript for important intellectual content. All authors are responsible for interpretation of the findings. All authors have read and agreed to the published version of the manuscript.

Funding: This research received no external funding.

Institutional Review Board Statement: This study was approved on 13 October 2014 by the Institutional Review Board (IRB) at the University General Hospital of Alexandroupolis.

Informed Consent Statement: Informed consent was obtained from all subjects involved in the study.

Data Availability Statement: Data Availability Statements are available upon request.

Conflicts of Interest: The authors declare no conflict of interest.

References

1. American Academy of Sleep Medicine. Sleep-related breathing disorders in adults: Recommendations for syndrome definition and measurement techniques in clinical research. The Report of an American Academy of Sleep Medicine Task Force. *Sleep* **1999**, *22*, 667–689. [CrossRef]
2. Peppard, P.E.; Young, T.; Barnet, J.H.; Palta, M.; Hagen, E.W.; Hla, K.M. Increased prevalence of sleep-disordered breathing in adults. *Am. J. Epidemiol.* **2013**, *177*, 1006–1014. [CrossRef]
3. Epstein, L.J.; Kristo, D.; Strollo, P.J., Jr.; Friedman, N.; Malhotra, A.; Patil, S.P.; Ramar, K.; Rogers, R.; Schwab, R.J.; Weaver, E.M.; et al. Clinical guideline for the evaluation, management and long-term care of obstructive sleep apnea in adults. *J. Clin. Sleep Med.* **2009**, *5*, 263–276.
4. Punjabi, N.M.; O'Hearn, D.J.; Neubauer, D.N.; Nieto, F.J.; Schwartz, A.R.; Smith, P.L.; Bandeen-Roche, K. Modeling hypersomnolence in sleep-disordered breathing. A novel approach using survival analysis. *Am. J. Respir. Crit. Care Med.* **1999**, *159*, 1703–1709. [CrossRef]
5. Garbarino, S.; Scoditti, E.; Lanteri, P.; Conte, L.; Magnavita, N.; Toraldo, D.M. Obstructive Sleep Apnea with or without Excessive Daytime Sleepiness: Clinical and Experimental Data-Driven Phenotyping. *Front. Neurol.* **2018**, *9*, 505. [CrossRef]
6. American Academy of Sleep Medicine. *International Classification of Sleep Disorders*, 3rd ed.; American Academy of Sleep Medicine: Darien, IL, USA, 2014.
7. Slater, G.; Steier, J. Excessive daytime sleepiness in sleep disorders. *J. Thorac. Dis.* **2012**, *4*, 608–616. [PubMed]
8. Herrmann, M.; Farrell, C.L.; Pusceddu, I.; Fabregat-Cabello, N.; Cavalier, E. Assessment of vitamin D status—A changing landscape. *Clin. Chem. Lab. Med.* **2017**, *55*, 3–26. [CrossRef]
9. Hussein, A.S.; Hamzah, S.H.; Rahman, S.K.A.S.A.; Zamri, Z.A. YouTube™ as a source of information on vitamin D: A content-quality analysis. *Dent. Med. Probl.* **2022**, *59*, 263–270. [CrossRef]
10. Pfeffer, P.E.; Hawrylowicz, C.M. Vitamin D and lung disease. *Thorax* **2012**, *67*, 1018–1020. [CrossRef]
11. Neighbors, C.L.P.; Noller, M.W.; Song, S.A.; Zaghi, S.; Neighbors, J.; Feldman, D.; Kushida, C.A.; Camacho, M. Vitamin D and obstructive sleep apnea: A systematic review and meta-analysis. *Sleep Med.* **2018**, *43*, 100–108. [CrossRef]
12. Liguori, C.; Izzi, F.; Mercuri, N.B.; Romigi, A.; Cordella, A.; Tarantino, U.; Placidi, F. Vitamin D status of male OSAS patients improved after long-term CPAP treatment mainly in obese subjects. *Sleep Med.* **2017**, *29*, 81–85. [CrossRef]
13. Guilleminault, C.; Brooks, S.N. Excessive daytime sleepiness: A challenge for the practising neurologist. *Brain* **2001**, *124*, 1482–1491. [CrossRef]
14. Tsara, V.; Serasli, E.; Amfilochiou, A.; Constantinidis, T.; Christaki, P. Greek version of the Epworth Sleepiness Scale. *Sleep Breath* **2004**, *8*, 91–95. [CrossRef]
15. Berry, R.B.; Budhiraja, R.; Gottlieb, D.J.; Gozal, D.; Iber, C.; Kapur, V.K.; Marcus, C.L.; Mehra, R.; Parthasarathy, S.; Quan, S.F.; et al. Rules for scoring respiratory events in sleep: Update of the 2007 AASM Manual for the Scoring of Sleep and Associated Events. Deliberations of the Sleep Apnea Definitions Task Force of the American Academy of Sleep Medicine. *J. Clin. Sleep Med.* **2012**, *8*, 597–619. [CrossRef]
16. World Medical Association. World Medical Association Declaration of Helsinki: Ethical principles for medical research involving human subjects. *JAMA* **2013**, *310*, 2191–2194. [CrossRef]
17. McCarty, D.E.; Reddy, A.; Keigley, Q.; Kim, P.Y.; Marino, A.A. Vitamin D, race, and excessive daytime sleepiness. *J. Clin. Sleep Med.* **2012**, *8*, 693–697. [CrossRef]
18. Archontogeorgis, K.; Nena, E.; Papanas, N.; Zissimopoulos, A.; Voulgaris, A.; Xanthoudaki, M.; Manolopoulos, V.; Froudarakis, M.; Steiropoulos, P. Vitamin D Levels in Middle-Aged Patients with Obstructive Sleep Apnoea Syndrome. *Curr. Vasc. Pharmacol.* **2018**, *16*, 289–297. [CrossRef]
19. Upala, S.; Sanguankeo, A. Association between 25-Hydroxyvitamin D and Obstructive Sleep Apnea: A Systematic Review and Meta-Analysis. *J. Clin. Sleep Med.* **2015**, *11*, 1347. [CrossRef]
20. Liguori, C.; Romigi, A.; Izzi, F.; Mercuri, N.B.; Cordella, A.; Tarquini, E.; Giambrone, M.P.; Marciani, M.G.; Placidi, F. Continuous Positive Airway Pressure Treatment Increases Serum Vitamin D Levels in Male Patients with Obstructive Sleep Apnea. *J. Clin. Sleep Med.* **2015**, *11*, 603–607. [CrossRef] [PubMed]
21. Theorell-Haglow, J.; Hoyos, C.M.; Phillips, C.L.; Yee, B.J.; Herrmann, M.; Brennan-Speranza, T.C.; Grunstein, R.R.; Liu, P.Y. Changes of vitamin D levels and bone turnover markers after CPAP therapy: A randomized sham-controlled trial. *J. Sleep Res.* **2018**, *27*, e12606. [CrossRef]

22. Kanclerska, J.; Wieckiewicz, M.; Nowacki, D.; Szymanska-Chabowska, A.; Poreba, R.; Mazur, G.; Martynowicz, H. Sleep architecture and vitamin D in hypertensives with obstructive sleep apnea: A polysomnographic study. *Dent. Med. Probl.* **2024**, *61*, 43–52. [CrossRef] [PubMed]
23. Mediano, O.; Barcelo, A.; de la Pena, M.; Gozal, D.; Agusti, A.; Barbe, F. Daytime sleepiness and polysomnographic variables in sleep apnoea patients. *Rev. Port. Pneumol.* **2007**, *13*, 896–898. [CrossRef] [PubMed]
24. Oksenberg, A.; Arons, E.; Nasser, K.; Shneor, O.; Radwan, H.; Silverberg, D.S. Severe obstructive sleep apnea: Sleepy versus nonsleepy patients. *Laryngoscope* **2010**, *120*, 643–648. [CrossRef] [PubMed]
25. Ben-Shoshan, M.; Amir, S.; Dang, D.T.; Dang, L.H.; Weisman, Y.; Mabjeesh, N.J. 1alpha,25-dihydroxyvitamin D3 (Calcitriol) inhibits hypoxia-inducible factor-1/vascular endothelial growth factor pathway in human cancer cells. *Mol. Cancer Ther.* **2007**, *6*, 1433–1439. [CrossRef]
26. Lu, D.; Li, N.; Yao, X.; Zhou, L. Potential inflammatory markers in obstructive sleep apnea-hypopnea syndrome. *Bosn. J. Basic Med. Sci.* **2017**, *17*, 47–53. [CrossRef]
27. McCarty, D.E.; Chesson, A.L., Jr.; Jain, S.K.; Marino, A.A. The link between vitamin D metabolism and sleep medicine. *Sleep Med. Rev.* **2014**, *18*, 311–319. [CrossRef]
28. Archontogeorgis, K.; Nena, E.; Papanas, N.; Steiropoulos, P. The role of vitamin D in obstructive sleep apnoea syndrome. *Breathe* **2018**, *14*, 206–215. [CrossRef]
29. Hayashida, K.; Inoue, Y.; Chiba, S.; Yagi, T.; Urashima, M.; Honda, Y.; Itoh, H. Factors influencing subjective sleepiness in patients with obstructive sleep apnea syndrome. *Psychiatry Clin. Neurosci.* **2007**, *61*, 558–563. [CrossRef]
30. Knorst, M.M.; Souza, F.J.; Martinez, D. Obstructive sleep apnea-hypopnea syndrome: Association with gender, obesity and sleepiness-related factors. *J. Bras. Pneumol.* **2008**, *34*, 490–496. [CrossRef]
31. Vgontzas, A.N. Excessive daytime sleepiness in sleep apnea: It is not just apnea hypopnea index. *Sleep Med.* **2008**, *9*, 712–714. [CrossRef]
32. Medeiros, C.; Bruin, V.; Ferrer, D.; Paiva, T.; Montenegro, R., Jr.; Forti, A.; Bruin, P. Excessive daytime sleepiness in type 2 diabetes. *Arq. Bras. Endocrinol. Metabol.* **2013**, *57*, 425–430. [CrossRef] [PubMed]
33. Inkster, B.; Riha, R.L.; Van Look, L.; Williamson, R.; McLachlan, S.; Frier, B.M.; Strachan, M.W.; Price, J.F.; Reynolds, R.M. Association between excessive daytime sleepiness and severe hypoglycemia in people with type 2 diabetes: The Edinburgh Type 2 Diabetes Study. *Diabetes Care* **2013**, *36*, 4157–4159. [CrossRef]
34. Archontogeorgis, K.; Papanas, N.; Rizos, E.C.; Nena, E.; Zissimopoulos, A.; Tsigalou, C.; Voulgaris, A.; Mikhailidis, D.P.; Elisaf, M.S.; Froudarakis, M.E.; et al. Reduced Serum Vitamin D Levels Are Associated with Insulin Resistance in Patients with Obstructive Sleep Apnea Syndrome. *Medicina* **2019**, *55*, 174. [CrossRef] [PubMed]
35. Kritikou, I.; Basta, M.; Vgontzas, A.N.; Pejovic, S.; Liao, D.; Tsaoussoglou, M.; Bixler, E.O.; Stefanakis, Z.; Chrousos, G.P. Sleep apnoea, sleepiness, inflammation and insulin resistance in middle-aged males and females. *Eur. Respir. J.* **2014**, *43*, 145–155. [CrossRef] [PubMed]
36. Nena, E.; Steiropoulos, P.; Papanas, N.; Tsara, V.; Fitili, C.; Froudarakis, M.E.; Maltezos, E.; Bouros, D. Sleepiness as a marker of glucose deregulation in obstructive sleep apnea. *Sleep Breath* **2012**, *16*, 181–186. [CrossRef]
37. Wang, M.; Zhou, T.; Li, X.; Ma, H.; Liang, Z.; Fonseca, V.A.; Heianza, Y.; Qi, L. Baseline Vitamin D Status, Sleep Patterns, and the Risk of Incident Type 2 Diabetes in Data From the UK Biobank Study. *Diabetes Care* **2020**, *43*, 2776–2784. [CrossRef]
38. Carlander, B.; Puech-Cathala, A.M.; Jaussent, I.; Scholz, S.; Bayard, S.; Cochen, V.; Dauvilliers, Y. Low vitamin D in narcolepsy with cataplexy. *PLoS ONE* **2011**, *6*, e20433. [CrossRef] [PubMed]
39. Dauvilliers, Y.; Evangelista, E.; Lopez, R.; Barateau, L.; Scholz, S.; Crastes de Paulet, B.; Carlander, B.; Jaussent, I. Vitamin D deficiency in type 1 narcolepsy: A reappraisal. *Sleep Med.* **2017**, *29*, 1–6. [CrossRef]
40. Sansa, G.; Iranzo, A.; Santamaria, J. Obstructive sleep apnea in narcolepsy. *Sleep Med.* **2010**, *11*, 93–95. [CrossRef]
41. Johns, M.W. Sensitivity and specificity of the multiple sleep latency test (MSLT), the maintenance of wakefulness test and the epworth sleepiness scale: Failure of the MSLT as a gold standard. *J. Sleep Res.* **2000**, *9*, 5–11. [CrossRef]
42. Lal, C.; Weaver, T.E.; Bae, C.J.; Strohl, K.P. Excessive Daytime Sleepiness in Obstructive Sleep Apnea, Mechanisms and Clinical Management. *Ann. Am. Thorac. Soc.* **2021**, *18*, 757–768. [CrossRef] [PubMed]

Disclaimer/Publisher's Note: The statements, opinions and data contained in all publications are solely those of the individual author(s) and contributor(s) and not of MDPI and/or the editor(s). MDPI and/or the editor(s) disclaim responsibility for any injury to people or property resulting from any ideas, methods, instructions or products referred to in the content.

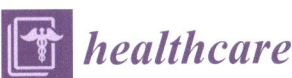

Article

Sleep Quality and Fatigue during Exam Periods in University Students: Prevalence and Associated Factors

Izolde Bouloukaki [1,2,*], Ioanna Tsiligianni [1], Giorgos Stathakis [2], Michail Fanaridis [2], Athina Koloi [2], Ekaterini Bakiri [2], Maria Moudatsaki [2], Eleptheria Pouladaki [2] and Sophia Schiza [2]

[1] Department of Social Medicine, School of Medicine, University of Crete, 71500 Heraklion, Greece; i.tsiligianni@uoc.gr

[2] Sleep Disorders Center, Department of Respiratory Medicine, School of Medicine, University of Crete, 71500 Heraklion, Greece; stathakisgg@gmail.com (G.S.); michfana@gmail.com (M.F.); athina_k45@hotmail.com (A.K.); aik.bakiri@gmail.com (E.B.); mariamoudatsaki@yahoo.gr (M.M.); elle.ria@hotmail.com (E.P.); schizas@uoc.gr (S.S.)

* Correspondence: izolthi@gmail.com; Tel.: +30-2810-394824

Abstract: The aim of our study was to assess university students' sleep quality and fatigue before and during the academic exam period and identify potential associated factors. A Web-based survey was completed by 940 students of 20 different Tertiary Institutions including demographics, sleep habits, exercise, caffeine, tobacco, alcohol use, subjective sleep quality (Pittsburgh Sleep Quality Index—PSQI), and fatigue (Fatigue severity scale—FSS) at the beginning of the semester and during the examination period. During the exam period, PSQI (8.9 vs. 6.1, $p < 0.001$) and FSS scores (36.9 vs. 32.7, $p < 0.001$) were significantly elevated compared to the pre-exam period. An increase in the PSQI score was associated with age ($\beta = 0.111$, $p = 0.011$), presence of chronic disease ($\beta = 0.914$, $p = 0.006$), and depressive symptoms ($\beta = 0.459$, $p = 0.001$). An increase in the FSS score was associated with female gender ($\beta = 1.658$, $p < 0.001$), age, ($\beta = 0.198$, $p = 0.010$), increase in smoking ($\beta = 1.7$, $p = 0.029$), coffee/energy drinks consumption ($\beta = 1.988$, $p < 0.001$), decreased levels of physical exercise ($\beta = 1.660$, $p < 0.001$), and depressive symptoms ($\beta = 2.526$, $p < 0.001$). In conclusion, our findings indicate that exam periods have a negative impact on the sleep quality and fatigue levels of university students. Potential factors were identified that could contribute to the formulation of strategies for improved sleep quality and wellness.

Keywords: sleep quality; fatigue; university students; exam period

1. Introduction

Adequate sleep duration has a critical role in promoting optimal physical health, immune function, mental health, and cognition [1]. According to consensus recommendations of the National Sleep Foundation and the American Academy of Sleep Medicine and Sleep Research Society guidelines, young adults should sleep 7 to 9 h per night on a regular basis for optimal sleep health [2,3]. Generally, deviating from the recommended sleep duration is associated with adverse health-related outcomes, including but not limited to poor attention, depression, obesity, and cardiovascular disease [4]. More specifically, sleep duration that deviates from the ideal range, either being excessively short or excessively long, appears to be linked to an elevated risk of all-cause mortality and cardiovascular events, with the risk being at its lowest when an individual sleeps for approximately 7 h per day [4]. Interestingly, earlier data suggests that inadequate sleep may be more concerning than excessive sleep in younger populations, as insufficient sleep durations were linked to poorer self-reported health in university students aged 17 to 30 years, while longer sleep durations were not related to self-reported health [5]. University students are considered as a population subset that is notably vulnerable to a shortened sleep duration and sleep disruptions [6,7]. Indeed, a young adult's life is going through numerous transitions during their time at university in which students have reduced parental support, increased stress from academic loads and lifestyle, and irregularities in the sleep–wake cycle, all resulting in shortened and delayed sleep [8]. These sleep disruptions are of particular concern due to their negative impact on mental and physical well-being, as well as cognitive abilities that are crucial for students' day-to-day performance and academic achievement [9–11]. Importantly, sleep quality in this population has been identified as the strongest predictor of well-being compared with physical activity, depression, and use of tobacco [12]. Attending university is also characterized by fatigue, which is often overlooked and also contributes to poor sleep [13].

Recent studies, representing different socio-cultural regions mainly from the US and China, have shown that sleep disturbances and dissatisfaction are particularly prevalent among university students, affecting 30 to 70% of this population [6,14–23]. During times of theorized greater stress, such as exams periods, students seem to demonstrate even worse sleep quality and less sleep than recommended [24]. However, these findings may not accurately represent sleep disorders rates among university students attending universities in Europe, which has distinct features associated with living arrangements, educational expenses, the application process, and facilities [25].

In Greece, research on sleep in university students remains scarce [26] and is mainly derived from studies during the COVID-19 pandemic [26–28]. Little is also known about how students' sleep patterns change before and during the academic exam period [29,30]. To elaborate further, there is a scarcity of evidence pointing towards compromised sleep quality and quantity during exam periods, which may cause impaired daytime functioning [28–30]. Therefore, the aim of our study was to assess changes in Greek university students' sleep quality and fatigue before (low stress) and during an academic exam (high stress) period and to identify possible associated factors.

2. Materials and Methods

2.1. Study Setting and Participants

A Web-based survey was conducted by university students of 20 different Tertiary Institutions (Medical/Health, Physics, Educational Sciences, Technical, Social sciences, Economic, etc.) in Crete, Greece, across 2 periods, at the beginning of the semester and during examination period in the academic year of 2018–2019 (before COVID-19 lockdown). The process of identifying and recruiting student participants involved two phases. The initial phase encompassed enlisting university professors and conveying the objectives of the current study on social media platforms. Subsequently, with the consent of their professors, university's public e-mail board and social media platforms were used to send online anonymous survey links to students.

The students were asked to answer questions about demographics, sleep habits, exercise habits, caffeine, tobacco and alcohol use, hours of technology use (cell phones, tablets, laptop computers), obstructive sleep apnea (OSA) and insomnia symptoms, excessive daytime sleepiness, subjective sleep quality (using the Pittsburgh Sleep Quality Index—PSQI), and fatigue (Fatigue severity scale—FSS). Depressive mood, excessive daytime sleepiness, insomnia, and OSA symptoms were assessed by yes/no single item questions ("Have you felt depressed or sad/sleepy or had insomnia/OSA symptoms much of the time in the past month?").

All procedures were approved by the University of Crete Research Ethics Committee and all participants gave their informed consent to participate prior to both survey administrations, using a digital form.

2.2. Study Tools and Outcomes

2.2.1. PSQI

A self-reported assessment of sleep was determined using the validated Greek version of the PSQI questionnaire, which is a standard instrument that has been validated as differentiating poor from good sleep [31,32]. The PSQI is a 19-item self-rated questionnaire that evaluates subjective sleep quality and quantity, sleep habits related to quality, and occurrence of sleep disturbances in adults over a 1-month interval. The 19 individual items are utilized in the generation of the following seven component scores: subjective sleep quality (one item), sleep latency (two items), sleep duration (one item), habitual sleep efficiency (three items), sleep disturbances (nine items), use of sleep medication (one item), and daytime dysfunction (two items). Each component score is equally weighted on a 0–3 scale, where 0 indicates no difficulty and 3 indicates severe difficulty. The aforementioned items, taken together, generate a score that reflects global subjective sleep quality, which varies between 0 and 21. The higher the score, the greater the negative impact on sleep quality. A global score of 6 or higher indicates poor sleep [33]. Previous studies have indicated adequate levels of internal consistency (Cronbach's alphas 0.70–0.83), and construct validity on this questionnaire in various populations [32–35].

2.2.2. FSS

In this scale, which is also translated and validated in Greek language [36,37], individuals rate their agreement (range, 1–7) with 9 statements concerning the severity, frequency, and impact of fatigue on daily life (physical functioning, exercise and work, and family or social life). Each item is rated on a 7-point Likert scale (1 'strongly disagree' to 7 'strongly agree'). The FSS score is determined by calculating the average of all item scores. A total score of less than 36 is considered normal. A score above that limit (maximum score 63) is suggestive of a significant negative impact of fatigue on daily life activities [38]. FSS psychometric properties have been assessed in different populations indicating sufficient concurrent validity and internal consistency (Cronbach's alphas 0.89–0.96) [36,37].

2.2.3. Outcomes

The primary outcome of the study was to compare the absolute change in students' global PSQI and FSS scores between a time of low stress (at the beginning of the semester) and a time of perceived high stress (academic exam period). Secondary outcomes involved identifying potential factors linked to baseline sleep quality, fatigue, and sleepiness, along with changes in sleep quality and fatigue among students.

2.3. Statistical Analysis

Our analysis was restricted to the subset of participants who gave responses in both the initial semester and exam period. Results are presented as mean ± standard deviation (SD) for continuous variables if normally distributed and as median (25–75th percentile) if not. Qualitative variables are presented as absolute number (percentage). To compare changes from the beginning of semester to exam period, the paired samples t-test (for normally distributed data) and the Wilcoxon Signed Rank test (for non-normally distributed data) were used. Changes of continuous variables from baseline to follow up were defined as baseline minus follow-up values. Factors associated with poor sleep quality and fatigue were analyzed with binomial logistic regression after adjustment for various potential explanatory variables, including age, gender, BMI, smoking status, presence of chronic disease, use of alcohol, caffeine, physical exercise, work, and use of technology. Multivariate linear regression analysis was used to examine any association of the previous potential confounders with changes in questionnaires scores (PSQI and FSS) during exam period. We checked multicollinearity among the predictors using collinearity statistics to ensure that collinearity between predictor variables was in the acceptable range as indicated by the tolerance value variance inflation factor. Internal consistency for PSQI and FSS was calculated with the Cronbach's alpha (α) coefficient and item-total correlations. Spearman's (rho) coefficients were used to calculate correlations between the questionnaire sub-scales. Test–retest reliability for the aforementioned questionnaires scores was explored with the intraclass correlation coefficient, ICC. Results were considered significant when p values were < 0.05. Data were analyzed using SPSS software (version 25, SPSS Inc., Chicago, IL, USA).

3. Results

3.1. Study Population

A total of 940 university students completed the questionnaire, of whom 60% were females (Table 1). Ages ranged from 17 to 48 years with a mean age of 21 years. Out of 940 participants, only a small fraction of 4 were above 40 years old and 9 were above 30 years old. Most of the participants were from Medical/Health (36%) and Physics (18%) universities. The majority of the participants were in the fourth year of education (50%) followed by the second (18%) and third (17%) years. Of note, 15% of students engaged in work and studies concurrently. Not a single participant reported having a family or young children.

Table 1. Characteristics of the participants (n = 940).

Characteristics	
Age (years)	21 ± 3
Gender, male (%)	371 (40%)
BMI (kg/m^2)	23.7 ± 4.8
BMI $\geq$ 30	65 (7%)
Current Smoking	242 (26%)
Type of education	
Medical/Health	343 (36%)
Physics	166 (18%)
Educational Sciences	79 (8%)
Technical	82 (9%)
Social sciences	92 (10%)
Economic	130 (14%)
Other	41 (4%)
Year of education	
1st	136 (15%)
2nd	168 (18%)
3rd	162 (17%)
4th +	474 (50%)
Working Students	136 (15%)

Data are presented as mean values ± SD or median (25–75th percentile), unless otherwise indicated. BMI, body mass index.

Further sample characteristics including exercise habits, caffeine, tobacco and alcohol use, and hours of technology use are presented in Table 2.

Table 2. Exercise habits, caffeine, tobacco and alcohol use, and hours of technology use.

Characteristics	
Alcohol consumption	
Low (0–3 drinks/week)	718 (76%)
Moderate (4–8 drinks/week)	166 (18%)
High ($\geq$9 drinks/week)	56 (6%)
Coffee/energy drinks consumption	
None	302 (32%)
Low (1–2 drinks/day)	557 (59%)
Moderate to high (>3 drinks/day)	81 (9%)
Physical activity	
None	328 (35%)
1–3/week	479 (51%)
>4/week	133 (14%)
Hours of technology use	
0–2 h/day	140 (15%)
2–5 h/day	449 (48/%)
5–8 h/day	230 (24%)
>8 h/day	121 (13%)

3.2. Sleep Patterns

Sleep patterns of the surveyed students are depicted in Table 3, where most students (75%) report late bedtimes. No significant difference was noted in the number of students' reported hours of sleep among all academic years ($p = 0.095$). Only 29 (3%) of the students reported frequently taking prescription medicine for insomnia.

Table 3. Daytime symptoms, sleep patterns, and disorders of university students (n = 940).

Symptoms	Pre-Exam Period	Exam Period	*p*-Value
Daytime symptoms			
FSS	32.7 ± 11.4	36.9 ± 12.3	<0.001
FSS ≥ 36	365 (39%)	473 (50%)	<0.001
Excessive Daytime Sleepiness			
(2 times or more per week)	168 (18%)	222 (24%)	<0.001
Depressive mood	391 (42%)	547 (58%)	<0.001
Sleep Characteristics			
Bedtime			
Between 9 pm and 12 am	238 (25%)	230 (25%)	
After 12 am	702 (75%)	710 (75%)	0.643
Wake up time			
Between 5 and 8 am	219 (23%)	222 (23%)	
Between 8 and 11 am	485 (52%)	553 (59%)	
After 11 am	236 (25%)	165 (18%)	<0.001
Sleep duration	7.4 ± 1.3	6.9 ± 2.9	<0.001
Frequent use of sleep medications			
(2 times or more per week)	29 (3%)	41 (4%)	0.031
PSQI	6.1 ± 1.8	8.9 ± 1.9	<0.001
PSQI > 5	435 (59%)	919 (98%)	<0.001
Insomnia symptoms			
(2 times or more per week)	417 (44%)	505 (54%)	<0.001
Obstructive Sleep Apnea symptoms			
(2 times or more per week)	122 (13%)	131 (14%)	0.256

According to the PSQI results, 554 (59%) out of 940 university students were classified as poor sleepers, a rate that remained similar across academic years ($p = 0.299$). On average, the PSQI global score of our sample was 6.1 ± 1.8 (Range: 1 to 14), which is above the cutoff for good sleepers (≤5), indicating that sleep quality was impaired. The ICC for the PSQI score was 0.717 and Cronbach's α value was 0.739. The global PSQI score was significantly correlated with each component ($p < 0.01$). Item-total Spearman's rho correlations ranged from 0.711 (component 1) to 0.838 (item 4).

Impaired sleep quality was independently associated with the female gender (OR = 1.524, 95% CI 1.086–2.138; $p = 0.015$), younger age (OR = 0.922, 95% CI 0.866–0.981; $p = 0.011$), high alcohol consumption (OR = 2.095, 95% CI 1.023–4.290; $p = 0.043$), lack of physical activity (OR = 0.566, 95% CI 0.338–0.946; $p = 0.030$), presence of a chronic disease (OR = 2.695, 95% CI 1.542–4.711; $p < 0.001$), depressive symptoms (OR = 3.232, 95% CI 2.311–4.519; $p < 0.001$), sleepiness (OR = 9.893, 95% CI 5.163–18.956; $p < 0.001$), and fatigue (FSS ≥ 36) (OR = 1.550, 95% CI 1.094–2.195; $p = 0.014$).

3.3. Daytime Functioning

On average, the FSS total score of our sample was 32.7 ± 11.4 (Range: 9–62) and 365 out of 940 university students (39%) reported suffering from fatigue. The prevalence of fatigue remained similar across academic years ($p = 0.754$). The ICC for the FSS score was 0.845 and Cronbach's α value was 0.868. The total FSS score was significantly correlated with each component ($p < 0.01$). Item-total Spearman's rho correlations ranged from 0.529 (item 3) to 0.770 (item 6).

Fatigue was independently associated with lack of physical activity (OR = 0.299, 95% CI 0.187–0.478; $p < 0.001$), presence of a chronic disease (OR = 1.619, 95% CI 1.080–2.426; $p = 0.020$), depressive (OR = 3.498, 95% CI 2.646–4.625; $p < 0.001$), and OSA symptoms (OR = 1.990, 95% CI 1.154–3.432; $p = 0.013$), sleepiness (OR = 1.911, 95% CI 1.333–2.739; $p < 0.001$), and impaired sleep quality (PSQI $\geq$ 6) (OR = 1.682, 95% CI 1.135–2.495; $p = 0.010$).

Regarding the frequency of excessive daytime sleepiness (two times or more per week), younger age (OR = 0.906, 95% CI 0.824–0.996; $p = 0.040$), presence of a chronic disease (OR = 2.071, 95% CI 1.145–3.747; $p = 0.016$), depressive symptoms (OR = 1.907, 95% CI 1.205–3.019; $p = 0.006$), presence of OSA symptoms (OR = 2.299, 95% CI 1.224–4.316; $p = 0.010$), and impaired sleep quality (OR = 14.565, 95% CI 6.166–34.042; $p < 0.001$) all significantly associated with more frequent reported sleepiness among students.

3.4. Changes in Sleep Quality and Fatigue during the Exam Period

During the exam period average sleep duration was significantly reduced (6.9 vs. 7.4, $p < 0.001$), 134 out of 242 (55%) smokers increased smoking, 489 out of 940 (52%) students increased coffee/energy drink consumption, 514 out of 940 (55%) decreased alcohol consumption and 474 (50%) decreased exercise. Insomnia symptoms, daytime sleepiness, and depressive symptoms were also more frequently reported in the exam period (Table 3).

PSQI global score was significantly elevated in the exam period compared to the pre-exam period (8.9 vs. 6.1, $p < 0.001$). Notably, all sub-scales of the PSQI contributed to the decline in sleep quality in the exam period (all $p < 0.05$). The increase in PSQI score (2.9 ± 1.6), which was similar in all years of education ($p = 0.109$), was independently associated with age ($\beta = 0.111$, $p = 0.011$), presence of chronic disease ($\beta = 0.914$, $p = 0.006$), worsening of FSS ($\beta = 0.048$, $p < 0.001$) depressive symptoms ($\beta = 0.459$, $p = 0.001$), and sleepiness ($\beta = 0.601$, $p < 0.001$). Furthermore, the prevalence of poor sleep quality (PSQI global score > 5) was also higher (98% vs. 59%) in this period.

FSS score was significantly elevated during the exam period compared to the pre-exam period (36.9 vs. 32.7, $p < 0.001$). Notably, all sub-scales of the FSS in the exam period were significantly elevated compared to the pre-exam period (all $p < 0.001$). This increase in FSS score (3.2 ± 6.4) was independently associated with the female gender ($\beta = 1.658$, $p < 0.001$), younger age, ($\beta = 0.198$, $p = 0.010$), increase in smoking ($\beta = 1.7$, $p = 0.029$), coffee/energy drinks consumption ($\beta = 1.988$, $p < 0.001$), decreased levels of physical exercise ($\beta = 1.660$, $p < 0.001$), depressive symptoms ($\beta = 2.526$, $p < 0.001$), sleepiness ($\beta = 1867$, $p < 0.001$), and worsening of PSQI ($\beta = 0.754$, $p < 0.001$). The prevalence of fatigue (FSS > 36) was also higher (50% vs. 39%, $p < 0.001$) in this period.

4. Discussion

The results of our study, obtained from students attending different Tertiary Institutions, showed that sleep quality and fatigue are frequent at the beginning of the semester and deteriorate during academic exam periods. Furthermore, this study provides a wide understanding of the factors that influence these observations during the demanding exam period. These factors include younger age, female gender, presence of chronic disease, decreased levels of physical exercise, depressive symptoms, and an increase in smoking and coffee/energy drinks consumption.

University students are recognized as a population group particularly affected by sleep problems and fatigue. In the present study, at the beginning of semester when stress would theoretically be low, about 60% of participants reported poor sleep quality with an average of 7.4 h of sleep per night, also indicating sleep deprivation among students. Increased autonomy, irregularities in the sleep–wake cycle, resulting from academic and social pressure at an age when the circadian rhythm is delayed and the central nervous system is still maturing, along with lifestyle and physical inactivity, increased caffeine and alcohol consumption may explain the poor sleep quality in this population [39–42]. Insomnia symptoms were also frequently reported, with similar [43] or higher rates compared to previous studies [44]. Potential factors that could contribute to poor sleep quality in our study were identified, such as being female, younger age, consuming high amounts of alcohol, not engaging in physical activity, and having a chronic disease, consistent with previous research [16,18,45–48]. Importantly, the presence of depressive symptoms was associated with an approximately threefold increase in the risk of reporting poor sleep. This association poses a significant concern for the mental well-being of students, given that sleep disruptions have been recognized as not only a risk factor for depression but also for other psychiatric disorders [49,50].

Academic responsibilities during university may also lead to fatigue, with concerning prevalence rates reported [51]. In our study, we found a fatigue prevalence of 39% in our university students at the beginning of semester, which is lower compared to a recent study (59.5%) [52] but higher compared to previous studies (16.7% and 13.7%) [53,54]. However, as a considerable proportion of our sample is from demanding disciplines like Medical/Health universities, a substantial prevalence of fatigue is anticipated. The level of fatigue was associated with the presence of chronic disease and depressive and OSA symptoms. At the same time, an inverse relationship was noted between fatigue and physical activity, in line with previous studies [52,55]. Consistent with previous research [52,55], poor sleep quality was also associated with fatigue, which could potentially have a more pronounced effect on university students' academic performance and mental health.

During periods of high stress, such as academic exam periods, university students are particularly affected by lower sleep duration and poor sleep quality [29,30]. In our study, shorter night sleeps during the exam period were reported compared with students' typical routines and PSQI scores were significantly worse, with the prevalence of poor sleep quality increasing from 59 to 98%. Although there are several studies in the literature on the topic of sleep quality in university students, few studies have examined changes in university students' sleep quality and fatigue across multiple time points (before and during an academic exam period) [24,29,30,56]. Based on recent research, university students exhibited negative outcomes, like deteriorating sleep quality [24,29,30], daytime dysfunction [29], and declining academic performance [30] during high-stress periods; however, the number of participants in previous studies was low (31–252 participants) [24, 29,30]. In support of this, students who adhered to a regular sleep–wake routine in the 2 weeks preceding their end-of-semester exams tended to perform better academically [56]. Notably, in our cohort, we also highlighted a significant relationship between worsening of sleep quality and age, chronic disease, and depressive symptoms.

Further, we found that students who reported worsening sleep quality also had a higher risk of fatigue, the prevalence of which was also significantly elevated during the exam period, from 39% to 50%. The female gender, age, depressive symptoms, increase in smoking, coffee/energy drinks consumption, and lower physical activity levels were significant predictors of fatigue during exam periods. However, although the level of fatigue has been found previously to be associated with female gender, caffeine intake, physical activity, and sleep duration [52,57,58], these relationships in university students during exam periods are not documented.

Considering that sleep disruption and fatigue potentially affect university students' academic performance, getting sufficient quality sleep, especially before exams, may be associated with better academic performance, and lower odds of course failures [59]. Importantly, in a recent study, evaluating cognitive performance in medical students with visual and auditory evoked potentials, sleep deprivation during previous 2–3 nights before exam session and psychosomatic fatigue were found to be closely related to cognitive abilities, which in turn adversely affected academic achievements [60]. In support of this, it has been shown that university students who reported sleeping less than seven hours per night had a higher risk of exhaustion and low professional efficacy [30,61]. It is noteworthy that our findings are consistent with prior research indicating a strong correlation between poor sleep, excessive daytime sleepiness, and poor academic achievements [59,62]. Thus, it is crucial for universities to attempt to enhance students' knowledge of how their lifestyle and sleeping behaviors can influence their academic performance. Such guidance along with recommendations for establishing good sleep hygiene would be valuable, particularly for first-year students and may enable students to improve sleep habits, not only in the university years but also in their later professional careers.

Our study has some limitations that deserve comments. First, the cross-sectional design of the current study precludes causal interpretations of the results. However, when examining the longitudinal portion of the research that examines the alterations in sleep quality, fatigue, excessive daytime sleepiness, and depression, it is possible to make some causal inferences about the impact of exam stress on the outcomes considered. Second, as this was a self-administered survey, it was prone to recall bias. Future studies including objective methods such as actigraphy or qualitative methods using semi-structured interviews and sleep diaries could obtain information that may have been overlooked due to the use of self-reported measures in the current study. Third, sleep quality and fatigue evaluation were taken from students studying in different institutions; therefore, factors such as academic demand and level of difficulty may potentially affect our results. Additionally, co-morbid mental health issues that could potentially impair sleep quality, such as anxiety, were not assessed and warrant consideration in future research. It should also be pointed out that this study did not account for participants who experienced a traumatic or highly stressful event between the two time points, such as a family member's death, which could have undermined the validity of our results. Lastly, taking into account that the participants included lived in Crete (south of Greece), sleep quality and fatigue levels may be different in other regions of Greece. Consequently, the generalization of our conclusions to all Greek university students should be made with caution.

5. Conclusions

Our results indicate that sleep quality and fatigue are frequent and deteriorate in university students during academic exam periods. Potential factors associated with the risk of inadequate sleep quality and increased fatigue were identified, such as female gender, younger age, presence of chronic disease, increase in smoking, coffee/energy drinks consumption, decreased levels of physical exercise, and depressive symptoms, which may assist in prevention strategies to promote a better quality of sleep. Future studies are desirable to identify the mechanisms behind sleeping problems and fatigue during exam stress.

Author Contributions: Conceptualization, G.S. and I.B.; methodology, I.B.; software, G.S. and M.F.; validation, A.K., E.B., E.P. and M.M.; formal analysis, I.B.; investigation, G.S. and M.F.; writing—original draft preparation, I.B.; writing—review and editing, I.B., I.T. and S.S.; visualization, I.B.; and supervision, S.S. and I.T. All authors have read and agreed to the published version of the manuscript.

Funding: This research received no external funding.

Institutional Review Board Statement: The study was conducted in accordance with the Declaration of Helsinki and approved by the University of Crete Research Ethics Committee (protocol code 4222/28 May 2018).

Informed Consent Statement: Informed consent was obtained from all subjects involved in the study.

Data Availability Statement: The datasets generated during and/or analyzed during the current study are available from the corresponding author on reasonable request.

Conflicts of Interest: The authors declare no conflict of interest.

References

1. Irwin, M.R. Why sleep is important for health: A psychoneuroimmunology perspective. *Annu. Rev. Psychol.* **2015**, *66*, 143–172. [CrossRef] [PubMed]
2. Hirshkowitz, M.; Whiton, K.; Albert, S.M.; Alessi, C.; Bruni, O.; Don Carlos, L.; Hazen, N.; Herman, J.; Katz, E.S.; Kheirandish-Gozal, L.; et al. National Sleep Foundation's sleep time duration recommendations: Methodology and results summary. *Sleep Health* **2015**, *1*, 40–43. [CrossRef]
3. Consensus Conference Panel; Watson, N.F.; Badr, M.S.; Belenky, G.; Bliwise, D.L.; Buxton, O.M.; Buysse, D.; Dinges, D.F.; Gangwisch, J.; Grandner, M.A.; et al. Recommended amount of sleep for a healthy adult: A joint consensus statement of the American Academy of Sleep Medicine and Sleep Research Society. *J. Clin. Sleep Med.* **2015**, *11*, 591–592. [CrossRef]
4. Yin, J.; Jin, X.; Shan, Z.; Li, S.; Huang, H.; Li, P.; Peng, X.; Peng, Z.; Yu, K.; Bao, W.; et al. Relationship of Sleep Duration With All-Cause Mortality and Cardiovascular Events: A Systematic Review and Dose-Response Meta-Analysis of Prospective Cohort Studies. *J. Am. Heart Assoc.* **2017**, *6*, e005947. [CrossRef]
5. Steptoe, A.; Peacey, V.; Wardle, J. Sleep duration and health in young adults. *Arch. Intern. Med.* **2006**, *166*, 1689–1692. [CrossRef]
6. Becker, S.P.; Jarrett, M.A.; Luebbe, A.M.; Garner, A.A.; Burns, G.L.; Kofler, M.J. Sleep in a large, multi-university sample of college students: Sleep problem prevalence, sex differences, and mental health correlates. *Sleep Health* **2018**, *4*, 174–181. [CrossRef]
7. Schlarb, A.A.; Claßen, M.; Hellmann, S.M.; Vögele, C.; Gulewitsch, M.D. Sleep and somatic complaints in university students. *J. Pain Res.* **2017**, *10*, 1189–1199. [CrossRef]
8. Chandler, L.; Patel, C.; Lovecka, L.; Gardani, M.; Walasek, L.; Ellis, J.; Meyer, C.; Johnson, S.; Tang, N.K.Y. Improving university students' mental health using multi-component and single-component sleep interventions: A systematic review and meta-analysis. *Sleep Med.* **2022**, *100*, 354–363. [CrossRef]
9. Buysse, D.J. Sleep health: Can we define it? Does it matter? *Sleep* **2014**, *37*, 9–17. [CrossRef]
10. Garbarino, S.; Lanteri, P.; Durando, P.; Magnavita, N.; Sannita, W.G. Co-Morbidity, Mortality, Quality of Life and the Healthcare/Welfare/Social Costs of Disordered Sleep: A Rapid Review. *Int. J. Environ. Res. Public. Health* **2016**, *13*, 831. [CrossRef]
11. Shochat, T.; Cohen-Zion, M.; Tzischinsky, O. Functional consequences of inadequate sleep in adolescents: A systematic review. *Sleep Med. Rev.* **2014**, *18*, 75–87. [CrossRef]
12. Ridner, S.L.; Newton, K.S.; Staten, R.R.; Crawford, T.N.; Hall, L.A. Predictors of well-being among college students. *J. Am. Coll. Health* **2016**, *64*, 116–124. [CrossRef]
13. Li, W.; Chen, J.; Li, M.; Smith, A.P.; Fan, J. The effect of exercise on academic fatigue and sleep quality among university students. *Front. Psychol.* **2022**, *13*, 1025280. [CrossRef]
14. Jahrami, H.; Dewald-Kaufmann, J.; Faris, M.A.-I.; AlAnsari, A.M.S.; Taha, M.; AlAnsari, N. Prevalence of sleep problems among medical students: A systematic review and meta-analysis. *J. Public Health* **2020**, *28*, 605–622. [CrossRef]
15. Schlarb, A.A.; Claßen, M.; Grünwald, J.; Vögele, C. Sleep disturbances and mental strain in university students: Results from an online survey in Luxembourg and Germany. *Int. J. Ment. Health Syst.* **2017**, *11*, 24. [CrossRef]
16. Alghwiri, A.A.; Almomani, F.; Alghwiri, A.A.; Whitney, S.L. Predictors of sleep quality among university students: The use of advanced machine learning techniques. *Sleep Breath.* **2021**, *25*, 1119–1126. [CrossRef]
17. Lund, H.G.; Reider, B.D.; Whiting, A.B.; Prichard, J.R. Sleep patterns and predictors of disturbed sleep in a large population of college students. *J. Adolesc. Health* **2010**, *46*, 124–132. [CrossRef]
18. Li, Y.; Bai, W.; Zhu, B.; Duan, R.; Yu, X.; Xu, W.; Wang, M.; Hua, W.; Yu, W.; Li, W.; et al. Prevalence and correlates of poor sleep quality among college students: A cross-sectional survey. *Health Qual. Life Outcomes* **2020**, *18*, 210. [CrossRef] [PubMed]
19. Wang, L.; Qin, P.; Zhao, Y.; Duan, S.; Zhang, Q.; Liu, Y.; Hu, Y.; Sun, J. Prevalence and risk factors of poor sleep quality among Inner Mongolia Medical University students: A cross-sectional survey. *Psychiatry Res.* **2016**, *244*, 243–248. [CrossRef]
20. Lemma, S.; Gelaye, B.; Berhane, Y.; Worku, A.; Williams, M.A. Sleep quality and its psychological correlates among university students in Ethiopia: A cross-sectional study. *BMC Psychiatry* **2012**, *12*, 237. [CrossRef] [PubMed]
21. Zhang, L.; Zheng, H.; Yi, M.; Zhang, Y.; Cai, G.; Li, C.; Zhao, L. Prediction of sleep quality among university students after analyzing lifestyles, sports habits, and mental health. *Front. Psychiatry* **2022**, *13*, 927619. [CrossRef]
22. Orzech, K.M.; Salafsky, D.B.; Hamilton, L.A. The state of sleep among college students at a large public university. *J. Am. Coll. Health* **2011**, *59*, 612–619. [CrossRef] [PubMed]
23. Cheng, S.H.; Shih, C.C.; Lee, I.H.; Hou, Y.W.; Chen, K.C.; Chen, K.T.; Yang, Y.K.; Yang, Y.C. A study on the sleep quality of incoming university students. *Psychiatry Res.* **2012**, *197*, 270–274. [CrossRef] [PubMed]
24. Mnatzaganian, C.L.; Atayee, R.S.; Namba, J.M.; Brandl, K.; Lee, K.C. The effect of sleep quality, sleep components, and environmental sleep factors on core curriculum exam scores among pharmacy students. *Curr. Pharm. Teach. Learn.* **2020**, *12*, 119–126. [CrossRef] [PubMed]
25. Romero, A., Jr. *U.S. vs. Europe in Higher Education*; The Edwardsville Intelligencer: Edwardsville, IL, USA, 2018; p. A3.
26. Pataka, A.; Sourla, E.; Anagnostopoulos, A.; Vareta, G.; Aggeli, N.; Koutoukoglou, P.; Biolakis, E.; Xida, S.; Vaitsi, E.; Paspala, A.; et al. Sleep habits among Greek university students. *ERJ* **2014**, *44* (Suppl. S58), P2385.
27. Eleftheriou, A.; Rokou, A.; Arvaniti, A.; Nena, E.; Steiropoulos, P. Sleep Quality and Mental Health of Medical Students in Greece During the COVID-19 Pandemic. *Front. Public Health* **2021**, *9*, 775374. [CrossRef]
28. Kaparounaki, C.K.; Patsali, M.E.; Mousa, D.V.; Papadopoulou, E.V.K.; Papadopoulou, K.K.K.; Fountoulakis, K.N. University students' mental health amidst the COVID-19 quarantine in Greece. *Psychiatry Res.* **2020**, *290*, 113111. [CrossRef]

29. Campbell, R.; Soenens, B.; Beyers, W.; Vansteenkiste, M. University students' sleep during an exam period: The role of basic psychological needs and stress. *Motiv. Emot.* **2018**, *42*, 671–681. [CrossRef]
30. Estevan, I.; Sardi, R.; Tejera, A.C.; Silva, A.; Tassino, B. Should I study or should I go (to sleep)? The influence of test schedule on the sleep behavior of undergraduates and its association with performance. *PLoS ONE* **2021**, *16*, e0247104. [CrossRef]
31. Mystakidou, K.; Parpa, E.; Tsilika, E.; Pathiaki, M.; Patiraki, E.; Galanos, A.; Vlahos, L. Sleep quality in advanced cancer patients. *J. Psychosom. Res.* **2007**, *62*, 527–533. [CrossRef]
32. Kotronoulas, G.C.; Papadopoulou, C.N.; Papapetrou, A.; Patiraki, E. Psychometric evaluation and feasibility of the Greek Pittsburgh Sleep Quality Index (GR-PSQI) in patients with cancer receiving chemotherapy. *Support. Care Cancer* **2011**, *9*, 1831–1840. [CrossRef] [PubMed]
33. Backhaus, J.; Junghanns, K.; Broocks, A.; Riemann, D.; Hohagen, F. Test-retest reliability and validity of the Pittsburgh Sleep Quality Index in primary insomnia. *J. Psychosom. Res.* **2002**, *53*, 737–740. [CrossRef] [PubMed]
34. Beck, S.L.; Schwartz, A.L.; Towsley, G.; Dudley, W.; Barsevick, A. Psychometric evalua-tion of the Pittsburgh sleep quality index in cancer patients. *J. Pain Symptom Manag.* **2004**, *27*, 140–148. [CrossRef] [PubMed]
35. Carpenter, J.S.; Andrykowski, M.A. Psychometric evaluation of the Pittsburgh Sleep Quality Index. *J. Psychosom. Res.* **1998**, *45*, 5–13. [CrossRef] [PubMed]
36. Ferentinos, P.; Kontaxakis, V.; Havaki-Kontaxaki, B.; Dikeos, D.; Lykouras, L. Psychometric evaluation of the Fatigue Severity Scale in patients with major depression. *Qual. Life Res.* **2011**, *20*, 457–465. [CrossRef]
37. Bakalidou, D.; Skordilis, E.K.; Giannopoulos, S.; Stamboulis, E.; Voumvourakis, K. Validity and reliability of the FSS in Greek MS patients. *SpringerPlus* **2013**, *2*, 304. [CrossRef]
38. Hjollund, N.H.; Andersen, J.H.; Bech, P. Assessment of fatigue in chronic disease: A bibliographic study of fatigue measurement scales. *Health Qual. Life Outcomes* **2007**, *5*, 12. [CrossRef]
39. Silva, R.M.D.; Costa, A.L.S.; Mussi, F.C.; Lopes, V.C.; Batista, K.M.; Santos, O.P.D. Health alterations in nursing students after a year from admission to the undergraduate course. *Rev. Esc. Enferm. USP* **2019**, *53*, e03450. [CrossRef]
40. Silva, V.M.; Magalhaes, J.E.M.; Duarte, L.L. Quality of sleep and anxiety are related to circadian preference in university students. *PLoS ONE* **2020**, *15*, e0238514. [CrossRef]
41. Ghrouz, A.K.; Noohu, M.M.; Dilshad Manzar, M.; Warren Spence, D.; BaHammam, A.S.; Pandi-Perumal, S.R. Physical activity and sleep quality in relation to mental health among college students. *Sleep Breath.* **2019**, *23*, 627–634. [CrossRef]
42. Kenney, S.R.; Paves, A.P.; Grimaldi, E.M.; La Brie, J.W. Sleep quality and alcohol risk in college students: Examining the moderating effects of drinking motives. *J. Am. Coll. Health* **2014**, *62*, 301–308. [CrossRef] [PubMed]
43. Sivertsen, B.; Vedaa, O.; Harvey, A.G.; Glozier, N.; Pallesen, S.; Aaro, L.E.; Lønning, K.J.; Hysing, M. Sleep patterns and insomnia in young adults: A national survey of Norwegian university students. *J. Sleep Res.* **2019**, *28*, e12790. [CrossRef] [PubMed]
44. Baglioni, C.; Battagliese, G.; Feige, B.; Spiegelhalder, K.; Nissen, C.; Voderholzer, U.; Lombardo, C.; Riemann, D. Insomnia as a predictor of depression: A meta-analytic evaluation of longitudinal epidemiological studies. *J. Affect. Disord.* **2011**, *135*, 10–19. [CrossRef] [PubMed]
45. Gui, Z.; Sun, L.; Zhou, C. Self-reported sleep quality and mental health mediate the relationship between chronic diseases and suicidal ideation among Chinese medical students. *Sci. Rep.* **2022**, *12*, 18835. [CrossRef] [PubMed]
46. Shaheen, A.M.; Alkaid Albqoor, M. Prevalence and Correlates of Sleep Quality Among Jordanian University Students: A Cross-Sectional National Study. *Eval. Health Prof.* **2022**, *45*, 176–182. [CrossRef] [PubMed]
47. Santos, M.; Sirtoli, R.; Rodrigues, R.; López-Gil, J.F.; Martínez-Vizcaíno, V.; Guidoni, C.M.; Mesas, A.E. Relationship between free-time physical activity and sleep quality in Brazilian university students. *Sci. Rep.* **2023**, *13*, 6652. [CrossRef]
48. Sanchez, S.E.; Martinez, C.; Oriol, R.A.; Yanez, D.; Castañeda, B.; Sanchez, E.; Gelaye, B.; Williams, M.A. Sleep Quality, Sleep Patterns and Consumption of Energy Drinks and Other Caffeinated Beverages among Peruvian College Students. *Health* **2013**, *5*, 26–35. [CrossRef]
49. Hertenstein, E.; Feige, B.; Gmeiner, T.; Kienzler, C.; Spiegelhalder, K.; Johann, A.; Jansson-Fröjmark, M.; Palagini, L.; Rücker, G.; Riemann, D.; et al. Insomnia as a predictor of mental disorders: A systematic review and meta-analysis. *Sleep Med. Rev.* **2019**, *43*, 96–105. [CrossRef]
50. Shim, E.J.; Noh, H.L.; Yoon, J.; Mun, H.S.; Hahm, B.J. A longitudinal analysis of the relationships among daytime dysfunction, fatigue, and depression in college students. *J. Am. Coll. Health* **2019**, *67*, 51–58. [CrossRef]
51. Güneş, M.; Demirer, B. A Comparison of Caffeine Intake and Physical Activity According to Fatigue Severity in University Students. *Eval. Health Prof.* **2023**, *46*, 92–99. [CrossRef]
52. Tanaka, M.; Mizuno, K.; Fukuda, S.; Shigihara, Y.; Watanabe, Y. Relationships between dietary habits and the prevalence of fatigue in medical students. *Nutrition* **2008**, *24*, 985–989. [CrossRef] [PubMed]
53. Yoshikawa, T.; Tanaka, M.; Ishii, A.; Watanabe, Y. Association of fatigue with emotional-eating behavior and the response to mental stress in food intake in a young adult population. *Behav. Med.* **2014**, *40*, 149–153. [CrossRef] [PubMed]
54. Strahler, J.; Doerr, J.M.; Ditzen, B.; Linnemann, A.; Skoluda, N.; Nater, U.M. Physical activity buffers fatigue only under low chronic stress. *Stress* **2016**, *19*, 535–541. [CrossRef] [PubMed]
55. Frederick, G.M.; O'Connor, P.J.; Schmidt, M.D.; Evans, E.M. Relationships between components of the 24-hour activity cycle and feelings of energy and fatigue in college students: A systematic review. *Ment. Health Phys. Act.* **2021**, *21*, 100409. [CrossRef]

56. Genzel, L.; Ahrberg, K.; Roselli, C.; Niedermaier, S.; Steiger, A.; Dresler, M.; Roenne-berg, T. Sleep timing is more important than sleep length or quality for medical school performance. *Chronobiol. Int.* **2013**, *30*, 766–771. [CrossRef]
57. Torquati, L.; Peeters, G.; Brown, W.J.; Skinner, T.L. A daily cup of tea or coffee may keep you moving: Association between tea and coffee consumption and physical activity. *Int. J. Environ. Res. Public Health* **2018**, *15*, 1812. [CrossRef]
58. Thabit, A.K.; Alsulami, A.A. Impact of Sleep Pattern of Pharmacy College Students on Academic Performance. *Sleep Vigil.* **2023**, *7*, 43–47. [CrossRef]
59. Janocha, A.; Molęda, A.; Sebzda, T. The influence of sleep deprivation on the cognitive processes in medical students during exam session. *Med. Pr.* **2023**, *74*, 27–40. [CrossRef]
60. Wolf, M.R.; Rosenstock, J.B. Inadequate sleep and exercise associated with burnout and depression among medical students *Acad. Psychiatry* **2017**, *41*, 174–179. [CrossRef]
61. Al Shammari, M.A.; Al Amer, N.A.; Al Mulhim, S.N.; Al Mohammedsaleh, H.N.; AlOmar, R.S. The quality of sleep and daytime sleepiness and their association with academic achievement of medical students in the eastern province of Saudi Arabia. *J. Fam. Community Med.* **2020**, *27*, 97–102. [CrossRef]
62. Rea, E.M.; Nicholson, L.M.; Mead, M.P.; Egbert, A.H.; Bohnert, A.M. Daily relations between nap occurrence, duration, and timing and nocturnal sleep patterns in college students. *Sleep Health* **2022**, *8*, 356–363. [CrossRef] [PubMed]

Disclaimer/Publisher's Note: The statements, opinions and data contained in all publications are solely those of the individual author(s) and contributor(s) and not of MDPI and/or the editor(s). MDPI and/or the editor(s) disclaim responsibility for any injury to people or property resulting from any ideas, methods, instructions or products referred to in the content.

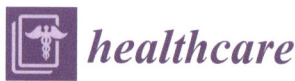 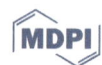

Article

Smoking-Induced Disturbed Sleep. A Distinct Sleep-Related Disorder Pattern?

Ioanna Grigoriou [1], Paschalia Skalisti [1], Ioanna Papagiouvanni [2], Anastasia Michailidou [3], Konstantinos Charalampidis [2], Serafeim-Chrysovalantis Kotoulas [4], Konstantinos Porpodis [5], Dionysios Spyratos [5] and Athanasia Pataka [1,*]

1. Respiratory Failure Clinic, Papanikolaou General Hospital, Aristotle University of Thessaloniki, 57010 Thessaloniki, Greece
2. Fourth Department of Internal Medicine, Hippokration General Hospital, Aristotle University of Thessaloniki, 54642 Thessaloniki, Greece
3. Second Propaedeutic Department of Internal Medicine, Hippokration General Hospital, Aristotle University of Thessaloniki, 54642 Thessaloniki, Greece
4. ICU, Hippokration General Hospital, Aristotle University of Thessaloniki, 54642 Thessaloniki, Greece
5. Pulmonology Department, Papanikolaou General Hospital, Aristotle University of Thessaloniki, 57010 Thessaloniki, Greece
* Correspondence: patakath@yahoo.gr

Abstract: The relationship between smoking and sleep disorders has not been investigated sufficiently yet. Many aspects, especially regarding non-obstructive sleep apnea–hypopnea (OSA)-related disorders, are still to be addressed. All adult patients who visited a tertiary sleep clinic and provided information about their smoking history were included in this cross-sectional study. In total, 4347 patients were divided into current, former and never smokers, while current and former smokers were also grouped, forming a group of ever smokers. Sleep-related characteristics, derived from questionnaires and sleep studies, were compared between those groups. Ever smokers presented with significantly greater body mass index (BMI), neck and waist circumference and with increased frequency of metabolic and cardiovascular co-morbidities compared to never smokers. They also presented significantly higher apnea–hypopnea index (AHI) compared to never smokers (34.4 ± 24.6 events/h vs. 31.7 ± 23.6 events/h, $p < 0.001$) and were diagnosed more frequently with severe and moderate OSA (50.3% vs. 46.9% and 26.2% vs. 24.8% respectively). Epworth sleepiness scale (ESS) ($p = 0.13$) did not differ between groups. Ever smokers, compared to never smokers, presented more frequent episodes of sleep talking (30.8% vs. 26.6%, $p = 0.004$), abnormal movements (31.1% vs. 27.7%, $p = 0.021$), restless sleep (59.1% vs. 51.6%, $p < 0.001$) and leg movements ($p = 0.002$) during sleep. Those were more evident in current smokers and correlated significantly with increasing AHI. These significant findings suggest the existence of a smoking-induced disturbed sleep pattern.

Keywords: obstructive sleep apnea; smoking; smoking-induced disturbed sleep pattern; obstructive sleep apnea–hypopnea

1. Introduction

Smoking is now considered a chronic relapsing disease, which is rather difficult to treat. According to the World Health Organization (WHO), smoking is a major cause of early death worldwide, responsible not only for health problems, but also for increasing the costs to healthcare systems [1]. Smoking-related diseases, such as ischemic heart disease, ischemic cerebral disease and lower respiratory tract diseases are responsible for a great proportion of deaths worldwide (12.9%, 11.4% and 5.9%, respectively) [2]. The relative risk attributed to smoking is estimated to be 26.7% for ischemic heart disease, 32.2% for ischemic cerebral disease and 72.2% for chronic obstructive pulmonary disease (COPD) [3].

Obstructive sleep apneas–hypopneas (OSA) affect 17% and 9% of middle-aged males and females, respectively [4], while obstructive sleep apnea–hypopnea syndrome (OSAHS), which is characterized by symptoms, such as excessive daytime sleepiness, affects 3–7% of the population worldwide [5]. OSAHS symptoms include excessive daytime sleepiness, snoring, non-refreshing sleep, gasping–choking episodes and awakenings during sleep. OSA can emerge in every sleep stage; however, the respiratory events are more often during rapid eye movement (REM) sleep, due to the decreased muscle tone. Dynamic narrowing of the upper airways during sleep causes repeated apneic episodes, leading to sleep fragmentation and excessive daytime sleepiness [6]. Additionally, repeated sleep apneas result in hypoxemia, hypercarbia, hypertension and increased sympathetic tone, increasing the risk of endothelial dysfunction [7]. Significant intrathoracic pressure swings and increased blood pressure during sleep are considered to augment the risk for cardiovascular events in patients with OSA [8]. Therefore, OSA, along with smoking, both constitute significant risk factors for cardiovascular disease.

Many studies have tried to prove the relationship between OSAHS and smoking, showing a higher prevalence of smoking in OSAHS patients [9,10]. Additionally, there is evidence that smoking might be a risk factor for apneas and snoring [11–13]. Smokers present decreased sleep quality with greater sleep latency and increased difficulty in maintaining sleep [14–16]. Smoking worsens chronic airway inflammation, contributing to OSAHS symptoms [17]. Active and passive smoking, as well as a history of smoking, have been correlated with snoring [12]. Nevertheless, evidence is still conflicting, failing to prove a definite and clinically significant correlation between smoking and OSAHS. Despite that, possible mechanisms by which smoking affects OSAHS include changes in sleep architecture, neuromuscular dysfunction of the upper airway, frequent awakenings and enhancement in upper-airway inflammation [13]. Additionally, non-treated OSAHS has been correlated with increased smoking addiction [18,19]. Yet, there is a need for more large-scale studies, in order to clarify the relationship of these two disorders.

Apart from OSAHS, there are also sleep disorders that are not directly related to apneic episodes during sleep. Sleep behaviors, such as sleep talking, sleepwalking, sleep paralysis, night terrors, nightmares, restless sleep, bruxism, sleep-related eating disorder, restless legs and abnormal movements during sleep, are a nuisance for a significant part of the general population; however, there is little understanding about the pathogenesis of these disorders. Smoking has been proposed to be one of the etiologic factors for these disorders, particularly in the form of second-hand smoke exposure during pregnancy or early childhood [20,21]. In addition to that, smoking has been associated with possible REM behavior disorder (RBD) [22,23], sleep-related eating disorder [24] and sleep paralysis [25]. However, other studies failed to prove a relationship between smoking and parasomnias in general [26].

The aim of this study was to assess possible relations between smoking history and OSAHS-related symptoms, sleep study findings and co-morbidities. Additionally, this study aimed to evaluate other non-OSAHS-related sleep disorders, in patients visiting a sleep clinic, in order to investigate a holistic relationship between smoking and sleep disturbances.

2. Materials and Methods

The protocol of this cross-sectional study was approved by the local ethics committee (reference number: 965/290618) and all participants gave their written informed consent. All adult patients who visited the sleep clinic in our hospital from September 2010 to September 2020 and consented to participate were considered eligible and were included in the analysis. The patients were divided by their smoking history as current smokers (adults who have smoked 100 cigarettes in their lifetime and who currently smoke cigarettes), former smokers (adults who have smoked at least 100 cigarettes in their lifetime but who had quit smoking at the time of interview) and never smokers (adults who have never smoked or who have smoked less than 100 cigarettes in their lifetime), according to the definitions of the National Health Interview Survey (NHIS) of the US Centers for Disease Control and Prevention (CDC) [27]. Current smokers and former smokers were also grouped together, creating the group of ever smokers. Eventually, 4347 participants (1498 never smokers, 1480 former smokers and 1369 current smokers) were included in the analysis.

The baseline characteristics of the participants were recorded and included their age, gender, family status, body mass index (BMI), neck, waist and hip circumference, Malampati score, SaO_2, heart rate and arterial blood pressure. The participants answered a questionnaire about their smoking status, i.e., their smoking history, the number of cigarettes smoked per day and the number of packyears. The medical history of the participants was also recorded (alcohol consumption, cardiovascular, respiratory, metabolic and psychiatric co-morbidities). In addition, questionnaires about night-time sleep and nap duration, sleep latency, questions regarding possible sleep disturbances (the existence of nightmares, sleep talking, abnormal movements, restless sleep or leg movements) and about OSA-related symptoms (dry mouth, morning fatigue, bad mood, headaches, heavy head, memory loss, dropping thing from hands, needing a passenger when driving to be kept awake, snoring frequency and loudness, choking–breathing pauses during sleep and night awakenings) were completed. Epworth sleepiness scale (ESS) [28], Berlin and STOP bang questionnaires [29,30], Athens insomnia scale (AIS) [31] and Rosenberg self-esteem scale [32] were also included

All patients that participated in the study were subjected to sleep studies: 186 underwent full polysomnography (PSG) (type 1 sleep study, including: electroencephalogram (EEG), electrooculogram (EOG), electromyogram (EMG), electrocardiogram (ECG), airflow, respiratory effort and oxygen saturation measurements) and the rest polygraphy (type 3 sleep study, including: respiratory movement, airflow, pulse rate and oxygen saturation measurements) [33]. The sleep studies were manually scored according to the American Academy of Sleep Medicine (AASM) criteria [34], by sleep technicians with more than 3 years of experience. Apnea hypopnea index (AHI) was used to evaluate OSA severity (no OSA: AHI < 5, mild OSA: AHI 5–15, moderate OSA: AHI 15–30, severe OSA: AHI > 30) [35,36].

Statistical analysis was performed using SPSS (version 20 IBM SPSS statistical software, Armonk, NY, USA). Continuous variables were presented as mean ± SD and categorical variables as number/total (%). $p < 0.05$ was accepted as statistically significant. To separate parametric from non-parametric variables, normality tests using the Kolmogorov–Smirnov test were performed. To detect significant differences between current, former and never smokers, a one-way ANOVA or a Kruskal–Wallis test was performed for parametric and non-parametric variables, respectively, followed by a post hoc analysis between pairs of groups, using the Bonferroni test or the Mann–Whitney U test for parametric and non-parametric variables, respectively. An independent samples *T* test or Mann–Whitney U test was performed for parametric and non-parametric variables, respectively, in order to detect significant differences between ever and never smokers. To detect significant differences for categorical variables, between current, former and never smokers or between ever and never smokers, a Chi-Square Test, using the Fisher's exact test where appropriate, was performed. A post hoc analysis, using the same tests, was performed between the pairs of groups of current, former and never smokers. Finally, to compare AHI among possible answers regarding abnormal sleep behaviors between ever and never smokers, the same parametric or non-parametric tests for continuous variables were used, where appropriate, in the same way as previously described.

3. Results

Comparison between former and current smokers showed that former smokers had a history of consumption of a significantly greater number of cigarettes per day and pack/years and that former smokers had quit 4.36 ± 7.84 years before study enrollment. Although former smokers were significantly older than never smokers, no significant age differences were established between ever and never smokers (53.3 ± 12.7 years vs. 53.7 ± 14.9 years, *p* = 0.26). The group of ever smokers included significantly more males compared to never smokers (78.1% vs. 58.6%, *p* < 0.001) with significantly higher BMI and larger neck and waist, but not hip, circumference (Table 1). Ever smokers were consuming more alcohol (*p* < 0.001) and suffered more frequently from diabetes mellitus (16.9% vs. 14.0%, *p* = 0.012), coronary heart disease (13.2% vs. 6.2%, *p* < 0.001), acute myocardial infarction (3.6% vs. 1.1%, *p* < 0.001), hyperlipidemia (18.0% vs. 15.0%, *p* = 0.014) and pulmonary disease (10.0% vs. 5.3%, *p* < 0.001), while the opposite was true for hypothyroidism (10.0% vs. 16.5%, *p* < 0.001) (Table 2).

Table 1. Baseline characteristics.

Characteristic		Smoking Status				Ever Smoker		
		Never Smoker	Former Smoker	Current Smoker	*p* (Value)	No	Yes	*p* (Value)
Age (years)		53.7 ± 14.9 (N = 1493)	57.5 ± 12.0 (N = 1478)	48.7 ± 11.7 (N = 1364)	<0.001	53.7 ± 14.9 (N = 1493)	53.3 ± 12.7 (N = 2842)	0.26
Gender	Female	619/1495 (41.4%)	322/1368 (23.5%)	301/1480 (20.3%)	<0.001	619/1495 (41.4%)	623/2848 (21.9%)	<0.001
	Male	876/1495 (58.6%)	1046/1368 (76.5%)	1179/1480 (79.7%)		876/1495 (58.6%)	2225/2848 (78.1%)	
Family status	Single	213/1213 (17.6%)	115/1199 (9.6%)	226/1157 (19.5%)	<0.001	213/1213 (17.6%)	341/2356 (14.5%)	0.013
	Married	969/1213 (79.9%)	1047/1199 (87.3%)	874/1157 (75.5%)		969/1213 (79.9%)	1921/2356 (81.5%)	
	Divorced	31/1213 (2.6%)	37/1199 (3.1%)	54/1157 (4.7%)		31/1213 (2.6%)	91/2356 (3.9%)	
Cigarettes per day		n/a	30.2 ± 19.9 (N = 1011)	21.5 ± 13.4 (N = 1345)	<0.001	n/a	25.3 ± 17.1 (N = 2356)	n/a
Packyears		n/a	42.6 ± 38.0 (N = 1011)	32.4 ± 25.0 (N = 1345)	<0.001	n/a	36.8 ± 31.6 (N = 2356)	n/a
BMI (kg/m^2)		32.9 ± 7.3 (N = 1451)	33.8 ± 6.9 (N = 1445)	33.1 ± 7.2 (N = 1350)	0.002	32.9 ± 7.3 (N = 1451)	33.5 ± 7.1 (N = 2795)	0.024
Neck circumference (cm)		41.1 ± 7.1 (N = 959)	42.6 ± 6.3 (N = 956)	41.9 ± 6.8 (N = 921)	<0.001	41.1 ± 7.1 (N = 959)	42.2 ± 6.5 (N = 1877)	<0.001
Waist circumference (cm)		110.7 ± 18.0 (N = 820)	112.4 ± 18.3 (N = 828)	114.9 ± 16.2 (N = 793)	<0.001	110.7 ± 18.0 (N = 820)	113.7 ± 17.3 (N = 1621)	<0.001
Hip circumference (cm)		112.3 ± 15.4 (N = 776)	113.5 ± 13.8 (N = 784)	112.1 ± 15.9 (N = 751)	0.16	112.3 ± 15.4 (N = 776)	112.8 ± 14.9 (N = 1535)	0.49
Malampati score		2.7 ± 0.7 (N = 95)	2.8 ± 0.6 (N = 92)	2.8 ± 0.6 (N = 104)	0.64	2.7 ± 0.7 (N = 95)	2.8 ± 0.6 (N = 196)	0.39
SaO$_2$ (%)		96.4 ± 2.2 (N = 981)	95.9 ± 2.9 (N = 999)	96.3 ± 1.8 (N = 937)	<0.001	96.4 ± 2.2 (N = 981)	96.1 ± 2.5 (N = 1936)	<0.001
Heart rate (beats/minute)		80.0 ± 13.5 (N = 980)	78.8 ± 13.0 (N = 996)	82.3 ± 13.0 (N = 933)	<0.001	80.0 ± 13.5 (N = 980)	80.5 ± 13.1 (N = 1929)	0.38
Systolic blood pressure (mmHg)		125.5 ± 17.1 (N = 273)	127.9 ± 15.5 (N = 312)	125.5 ± 16.8 (N = 262)	0.12	125.5 ± 17.1 (N = 273)	126.8 ± 16.2 (N = 574)	0.29
Diastolic blood pressure (mmHg)		76.3 ± 9.7 (N = 272)	77.5 ± 10.0 (N = 309)	77.2 ± 10.3 (N = 261)	0.34	76.3 ± 9.7 (N = 272)	77.4 ± 10.2 (N = 570)	0.16

N = number, n/a = not applicable, m = meters, Kg = kilograms, cm = centimeters, mmHg = millimeters of Mercury.

Table 2. Co-morbidities.

Co-Morbidity		Smoking Status				Ever Smoker		
		Never Smoker	Former Smoker	Current Smoker	p (Value)	No	Yes	p (Value)
Alcohol	Almost never	685/1469 (46.6%)	442/1452 (30.4%)	386/1343 (28.7%)	<0.001	685/1469 (46.6%)	828/2795 (29.6%)	<0.001
	A few times per month	685/1469 (46.6%)	829/1452 (57.1%)	729/1343 (54.3%)		685/1469 (46.6%)	1558/2795 (55.7%)	
	1–2 times per week	57/1469 (3.9%)	83/1452 (5.7%)	109/1343 (8.1%)		57/1469 (3.9%)	192/2795 (6.9%)	
	3–5 times per week	23/1469 (1.6%)	53/1452 (3.7%)	67/1343 (5.0%)		23/1469 (1.6%)	120/2795 (4.3%)	
	Every day	19/1469 (1.3%)	45/1452 (3.1%)	52/1343 (3.9%)		19/1469 (1.3%)	97/2795 (3.5%)	
Hypertension		630/1498 (42.1%)	683/1480 (46.1%)	450/1369 (32.9%)	<0.001	630/1498 (42.1%)	1133/2849 (39.8%)	0.14
Diabetes Mellitus		209/1498 (14.0%)	311/1480 (21.0%)	170/1369 (12.4%)	<0.001	209/1498 (14.0%)	481/2849 (16.9%)	0.012
Coronary disease		93/1498 (6.2%)	266/1480 (18.0%)	109/1369 (8.0%)	<0.001	93/1498 (6.2%)	375/2849 (13.2%)	<0.001
Acute myocardial infarction		17/1498 (1.1%)	68/1480 (4.6%)	33/1369 (2.4%)	<0.001	17/1498 (1.1%)	101/2849 (3.6%)	<0.001
Heart failure		12/1498 (0.8%)	19/1480 (1.3%)	5/1369 (0.4%)	0.026	12/1498 (0.8%)	24/2849 (0.8%)	0.89
Arrythmia		195/1498 (13.0%)	256/1480 (17.3%)	122/1369 (8.9%)	<0.001	195/1498 (13.0%)	378/2849 (13.3%)	0.82
Hyperlipidemia		225/1498 (15.0%)	309/1480 (20.9%)	203/1369 (14.8%)	<0.001	225/1498 (15.0%)	512/2849 (18.0%)	0.014
Ischemic stroke		41/1498 (2.7%)	47/1480 (3.2%)	39/1369 (2.9%)	0.76	41/1498 (2.7%)	86/2849 (3.0%)	0.60
Pulmonary disease		79/1498 (5.3%)	193/1480 (13.0%)	93/1369 (6.8%)	<0.001	79/1498 (5.3%)	286/2849 (10.0%)	<0.001
Hypothyroidism		247/1498 (16.5%)	168/1480 (11.4%)	117/1369 (8.6%)	<0.001	247/1498 (16.5%)	285/2849 (10.0%)	<0.001
Depression		27/1498 (1.8%)	31/1480 (2.1%)	45/1369 (3.3%)	0.023	27/1498 (1.8%)	76/2849 (2.7%)	0.08

From the data from sleep questionnaires, never smokers presented significantly higher night-sleep duration compared to ever smokers (3.18 ± 0.78 h vs. 3.13 ± 0.77 h, $p = 0.044$), who, on the other hand, presented longer nap duration (2.95 ± 0.58 h vs. 2.86 ± 0.61 h, $p < 0.001$). Never smokers had higher self-esteem, with a significantly higher score in the Rosenberg self-esteem scale (22.2 ± 4.8 vs. 21.8 ± 4.8, $p = 0.035$). Berlin and STOP Bang questionnaires predicted higher risk for OSAHS in ever smokers compared to never smokers (87.1% vs. 84.6%, $p = 0.024$ and 96.2% vs. 93.0%, $p < 0.001$, respectively). However, there were no significant differences between the two groups regarding ESS and AIS ($p = 0.13$, $p = 0.83$, respectively). Yet, ever smokers, compared to never smokers, presented significantly more frequent episodes of sleep talking (30.8% vs. 26.6%, $p = 0.004$), abnormal movements (31.1% vs. 27.7%, $p = 0.021$), restless sleep (59.1% vs. 51.6%, $p < 0.001$) and leg movements ($p = 0.002$), especially the group of current smokers (Table 3) ($p < 0.001$ for all comparisons between never and current smokers in the post hoc analysis).

Table 3. Sleep symptoms and sleep questionnaires according to the smoking status of the participants.

Characteristic		Smoking Status			p (Value)	Ever Smoker		p (Value)
		Never Smoker	Former Smoker	Current Smoker		No	Yes	
Epworth sleepiness scale		9.6 ± 4.7 (N = 1473)	9.9 ± 4.5 (N = 1459)	9.7 ± 4.7 (N = 1352)	0.23	9.6 ± 4.7 (N = 1473)	9.8 ± 4.6 (N = 2811)	0.13
Athens insomnia scale		17.1 ± 5.5 (N = 1241)	17.0 ± 5.6 (N = 1250)	17.2 ± 5.2 (N = 1181)	0.66	17.1 ± 5.5 (N = 1241)	17.1 ± 5.4 (N = 2431)	0.83
Rosenberg self-esteem scale		22.2 ± 4.8 (N = 758)	22.1 ± 4.8 (N = 788)	21.5 ± 4.8 (N = 806)	0.003	22.2 ± 4.8 (N = 758)	21.8 ± 4.8 (N = 1594)	0.035
Berlin questionnaire	Low risk	226/1469 (15.4%)	181/1452 (12.5%)	179/1344 (13.3%)	0.06	226/1469 (15.4%)	360/2796 (12.9%)	0.024
	High risk	1243/1469 (84.6%)	1271/1452 (87.5%)	1165/1344 (86.7%)		1243/1469 (84.6%)	2436/2796 (87.1%)	
Stop bang questionnaire	Low risk	66/939 (7.0%)	43/900 (4.8%)	27/938 (2.9%)	<0.001	66/939 (7.0%)	70/1838 (3.8%)	<0.001
	High risk	873/939 (93.0%)	857/900 (95.2%)	911/938 (97.1%)		873/939 (93.0%)	1768/1838 (96.2%)	
Nightmares		430/1498 (28.7%)	412/1480 (27.8%)	378/1369 (27.6%)	0.79	430/1498 (28.7%)	790/2849 (27.7%)	0.50
Sleep talking		398/1498 (26.6%)	421/1480 (28.5%)	456/1369 (33.3%)	<0.001	398/1498 (26.6%)	877/2849 (30.8%)	0.004
Abnormal movements during sleep		415/1498 (27.7%)	433/1480 (29.3%)	452/1369 (33.0%)	0.006	415/1498 (27.7%)	885/2849 (31.1%)	0.021
Restless sleep		773/1498 (51.6%)	872/1480 (58.9%)	811/1369 (59.2%)	<0.001	773/1498 (51.6%)	1683/2849 (59.1%)	<0.001
Legs movements	Do not know	60/1481 (4.1%)	58/1462 (4.0%)	54/1357 (4.0%)	<0.001	60/1481 (4.1%)	112/2819 (4.0%)	0.002
	Never	402/1481 (27.1%)	384/1462 (26.3%)	326/1357 (24.0%)		402/1481 (27.1%)	710/2819 (25.2%)	
	Rarely	93/1481 (6.3%)	91/1462 (6.2%)	105/1357 (7.7%)		93/1481 (6.3%)	196/2819 (7.0%)	
	Sometimes	447/1481 (30.2%)	405/1462 (27.7%)	327/1357 (24.1%)		447/1481 (30.2%)	732/2819 (26.0%)	
	Usually	407/1481 (27.5%)	440/1462 (30.1%)	439/1357 (32.4%)		407/1481 (27.5%)	879/2819 (31.2%)	
	Always	72/1481 (4.9%)	84/1462 (5.8%)	106/1357 (7.8%)		72/1481 (4.9%)	190/2819 (6.7%)	

In terms of OSA-related symptoms, there were no differences between ever and never smokers in the presence of symptoms, such as dry mouth, morning fatigue, bad mood, memory loss or dropping things from hands. Never smokers declared significantly more frequent headaches and/or heavy head compared to ever smokers ($p < 0.001$ in both), while the opposite applied for the need of the presence of a passenger when driving to be kept awake (19.9% vs. 15.4%, $p < 0.001$). Ever smokers also presented significantly more frequent breathing pauses during sleep ($p = 0.011$), while their snoring was louder ($p = 0.008$), especially the current smokers (Table 4).

Table 4. Sleep-apnea-related symptoms according to the smoking status of the participants.

Symptom		Smoking Status			p (Value)	Ever Smoker		p (Value)
		Never Smoker	Former Smoker	Current Smoker		No	Yes	
Dry mouth	Do not Know	2/1479 (0.1%)	4/1465 (0.3%)	2/1360 (0.2%)	0.74	2/1479 (0.1%)	6/2825 (0.2%)	0.55
	Almost never	411/1479 (27.8%)	423/1465 (28.9%)	388/1360 (28.5%)		411/1479 (27.8%)	811/2825 (28.7%)	
	1–2 times per month	14/1479 (1.0%)	12/1465 (0.8%)	6/1360 (0.4%)		14/1479 (1.0%)	18/2825 (0.6%)	
	1–2 times per week	19/1479 (1.3%)	28/1465 (1.9%)	24/1360 (1.8%)		19/1479 (1.3%)	52/2825 (1.8%)	
	3–4 times per week	38/1479 (2.6%)	38/1465 (2.6%)	29/1360 (2.1%)		38/1479 (2.6%)	67/2825 (2.4%)	
	Daily	995/1479 (67.3%)	960/1465 (65.5%)	911/1360 (67.0%)		995/1479 (67.3%)	1871/2825 (66.2%)	
Morning fatigue	Do not Know	1/1483 (0.1%)	4/1467 (0.3%)	2/1361 (0.2%)	0.035	1/1483 (0.1%)	6/2828 (0.2%)	0.38
	Almost never	416/1483 (28.1%)	468/1467 (31.9%)	369/1361 (27.1%)		416/1483 (28.1%)	837/2828 (29.6%)	
	1–2 times per month	15/1483 (1.0%)	21/1467 (1.4%)	16/1361 (1.2%)		15/1483 (1.0%)	37/2828 (1.3%)	
	1–2 times per week	47/1483 (3.2%)	39/1467 (2.7%)	29/1361 (2.1%)		47/1483 (3.2%)	68/2828 (2.4%)	
	3–4 times per week	63/1483 (4.3%)	64/1467 (4.4%)	46/1361 (3.4%)		63/1483 (4.3%)	110/2828 (3.9%)	
	Daily	941/1483 (63.5%)	871/1467 (59.4%)	899/1361 (66.1%)		941/1483 (63.5%)	1770/2828 (62.6%)	
Bad mood	Almost never	414/1483 (27.9%)	469/1467 (32.0%)	369/1361 (27.1%)	0.034	414/1483 (27.9%)	838/2828 (29.6%)	0.60
	1–2 times per month	17/1483 (1.2%)	21/1467 (1.4%)	15/1361 (1.1%)		17/1483 (1.2%)	36/2828 (1.3%)	
	1–2 times per week	48/1483 (3.2%)	38/1467 (2.6%)	35/1361 (2.6%)		48/1483 (3.2%)	73/2828 (2.6%)	
	3–4 times per week	70/1483 (4.7%)	67/1467 (4.6%)	53/1361 (3.9%)		70/1483 (4.7%)	120/2828 (4.2%)	
	Almost daily	933/1483 (62.9%)	868/1467 (59.2%)	889/1361 (65.3%)		933/1483 (62.9%)	1757/2828 (62.1%)	
	Daily	1/1483 (0.1%)	4/1467 (0.3%)	0/1361 (0.0%)		1/1483 (0.1%)	4/2828 (0.1%)	
Headache	Do not Know	3/1483 (0.2%)	1/1467 (0.1%)	0/1360 (0.0%)	<0.001	3/1483 (0.2%)	1/2827 (0.0%)	<0.001
	Almost never	841/1483 (56.7%)	942/1467 (64.2%)	845/1360 (62.1%)		841/1483 (56.7%)	1787/2827 (63.2%)	
	1–2 times per month	68/1483 (4.6%)	52/1467 (3.6%)	41/1360 (3.0%)		68/1483 (4.6%)	93/2827 (3.3%)	
	1–2 times per week	75/1483 (5.1%)	73/1467 (5.0%)	90/1360 (6.6%)		75/1483 (5.1%)	163/2827 (5.8%)	
	3–4 times per week	109/1483 (7.4%)	81/1467 (5.5%)	69/1360 (5.1%)		109/1483 (7.4%)	150/2827 (5.3%)	
	Daily	387/1483 (26.1%)	318/1467 (21.7%)	315/1360 (23.2%)		387/1483 (26.1%)	633/2827 (22.4%)	

Table 4. Cont.

Symptom		Smoking Status			p (Value)	Ever Smoker		p (Value)
		Never Smoker	Former Smoker	Current Smoker		No	Yes	
Heavy head	Do not Know	2/1482 (0.1%)	2/1467 (0.1%)	2/1361 (0.2%)	0.001	2/1482 (0.1%)	4/2828 (0.1%)	<0.001
	Almost never	827/1482 (55.8%)	928/1467 (63.3%)	841/1361 (61.8%)		827/1482 (55.8%)	1769/2828 (62.6%)	
	1–2 times per month	67/1482 (4.5%)	47/1467 (3.2%)	34/1361 (2.5%)		67/1482 (4.5%)	81/2828 (2.9%)	
	1–2 times per week	73/1482 (4.9%)	67/1467 (4.6%)	77/1361 (5.7%)		73/1482 (4.9%)	144/2828 (5.1%)	
	3–4 times per week	111/1482 (7.5%)	89/1467 (6.1%)	68/1361 (5.0%)		111/1482 (7.5%)	157/2828 (5.6%)	
	Daily	402/1482 (27.1%)	334/1467 (22.8%)	339/1361 (24.9%)		402/1482 (27.1%)	673/2828 (23.8%)	
Need a passenger when driving to be kept awake		231/1498 (15.4%)	299/1480 (20.2%)	269/1369 (19.7%)	0.001	231/1498 (15.4%)	568/2849 (19.9%)	<0.001
Snoring frequency	Never	15/1498 (1.0%)	14/1480 (1.0%)	9/1369 (0.7%)	0.31	15/1498 (1.0%)	23/2849 (0.8%)	0.20
	Almost never	46/1498 (3.1%)	44/1480 (3.0%)	25/1369 (1.8%)		46/1498 (3.1%)	69/2849 (2.4%)	
	1–2 times per month	5/1498 (0.3%)	3/1480 (0.2%)	3/1369 (0.2%)		5/1498 (0.3%)	6/2849 (0.2%)	
	1–2 times per week	9/1498 (0.6%)	3/1480 (0.2%)	6/1369 (0.4%)		9/1498 (0.6%)	9/2849 (0.3%)	
	3–4 times per week	13/1498 (0.9%)	7/1480 (0.5%)	7/1369 (0.5%)		13/1498 (0.9%)	14/2849 (0.5%)	
	Every night	1393/1498 (93.0%)	1385/1480 (93.6%)	1296/1369 (94.7%)		1393/1498 (93.0%)	2681/2849 (94.1%)	
	Many times per night	17/1498 (1.1%)	24/1480 (1.6%)	23/1369 (1.7%)		17/1498 (1.1%)	47/2849 (1.7%)	
Breathing pauses during sleep	Almost never	171/1479 (11.6%)	137/1463 (9.4%)	123/1357 (9.1%)	0.06	171/1479 (11.6%)	260/2820 (9.2%)	0.011
	1–2 times per month	7/1479 (0.5%)	6/1463 (0.4%)	4/1357 (0.3%)		7/1479 (0.5%)	10/2820 (0.4%)	
	1–2 times per week	15/1479 (1.0%)	9/1463 (0.6%)	14/1357 (1.0%)		15/1479 (1.0%)	23/2820 (0.8%)	
	3–4 times per week	28/1479 (1.9%)	16/1463 (1.1%)	21/1357 (1.6%)		28/1479 (1.9%)	37/2820 (1.3%)	
	Every night	1056/1479 (71.4%)	1125/1463 (76.9%)	1036/1357 (76.4%)		1056/1479 (71.4%)	2161/2820 (76.6%)	
	Many times per night	202/1479 (13.7%)	170/1463 (11.6%)	159/1357 (11.7%)		202/1479 (13.7%)	329/2820 (11.7%)	
Night awakenings	Almost never	315/1477 (21.3%)	255/1466 (17.4%)	365/1357 (26.9%)	<0.001	315/1477 (21.3%)	620/2823 (22.0%)	0.51
	1–2 times per month	12/1477 (0.8%)	16/1466 (1.1%)	16/1357 (1.2%)		12/1477 (0.8%)	32/2823 (1.1%)	
	1–2 times per week	49/1477 (3.3%)	35/1466 (2.4%)	41/1357 (3.0%)		49/1477 (3.3%)	76/2823 (2.7%)	
	3–4 times per week	1018/1477 (68.9%)	1074/1466 (73.3%)	881/1357 (64.9%)		1018/1477 (68.9%)	1955/2823 (69.3%)	
	Every night	83/1477 (5.6%)	86/1466 (5.9%)	54/1357 (4.0%)		83/1477 (5.6%)	140/2823 (5.0%)	

From the data collected from the sleep studies, ever smokers had significantly higher AHI and ODI compared to never smokers (34.4 ± 24.6 events/h vs. 31.7 ± 23.6 events/h, $p < 0.001$ and 33.9 ± 25.0 events/h vs. 31.0 ± 23.9 events/h, $p < 0.001$) and significantly lower mean SaO$_2$ (91.8 ± 3.4% vs. 92.2 ± 3.9%, $p < 0.001$). Furthermore, they suffered more frequently from moderate and severe OSAHS compared to never smokers (50.3% vs. 46.9% and 26.2% vs. 24.8%, respectively), who were more frequently diagnosed with no or mild disease (13.1% vs. 12.7% and 15.3% vs. 10.8%, respectively, $p < 0.001$) (Table 5).

Table 5. Sleep study parameters according to the smoking status of the participants.

Parameter		Smoking Status				Ever Smoker		
		Never Smoker	Former Smoker	Current Smoker	p (Value)	No	Yes	p (Value)
Total sleep time (minutes)		270.1 ± 73.0 (N = 70)	239.3 ± 81.6 (N = 63)	248.3 ± 82.2 (N = 70)	0.07	270.1 ± 73.0 (N = 70)	244.0 ± 81.8 (N = 133)	0.022
% REM sleep time (%)		25.1 ± 14.0 (N = 63)	24.2 ± 14.5 (N = 58)	20.8 ± 12.1 (N = 65)	0.17	25.1 ± 14.0 (N = 63)	22.4 ± 13.4 (N = 123)	0.20
% Non-REM sleep time (%)		74.9 ± 14.0 (N = 63)	75.8 ± 14.5 (N = 58)	79.2 ± 12.1 (N = 65)	0.17	74.9 ± 14.0 (N = 63)	77.6 ± 13.4 (N = 123)	0.20
Night sleep duration (hours)		3.18 ± 0.78 (N = 1482)	3.15 ± 0.79 (N = 1465)	3.12 ± 0.76 (N = 1361)	0.06	3.18 ± 0.78 (N = 1482)	3.13 ± 0.77 (N = 2826)	0.044
Sleep latency (minutes)		12.19 ± 1.20 (N = 1480)	12.11 ± 1.16 (N = 1463)	12.12 ± 1.17 (N = 1359)	0.17	12.19 ± 1.20 (N = 1480)	12.12 ± 1.16 (N = 2822)	0.07
Nap duration (hours)		2.86 ± 0.61 (N = 895)	2.92 ± 0.59 (N = 975)	2.99 ± 0.56 (N = 806)	<0.001	2.86 ± 0.61 (N = 895)	2.95 ± 0.58 (N = 1781)	<0.001
AHI (events/hour)		31.7 ± 23.6 (N = 1498)	35.5 ± 23.8 (N = 1480)	33.3 ± 25.4 (N = 1369)	<0.001	31.7 ± 23.6 (N = 1498)	34.4 ± 24.6 (N = 2849)	<0.001
Central apneas (events/hour)		0.7 ± 3.3 (N = 1488)	0.7 ± 2.6 (N = 1468)	0.5 ± 2.3 (N = 1355)	0.05	0.7 ± 3.3 (N = 1488)	0.6 ± 2.5 (N = 2823)	0.26
Mean SaO$_2$ (%)		92.2 ± 3.9 (N = 1498)	91.6 ± 3.4 (N = 1480)	91.9 ± 3.3 (N = 1369)	<0.001	92.2 ± 3.9 (N = 1498)	91.8 ± 3.4 (N = 2849)	<0.001
Minimum SaO$_2$ (%)		79.1 ± 9.8 (N = 1496)	78.0 ± 9.6 (N = 1477)	79.1 ± 9.5 (N = 1369)	0.001	79.1 ± 9.8 (N = 1496)	78.5 ± 9.6 (N = 2846)	0.08
ODI (events/hour)		31.0 ± 23.9 (N = 1498)	35.1 ± 24.6 (N = 1477)	32.7 ± 25.3 (N = 1368)	<0.001	31.0 ± 23.9 (N = 1498)	33.9 ± 25.0 (N = 2845)	<0.001
Mean apnea duration (seconds)		22.1 ± 7.8 (N = 1201)	22.3 ± 7.1 (N = 1197)	21.6 ± 7.5 (N = 1127)	0.06	22.1 ± 7.8 (N = 1201)	22.0 ± 7.3 (N = 2324)	0.55
Maximum apnea duration (seconds)		47.5 ± 24.0 (N = 985)	50.1 ± 24.6 (N = 991)	47.0 ± 23.0 (N = 936)	0.009	47.5 ± 24.0 (N = 985)	48.6 ± 23.9 (N = 1927)	0.22
OSA diagnosis	Absent (AHI < 5)	229/1498 (15.3%)	124/1480 (8.4%)	184/1369 (13.4%)	<0.001	229/1498 (15.3%)	308/2849 (10.8%)	<0.001
	Mild (AHI 5–15)	196/1498 (13.1%)	176/1480 (11.9%)	186/1369 (13.6%)		196/1498 (13.1%)	362/2849 (12.7%)	
	Moderate (AHI 15–30)	371/1498 (24.8%)	394/1480 (26.6%)	352/1369 (25.7%)		371/1498 (24.8%)	746/2849 (26.2%)	
	Severe (AHI > 30)	702/1498 (46.9%)	786/1480 (53.1%)	647/1369 (47.3%)		702/1498 (46.9%)	1433/2849 (50.3%)	

N = number, REM = rapid eye movement, AHI = apnea hypopnea index, ODI = oxygen desaturation index, OSA = obstructive sleep apnea–hypopnea syndrome.

Finally, in both ever and never smokers who reported increased frequency of leg movements and other abnormal sleep behaviors, including sleep talking, abnormal movements and restless sleep, AHI was significantly higher ($p < 0.001$ in all of them), with the exception of nightmares ($p = 0.52$ in ever and $p = 0.31$ in never smokers) (Table 6).

Table 6. Comparison of AHI and abnormal sleep behaviors according to smoking history.

Abnormal Sleep Behavior		Never Smokers		Ever Smoker	
		AHI	p (Value)	AHI	p (Value)
Nightmares	Yes	32.7 ± 23.6 (N = 430)	0.31	34.9 ± 25.3 (N = 790)	0.52
	No	31.3 ± 23.6 (N = 1068)		34.2 ± 24.3 (N = 2059)	
Sleep talking	Yes	36.9 ± 24.8 (N = 398)	<0.001	38.6 ± 25.9 (N = 877)	<0.001
	No	29.8 ± 22.9 (N = 1100)		32.6 ± 23.7 (N = 1972)	
Abnormal movements during sleep	Yes	35.4 ± 24.6 (N = 415)	<0.001	38.3 ± 25.9 (N = 885)	<0.001
	No	30.3 ± 23.1 (N = 1083)		32.7 ± 23.8 (N = 1964)	
Restless sleep	Yes	34.4 ± 24.3 (N = 773)	<0.001	36.6 ± 25.1 (N = 1683)	<0.001
	No	28.9 ± 22.6 (N = 725)		31.3 ± 23.6 (N = 1166)	
Legs movements	Do not know	24.5 ± 20.4 (N = 60)	<0.001	28.8 ± 24.5 (N = 112)	<0.001
	Never	27.1 ± 23.6 (N = 402)		31.0 ± 24.2 (N = 710)	
	Rarely	29.5 ± 22.7 (N = 93)		33.8 ± 23.9 (N = 196)	
	Sometimes	33.6 ± 23.5 (N = 447)		34.3 ± 22.7 (N = 732)	
	Usually	34.1 ± 22.7 (N = 407)		36.6 ± 25.3 (N = 879)	
	Always	41.6 ± 27.7 (N = 72)		41.8 ± 27.6 (N = 190)	

4. Discussion

In this large-scale cross-sectional study, it was found that the severity of OSAHS was significantly greater in ever smokers compared to never smokers; Berlin and STOP Bang questionnaires predicted higher risk for OSAHS in ever smokers compared to never smokers. Additionally, there was a significant correlation between positive smoking history and sleep talking, and restless sleep and leg movements during sleep.

To the best of our knowledge, this is one of the largest observational studies—with a total of 4347 participants—which investigated the relationship between smoking and OSAHS. A recently published meta-analysis included a higher number of patients, but the data were derived from 13 distinct studies, and each one included a lower number of participants compared to ours [37]. Similar to previously published data, the present study also found that AHI was significantly higher in ever smokers compared to never smokers and that smoking is associated with OSA severity [9,13,37–39]. However, ESS and minimum SaO_2 did not differ between these two groups, whereas ODI and mean SaO_2 did [37]. Excessive daytime sleepiness was not found to differ between the two groups, which is in accordance with the fact that both groups presented similar prevalence in the majority of OSA-related symptoms, such as morning fatigue, bad mood, memory loss and falling asleep during reading.

Another interesting finding in the present research was that OSAHS patients in the ever-smoker group exhibited a significantly higher prevalence of co-morbidities, such as diabetes mellitus, hyperlipidemia, coronary disease, acute myocardial infarction and pulmonary disease. Previous studies have shown that untreated OSAHS, especially severe, significantly increases the incidence of diabetes mellitus, ischemic heart disease and acute myocardial infarction [40]. Therefore, smoking could contribute to the pathogenesis of these diseases, both directly, with its well-known mechanisms of action on the vascular endothelium, and indirectly, by increasing OSAHS severity.

Apart from OSAHS-related findings, this study also demonstrated that smoking had an impact on other non-OSAHS-related sleep parameters. Previous studies have shown that sleep quality might be worse in smokers, with increased sleep latency, higher prevalence of awakenings and difficulty in waking up [14–16,41]. In our study, sleep latency and reported awakenings did not differ significantly between ever and never smokers. However, night-sleep duration was significantly shorter in ever smokers, who presented longer nap duration during the daytime. These findings are in accordance with those of previous studies [42,43] in populations other than OSAHS, who had not been evaluated for sleep apnea with sleep studies. In addition to that, in the present study, abnormal sleep behaviors, such as sleep talking, abnormal movements, restless sleep and leg movements during sleep, were significantly more frequent in ever smokers and particularly in current smokers. This phenomenon has been observed, with second-hand smoke exposure during pregnancy or early childhood [20,21], or even with adult smoking [22–25], but not in all studies [26], none of which included OSAHS patients. Furthermore, abnormal sleep behaviors have also been related to increasing AHI [44–46]. Yet, to the best of our knowledge, our study is the first one to demonstrate that in a population of patients with OSAHS, there might be a significant correlation between positive smoking history and both abnormal sleep behaviors and increasing AHI. Thus, it is plausible to suggest that there might be a positive correlation between smoking history and abnormal sleep behaviors, not only directly but also indirectly, by increased AHI in ever smokers.

This study presents several limitations. It is a cross-sectional study and one cannot establish a cause-and-effect relationship between smoking and sleep disorders because the temporal sequence between the two cannot be determined. Furthermore, there were significant differences between ever and never smokers in baseline characteristics, such as BMI, neck and waist circumference, that might be responsible for the more severe presentation of OSAHS in these groups. Additional confounding factors contributing to more severe OSAHS in the group of ever smokers include increased alcohol consumption and a higher frequency of pulmonary and cardiovascular co-morbidities. On the other hand, cardiovascular disease may be the result of the more severe presentation of OSAHS, instead of the cause, creating a cause-and-effect loop. In any case, the population in our study represents a "real-life" patient group, visiting a sleep clinic, and the results should be interpreted under this spectrum. Another limitation is that full PSG was conducted in a minority of patients, while the majority was assessed with type 3 sleep studies, preventing a detailed evaluation of sleep architecture. Moreover, the presence of sleep behaviors was not based on objective means, but was made subjectively by the patients or their partners, leading to a potential recall bias.

Despite its limitations, the current study demonstrated a more severe presentation of OSAHS in smokers, with more frequent metabolic and cardiovascular co-morbidities, although it did not confirm the presence of the excessive daytime sleepiness of previous studies in this group of patients. More importantly, to the best of our knowledge, this is the first large-scale cross-sectional study that reported a significantly higher frequency of different sleep behaviors in smokers compared to non-smokers in patients with OSAHS. Hence, taking into consideration the findings of this study, the term "smoking obstructive sleep apnea" could be considered as a distinctive phenotype [38]. Future studies, more focused on additional sleep symptoms and disorders, are necessary in order to evaluate, in more detail, smoking-induced disturbed sleep patterns.

Author Contributions: Conceptualization, I.G., P.S., I.P., A.M., S.-C.K., K.P., D.S. and A.P.; methodology, I.G., P.S., I.P., A.M., K.C., S.-C.K., K.P., D.S. and A.P.; software, S.-C.K.; validation, I.G., P.S., K.C., S.-C.K., K.P., and A.P.; formal analysis, I.G., P.S., I.P., A.M., K.C., S.-C.K. and K.P.; investigation, I.G., P.S., I.P., A.M., K.P., D.S. and A.P.; resources, S.-C.K.; writing—original draft preparation, I.G., P.S., S.-C.K., K.P. and A.P.; writing—review and editing, I.P., A.M., K.C. and S.-C.K.; supervision, S.-C.K., D.S. and A.P.; project administration, A.P. All authors have read and agreed to the published version of the manuscript.

Funding: This research received no external funding.

Institutional Review Board Statement: The study was conducted in accordance with the Declaration of Helsinki and approved by the local Ethics Committee.

Informed Consent Statement: Written informed consent was obtained from all participants involved in the study.

Data Availability Statement: Data used in the present study are available upon request from the corresponding author.

Conflicts of Interest: The authors declare no conflict of interest.

References

1. World Health Organization. *Guidelines for Controlling and Monitoring the Tobacco Epidemic*; World Health Organization: Geneva, Switzerland, 1998; Available online: http://www.who.int/iris/handle/10665/42049 (accessed on 16 September 2022).
2. Kim, S.-H.; Lee, J.-A.; Kim, K.-U.; Cho, H.-J. Results of an Inpatient Smoking Cessation Program: 3-Month Cessation Rate and Predictors of Success. *Korean J. Fam. Med.* **2015**, *36*, 50–59. [CrossRef] [PubMed]
3. Jee, S.H.; Yun, J.E.; Park, J.Y.; Sull, J.W.; Kim, I.S. Smoking and cause of death in Korea: 11 years follow-up prospective study. *Korean J. Epidemiol.* **2005**, *27*, 182–190.
4. Peppard, P.E.; Young, T.; Barnet, J.H.; Palta, M.; Hagen, E.W.; Hla, K.M. Increased Prevalence of Sleep-Disordered Breathing in Adults. *Am. J. Epidemiol.* **2013**, *177*, 1006–1014. [CrossRef] [PubMed]
5. Pataka, A.; Riha, R.L. The obstructive sleep apnoea/hypopnoea syndrome—An overview. *Respir. Med. CME* **2009**, *2*, 111–117. [CrossRef]
6. Jennum, P.; Riha, R.L. Epidemiology of sleep apnoea/hypopnoea syndrome and sleep-disordered breathing. *Eur. Respir. J.* **2009**, *33*, 907–914. [CrossRef]
7. Gami, A.S.; Howard, D.E.; Olson, E.J.; Somers, V.K. Day–Night Pattern of Sudden Death in Obstructive Sleep Apnea. *N. Engl. J. Med.* **2005**, *352*, 1206–1214. [CrossRef] [PubMed]
8. Marshall, N.S.; Wong, K.K.H.; Cullen, S.R.; Knuiman, M.; Grunstein, R.R. Sleep Apnea and 20-Year Follow-Up for All-Cause Mortality, Stroke, and Cancer Incidence and Mortality in the Busselton Health Study Cohort. *J. Clin. Sleep Med.* **2014**, *10*, 355–362. [CrossRef]
9. Bielicki, P.; Trojnar, A.; Sobieraj, P.; Wąsik, M. Smoking Status in Relation to Obstructive Sleep Apnea Severity (OSA) And Cardiovascular Comorbidity in Patients with Newly Diagnosed OSA. *Adv. Respir. Med.* **2019**, *87*, 103–109. [CrossRef]
10. Deleanu, O.-C.; Pocora, D.; Mihălcuţă, S.; Ulmeanu, R.; Zaharie, A.-M.; Mihălţan, F.D. Influence of smoking on sleep and obstructive sleep apnea syndrome. *Pneumologia* **2016**, *65*, 28–35.
11. Bearpark, H.; Elliott, L.; Grunstein, R.; Cullen, S.; Schneider, H.; Althaus, W.; Sullivan, C. Snoring and sleep apnea. A population study in Australian men. *Am. J. Respir. Crit. Care Med.* **1995**, *151*, 1459–1465. [CrossRef]
12. Franklin, K.A.; Gíslason, T.; Omenaas, E.; Jögi, R.; Jensen, E.J.; Lindberg, E.; Gunnbjörnsdóttir, M.; Nyström, L.; Laerum, B.N.; Björnsson, E.; et al. The Influence of Active and Passive Smoking on Habitual Snoring. *Am. J. Respir. Crit. Care Med.* **2004**, *170*, 799–803. [CrossRef] [PubMed]
13. Krishnan, V.; Dixon-Williams, S.; Thornton, J.D. Where there is smoke there is sleep apnea: Exploring the relationship between smoking and sleep apnea. *Chest* **2014**, *146*, 1673–1680. [CrossRef] [PubMed]
14. Phillips, B.A.; Danner, F.J. Cigarette smoking and sleep disturbance. *Arch. Intern. Med.* **1995**, *155*, 734–737. [CrossRef] [PubMed]
15. Soldatos, C.R.; Kales, J.D.; Scharf, M.B.; Bixler, E.O.; Kales, A. Cigarette Smoking Associated with Sleep Difficulty. *Science* **1980**, *207*, 551–553. [CrossRef] [PubMed]
16. Zhang, L.; Samet, J.; Caffo, B.; Punjabi, N.M. Cigarette Smoking and Nocturnal Sleep Architecture. *Am. J. Epidemiol.* **2006**, *164*, 529–537. [CrossRef]
17. Kim, K.S.; Kim, J.H.; Park, S.Y.; Won, H.-R.; Lee, H.-J.; Yang, H.S.; Kim, H.J. Smoking Induces Oropharyngeal Narrowing and Increases the Severity of Obstructive Sleep Apnea Syndrome. *J. Clin. Sleep Med.* **2012**, *8*, 367–374. [CrossRef]
18. Schrand, J.R. Is sleep apnea a predisposing factor for tobacco use? *Med. Hypotheses* **1996**, *47*, 443–448. [CrossRef]
19. Wetter, D.W.; Young, T.B.; Bidwell, T.R.; Badr, M.S.; Palta, M. Smoking as a risk factor for sleep-disordered breathing. *Arch. Intern. Med.* **1994**, *154*, 2219–2224. [CrossRef]

20. O'Callaghan, F.; O'Callaghan, M.; Scott, J.G.; Najman, J.; Mamun, A. Effect of maternal smoking in pregnancy and childhood on child and adolescent sleep outcomes to 21 years: A birth cohort study. *BMC Pediatr.* **2019**, *19*, 70. [CrossRef]
21. Lin, L.-Z.; Xu, S.-L.; Wu, Q.-Z.; Zhou, Y.; Ma, H.-M.; Chen, D.-H.; Dong, P.-X.; Xiong, S.-M.; Shen, X.-B.; Zhou, P.-E.; et al. Exposure to second-hand smoke during early life and subsequent sleep problems in children: A population-based cross-sectional study. *Environ. Health* **2021**, *20*, 127. [CrossRef]
22. Yao, C.; Fereshtehnejad, S.M.; Keezer, M.R.; Wolfson, C.; Pelletier, A.; Postuma, R.B. Risk factors for possible REM sleep behavior disorder: A CLSA population-based cohort study. *Neurology* **2018**, *92*, e475–e485. [CrossRef]
23. Postuma, R.B.; Montplaisir, J.Y.; Pelletier, A.; Dauvilliers, Y.; Oertel, W.; Iranzo, A.; Strambi, L.F.; Arnulf, I.; Högl, B.; Manni, R.; et al. Environmental risk factors for REM sleep behavior disorder: A multicenter case-control study. *Neurology* **2012**, *79*, 428–434. [CrossRef]
24. Matsui, K.; Komada, Y.; Nishimura, K.; Kuriyama, K.; Inoue, Y. Prevalence and Associated Factors of Nocturnal Eating Behavior and Sleep-Related Eating Disorder-Like Behavior in Japanese Young Adults: Results of an Internet Survey Using Munich Parasomnia Screening. *J. Clin. Med.* **2020**, *9*, 1243. [CrossRef]
25. Wróbel-Knybel, P.; Flis, M.; Rog, J.; Jalal, B.; Wołkowski, L.; Karakuła-Juchnowicz, H. Characteristics of Sleep Paralysis and Its Association with Anxiety Symptoms, Perceived Stress, PTSD, and Other Variables Related to Lifestyle in Selected High Stress Exposed Professions. *Int. J. Environ. Res. Public Health* **2022**, *19*, 7821. [CrossRef]
26. Oluwole, O.S. Lifetime prevalence and incidence of parasomnias in a population of young adult Nigerians. *J. Neurol.* **2010**, *257*, 1141–1147. [CrossRef]
27. CDC/National Center for Health Statistics, 29 August 2017. Adult Tobacco Use Information. Available online: https://www.cdc.gov/nchs/nhis/tobacco/tobacco_glossary.htm (accessed on 29 August 2019).
28. Johns, M.W. A New Method for Measuring Daytime Sleepiness: The Epworth Sleepiness Scale. *Sleep* **1991**, *14*, 540–545. [CrossRef]
29. Netzer, N.C.; Stoohs, R.A.; Netzer, C.M.; Clark, K.; Strohl, K.P. Using the Berlin Questionnaire To Identify Patients at Risk for the Sleep Apnea Syndrome. *Ann. Intern. Med.* **1999**, *131*, 485–491. [CrossRef]
30. Chung, F.; Yegneswaran, B.; Liao, P.; Chung, S.A.; Vairavanathan, S.; Islam, S.; Shapiro, C.M. STOP questionnaire: A tool to screen patients for obstructive sleep apnea. *Anesthesiology* **2008**, *108*, 812–821. [CrossRef]
31. Soldatos, C.R.; Dikeos, D.G.; Paparrigopoulos, T.J. Athens Insomnia Scale: Validation of an instrument based on ICD-10 criteria. *J. Psychosom. Res.* **2000**, *48*, 555–560. [CrossRef]
32. Martín-Albo, J.; Núñez, J.L.; Navarro, J.G.; Grijalvo, F. The Rosenberg Self-Esteem Scale: Translation and Validation in University Students. *Span. J. Psychol.* **2007**, *10*, 458–467. [CrossRef]
33. Tsara, V.; Amfilochiou, A.; Papagrigorakis, M.J.; Georgopoulos, D.; Liolios, E. Guidelines for diagnosis and treatment of sleep-related breathing disorders in adults and children. Definition and classification of sleep related breathing disorders in adults: Different types and indications for sleep studies (Part 1). *Hippokratia* **2009**, *13*, 187–191.
34. Berry, R.B.; Brooks, R.; Gamaldo, C.; Harding, S.M.; Lloyd, R.M.; Quan, S.F.; Troester, M.T.; Vaughn, B.V. AASM Scoring Manual Updates for 2017 (Version 2.4). *J. Clin. Sleep Med.* **2017**, *13*, 665–666. [CrossRef]
35. Ruehland, W.R.; Rochford, P.D.; O'Donoghue, F.J.; Pierce, R.J.; Singh, P.; Thornton, A.T. The New Aasm Criteria for Scoring Hypopneas: Impact on the Apnea Hypopnea Index. *Sleep* **2009**, *32*, 150–157. [CrossRef]
36. Mbata, G.; Chukwuka, J. Obstructive sleep apnea hypopnea syndrome. *Ann. Med. Health Sci. Res.* **2012**, *2*, 74–77. [CrossRef]
37. Zeng, X.; Ren, Y.; Wu, K.; Yang, Q.; Zhang, S.; Wang, D.; Luo, Y.; Zhang, N. Association Between Smoking Behavior and Obstructive Sleep Apnea: A Systematic Review and Meta-Analysis. *Nicotine Tob. Res.* **2022**, ntac126. [CrossRef]
38. Oțelea, M.R.; Trenchea, M.; Rașcu, A.; Antoniu, S.; Zugravu, C.; Busnatu, Ș.; Simionescu, A.A.; Arghir, O.C. Smoking Obstructive Sleep Apnea: Arguments for a Distinctive Phenotype and a Personalized Intervention. *J. Pers. Med.* **2022**, *12*, 293. [CrossRef]
39. Ioannidou, D.; Kalamaras, G.; Kotoulas, S.-C.; Pataka, A. Smoking and Obstructive Sleep Apnea: Is There An Association between These Cardiometabolic Risk Factors?—Gender Analysis. *Medicina* **2021**, *57*, 1137. [CrossRef]
40. Dodds, S.; Williams, L.J.; Roguski, A.; Vennelle, M.; Douglas, N.J.; Kotoulas, S.-C.; Riha, R.L. Mortality and morbidity in obstructive sleep apnoea–hypopnoea syndrome: Results from a 30-year prospective cohort study. *ERJ Open Res.* **2020**, *6*, 00057–2020. [CrossRef]
41. Wetter, D.; Young, T. The Relation Between Cigarette Smoking and Sleep Disturbance. *Prev. Med.* **1994**, *23*, 328–334. [CrossRef]
42. Metse, A.P.; Clinton-McHarg, T.; Skinner, E.; Yogaraj, Y.; Colyvas, K.; Bowman, J. Associations between Suboptimal Sleep and Smoking, Poor Nutrition, Harmful Alcohol Consumption and Inadequate Physical Activity ('SNAP Risks'): A Comparison of People with and without a Mental Health Condition in an Australian Community Survey. *Int. J. Environ. Res. Public Health* **2021**, *18*, 5946. [CrossRef]
43. Cheng, G.H.-L.; Chan, A.; Lo, J.C. Factors of nocturnal sleep and daytime nap durations in community-dwelling elderly: A longitudinal population-based study. *Int. Psychogeriatr.* **2017**, *29*, 1335–1344. [CrossRef]
44. Verbraecken, J. More than sleepiness: Prevalence and relevance of nonclassical symptoms of obstructive sleep apnea. *Curr. Opin. Pulm. Med.* **2022**, *28*, 552–558. [CrossRef]

45. Baran, A.S.; Richert, A.C.; Douglass, A.B.; May, W.; Ansarin, K. Change in Periodic Limb Movement Index During Treatment of Obstructive Sleep Apnea with Continuous Positive Airway Pressure. *Sleep* **2003**, *26*, 717–720. [CrossRef]
46. Massahud, M.L.B.; Bruzinga, F.F.B.; Diniz, S.A.M.; Seraidarian, K.K.A.; Lopes, R.M.; Barros, V.M.; Seraidarian, P.I. Association between sleep bruxism, use of antidepressants, and obstructive sleep apnea syndrome: A cross-sectional study. *J. Oral Rehabil.* **2022**, *49*, 505–513. [CrossRef]

Disclaimer/Publisher's Note: The statements, opinions and data contained in all publications are solely those of the individual author(s) and contributor(s) and not of MDPI and/or the editor(s). MDPI and/or the editor(s) disclaim responsibility for any injury to people or property resulting from any ideas, methods, instructions or products referred to in the content.

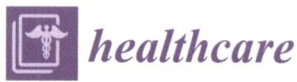

Article

Knowledge and Attitude towards Obstructive Sleep Apnea among Primary Care Physicians in Northern Regions of Saudi Arabia: A Multicenter Study

Abdullah N. Al-Rasheedi [1,*], Ashokkumar Thirunavukkarasu [2], Abdulhakeem Almutairi [3], Sultan Alruwaili [4], Hatem Alotaibi [4], Wasan Alzaid [4], Faisal Albalawi [4], Osama Alwadani [4] and Ahmed Dilli [4]

1. Department of Otolaryngology and Head and Neck Surgery, College of Medicine, Jouf University, Sakaka 72388, Saudi Arabia
2. Department of Community and Family Medicine, College of Medicine, Jouf University, Sakaka 72388, Saudi Arabia
3. Department of Otolaryngology, Head and Neck Surgery, College of Medicine, Qassim University, Qassim 52571, Saudi Arabia
4. College of Medicine, Jouf University, Sakaka 72388, Saudi Arabia
* Correspondence: analrasheedi@ju.edu.sa; Tel.: +966-591009005

Abstract: Obstructive sleep apnea (OSA) is a serious and often underreported condition, despite its highly prevalent distribution. Primary care physicians (PCPs) play an integral role in screening and managing patients with a high risk of developing OSA. This northern Saudi Arabian cross-sectional survey assessed the knowledge and attitude towards OSA among 264 randomly selected PCPs using the OSA Knowledge and Attitude (OSAKA) questionnaire. Among the participating PCPs, 43.9% and 45.1% had low scores in the knowledge and attitude categories, respectively. More than three-fourths (78%) of them recognized that an overnight sleep study is the gold standard for diagnosing OSA. Regarding referral, 39.4% of the OSA patients encountered by the PCPs were referred to ENT specialists, while 21% were referred to sleep clinics, and 18.2% were referred to pulmonologists. Nearly half (50.8%) of the participants recognized OSA as an important clinical disease, and 56.8% were confident in caring for OSA patients. Spearman's correlation of the current study identified a positive correlation between knowledge scores and attitude scores (rho—0.151, $p = 0.017$). It is important to improve PCPs' knowledge regarding OSA and the necessity for referral through different training methods. Furthermore, the study findings emphasize the need to include appropriate OSA programs and continuing medical education for PCPs.

Keywords: primary care physicians; Saudi; knowledge; attitude; obstructive sleep apnea; referral

1. Introduction

Sleep disorders are major public health issues, and their prevalence is increasing both in Saudi Arabia and globally [1,2]. Previous studies from Saudi Arabia observed a high prevalence of obstructive sleep apnea (OSA) among the general Saudi population, around 9%, and much higher among the special segment population, such as pregnant women. In general, the prevalence of OSA was higher in males than females [3–6]. This high prevalence of OSA correlates with the increasing obesity prevalence of about 35.6% among Saudi Arabians [3].

Sleep disruption is correlated with various daytime symptoms, such as daytime sleepiness, fatigue, and poor concentration. Furthermore, sufferers of OSA face higher risks of obesity and diabetes, as well as serious complications such as cardiovascular and cerebrovascular events [7,8]. A recent analysis estimated that 936 million individuals of both genders aged 30–69 years were found to have obstructive sleep apnea worldwide [9]. In Saudi Arabia, clinically diagnosed sleep apnea affects 8.5% of the population [3].

OSA is a serious and often underreported condition, despite its highly prevalent distribution. OSA's rising prevalence is progressively emerging as a global health epidemic, primarily as a result of the prevailing obesity epidemic [10]. A recent systematic review of 24 studies reported a wide range of OSA prevalence (apnea–hypopnea index, AHI ≥ 5) ranging from 9 to 38% [11]. Moreover, Chung et al. suggested that primary care physicians (PCPs) had insufficient knowledge of OSA, resulting in the underestimation and underdiagnosis of OSA [12].

PCPs are integral in screening and managing patients with several diseases, including OSA [13]. Patients with OSA symptoms often present in primary health care settings such as primary health centers (PHC) [14,15]. As such, many studies have been performed to assess PCPs' knowledge, attitude, and practice (KAP) regarding OSA, which showed variable results ranging from good to poor knowledge and attitudes. Furthermore, the ability to manage OSA among PCPs, even in those with good knowledge, was inadequate [14,16].

Several studies have been conducted to evaluate physicians' knowledge of OSA in several respects. Knowledge scores varied according to different specialties, where the highest score of 88.9% was seen among otolaryngology-head and neck surgery residents [17] and the lowest score of 64% was seen in PCPs [14]. Furthermore, Al-Khafaji et al., 2021, reported that higher knowledge scores were accomplished by physicians who have access to sleep centers (13.2 SD 2.2, $p < 0.001$) [16]. In a previous study in Saudi Arabia, Al-Saleem et al., 2020, estimated PCPs' knowledge level of OSA from the Al-Hasa region, which was about 55% [18].

The steps used to reach the diagnosis and initiation of treatment of OSA usually start in a PHC setting, followed by referral to secondary care, as OSA usually requires specialist input [19]. Devani et al., 2020, introduced a model for collaboration across primary and secondary care for patients with suspected OSA. This pathway allows patients to undergo a preliminary assessment and receive a sleep study device at a PHC setting while maintaining specialist input through a virtual multidisciplinary team [19].

Many studies have emphasized the importance of assessing PCPs' knowledge regarding OSA [15,16]. Therefore, investigating the gaps in this knowledge is important in the design of educational strategies. There is a wide variation in sociocultural and health-related characteristics among the Saudi population, as well as in different regions. Furthermore, most training programs are conducted in major cities. Hence, PCPs in the northern region might not have sufficient opportunities to attend the required training programs related to obesity and OSA. There has been an alarming increase in the prevalence of obesity in the Middle East, and OSA is one of the major complications that needs timely attention from PCPs. From our extensive literature search in major databases, the authors could not find sufficient data in this context in the northern regions of Saudi Arabia. Considering the need for region-specific data for formulating a necessary policy for the required training program related to OSA, the present study was conducted. The current study explores the knowledge and attitude towards OSA among PCPs in the northern regions of Saudi Arabia.

2. Materials and Methods

2.1. Study Description

The present survey is an analytical, cross-sectional study that was carried out in PHC settings in the Aljouf, Northern Borders, and Tabuk regions of Saudi Arabia. PCPs (i.e., general practitioners, family doctors, and family residents) were invited to participate in the study. This study was carried out from 1 February 2022 to 30 August 2022.

2.2. Inclusion and Exclusion Criteria

All PCPs working at PHCs in these regions and willing to participate in the study were included in the study. The PCPs who were on vacation and unwilling to participate were excluded from the study.

2.3. Sample Size

The present study utilized Cochran's sample size equation ($n = z^2 pq/e^2$), a widely used sample size estimation formula [20]. The sample size was calculated based on the level of sufficient knowledge of OSA among PCPs, representing 50% with a 5% margin of error and 95% confidence interval, as well as 80% power for the study. The estimated sample size was 384 participants. However, after applying it to the total number of PCPs in these three regions (a finite population), the final estimated minimum required sample size was 264. A systematic random sampling strategy was incorporated to select the necessary participants. The sampling strategy utilized in the present cross-sectional study is described in the flow chart below (Figure 1).

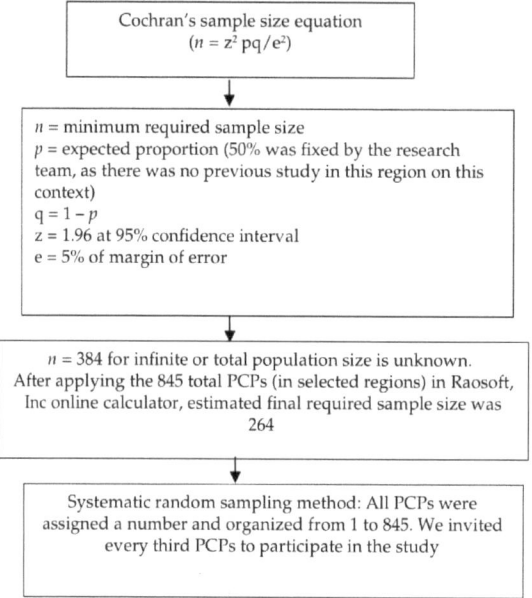

Figure 1. Sampling strategy flowchart.

2.4. Data Collection

We collected data after obtaining an ethical approval letter from a regional health affairs ethics committee (Qurrayat, Wide approval no. 120). All the PCPs agreed to participate in the present study through informed consent. This study was conducted using a self-administered questionnaire comprising two parts.

2.4.1. Part I: Personal Information

This part of the questionnaire contains sociodemographic data, including age, gender, nationality, highest qualification, current position, years in practice, number of OSA cases encountered during the past year, and the referring department.

2.4.2. Part II: The Obstructive Sleep Apnea Knowledge and Attitude (OSAKA) Questionnaire

We used the English version of the OSAKA questionnaire to assess PCPs' knowledge and attitudes towards OSA. This data-collection instrument was initially constructed and validated in the United States to assess physicians' knowledge and attitudes regarding the identification and management of patients with OSA [21]. The OSAKA questionnaire is a self-administered survey that takes only a few minutes to complete. It comprises the following parts:

The first part: This contains eighteen questions that assess five domains (epidemiology, pathophysiology, symptoms, diagnosis, and treatments). Knowledge items are presented as yes, no, and do not know options. The score for the correct answer was given as one; the other choices were marked as zero.

The second part: This constituted five items. The first is developed to measure the importance of OSA as an important clinical disease. The second item assessed the importance of identifying OSA patients by their PCPs. The remaining three items measured the self-confidence of PCPs in the management of OSA patients. The participants responded to these three items on a 5-point Likert scale, ranging from 1 to 5 (1—strongly disagree to 5—strongly agree). Both knowledge and attitude scores were further classified into low (<60% of the overall score), average (60 to 79% of the overall score), and high ($\geq$80% of the overall score). This category was included according to Bloom's criteria and has been used by several studies in the past [22,23].

2.5. Statistical Analysis

We used the statistical package for social sciences (SPSS), V.21 (IBM, SPSS Inc., Chicago, IL, USA) for data entry, coding, and analysis. The present study used frequency with proportion to show categorical data and mean and median to depict quantitative data. The Shapiro–Wilk test was used to test the data's normality assumption. We applied Spearman's analysis to find the correlation between knowledge and attitude scores. Furthermore, we executed a Chi-square test for categorical background characteristics of the PCPs and a Wilcoxon rank sum test for age and practice duration of the PCPs to find the association between the knowledge categories. We have set the *p*-value of less than 0.05 as a significant value. Finally, all of the statistical tests that were run were two-tailed.

3. Results

The total number of PCPs who participated in this study was 264, and these participants were selected using a systematic sampling strategy. The present survey's participants' demographic characteristics and education details are described in Table 1. Among the PCPs who participated, 48.1% were males and 51.9% were females, with a mean (SD) age of 33 (8.01). Nearly half (47.7%) of them had only undergraduate (MBBS) qualifications, and 57.9% of them were residents with a mean (SD) practice duration of 8 (6.6) years.

Table 1. Demographics and participants' characteristics (*n* = 264).

Characteristic	Frequency	Percentage
Gender		
Male	127	48.1
Female	137	51.9
Age in years, mean (SD)	33 (8.01)	
Regions		
Aljouf	59	22.3
Tabuk	89	33.7
Northern border	116	43.9
Latest qualification		
MBBS	126	47.7
MD	69	26.1
Board certified	42	15.9
Others	27	10.2
Current position		
Residents	153	57.9
Specialists/Registrars	63	23.9
Consultants	48	18.2
Practice duration in years, mean (SD)	8 (6.6)	
Rate OSA Cases encountered Mean (SD)	2.63 (2.22)	

Regarding referral patterns, 104 (39.4%) OSA patients encountered by the physicians were referred to ENT specialists, 21.0% were referred to a sleep clinic, and 18.2% of patients were referred to pulmonologists (Table 2).

Table 2. Referral patterns of primary care physicians ($n = 264$).

Specialty	Frequency	Percentage
ENT	104	39.4
Sleep clinic	57	21.0
Respiratory	48	18.2
Neurology	13	4.9
Pediatrics	4	1.5
Others	25	9.5
None	13	4.9

Figure 2 shows the categories of knowledge and attitude scores, as per Bloom's category. Among the sampled physicians, 43.9% had a low score in knowledge, while 18.9% had high scores. Regarding attitude, 45.1% had a low score and only 2.7% had a high score.

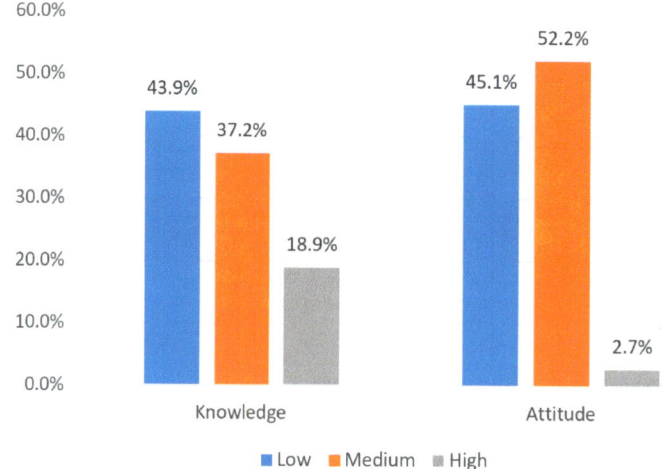

Figure 2. Knowledge and Attitude Categories ($n = 264$).

Table 3 depicts the proportion of correct answers given by the studied PCPs. The current survey found that the highest proportion of the correct answer was found for the statement "In children, adenoids and large tonsils most commonly cause OSA (81.8%)", followed by the statement "Snoring is present in most of the patients with OSA (81.4%)", and "An overnight sleep study is a gold standard for diagnosing OSA (78.0%)".

Table 3. Proportion of correct answers given by the study participants for each knowledge section item.

Question Number	OSAKA Questions	Correct Answer n (%)
1	Females with OSA (obstructive sleep apnea) may have only fatigue	149 (56.45)
2	Uvulopalatopharyngoplasty is a cure for most patients with OSA	130 (50.8)
3	Adult OSA prevalence is estimated to be between 2 and 10%	108 (40)
4	Snoring is present in most of the patients with OSA	215 (81.4)
5	OSA has an association with hypertension	175 (66.3)
6	The gold standard for the diagnosis of OSA is overnight sleep study	206 (78)
7	CPAP therapy may lead to nasal congestion	163 (61.7)
8	Laser-assisted uvuloplasty is an appropriate treatment for severe OSA	134 (50.8)
9	OSA may be due to a loss of upper airway muscle tone during sleep	184 (69.7)
10	In children, adenoids and large tonsils most commonly cause OSA	216 (81.8)
11	A useful examination in suspected OSA is a craniofacial and oropharyngeal examination	193 (73.1)
12	Alcohol at bedtime improves OSA	81 (30.7)
13	Untreated OSA has an association with a higher incidence of car related accidents	180 (68.2)
14	A collar size greater than 17 is associated with OSA in males	108 (40.9)
15	Females suffer from OSA more than males	141 (53.4)
16	CPAP is the first therapy for severe OSA	92 (34.8)
17	In adults, it is normal to have five apneas or hypopneas in one hour	95 (36)
18	There may be an association between untreated OSA and arrhythmias of the heart	171 (64.8)
	Median (IQR) of the correct answer (%) in the knowledge category	59.14 (33.3%)

When assessing the association between PCPs' sociodemographic and background characteristics, we found a significant association among different regions ($p = 0.002$) in terms of knowledge categories. No other factors were significantly associated with the knowledge categories (Table 4).

Table 4. Relationship between knowledge and background characteristics of the PCPs ($n = 264$).

		Knowledge		
	Total (264)	Low/Average (214) n (%)	High (50) n (%)	p-Value
Gender *				
Male	127	107 (84.3)	20 (15.7)	0.213
Female	137	107 (78.1)	30 (21.9)	
Age in years: Mean (SD) **		33.40 (8.41)	32.98 (8.11)	0.744
Regions *				
Aljouf	59	51 (86.4)	8 (13.6)	0.002 ***
Tabuk	89	81 (91.0)	8 (9.0)	
Northern border	116	81 (70.7)	34 (29.3)	
Latest qualification*				
MBBS	126	97 (77.0)	29 (23.0)	0.056
MD/MS	69	58 (84.1)	11 (15.9)	
Saudi Board certified	42	33 (78.6)	9 (21.4)	
Others (Fellowship, PhD)	27	26 (96.3)	1 (2.0)	
Current position *				
Residents	153	121 (79.1)	32 (20.9)	0.585
Specialists/Registrars	63	52 (82.5)	11 (17.5)	
Consultants	48	41 (85.4)	7 (14.6)	
Practice duration in years, mean (SD) **		7.99 (6.55)	6.82 (5.68)	0.267

* Chi-square test applied; ** independent t test applied; *** Significant association.

Regarding the importance of the attitude section, nearly half (50.8%) of the participants recognized OSA as an important or very important clinical disease. Additionally, 51.5% of the PCPs considered identifying people with OSA to be very critical. Regarding self-confidence, 73.9% of the participants were confident in finding people with OSA, and 56.8% were confident in caring for OSA patients (Table 5).

Table 5. PCPs' responses and associated factors in the attitude section (*n* = 264).

Item	Frequency	Proportion
Importance of identifying OSA patients (data shown are either important or very importance)		
OSA is an important disease	134	50.8
Diagnosis of people with OSA is very much essential	136	51.5
Self-confidence (data shown are either agree or strongly agree)		
Confident in diagnosing patients with a high risk of developing OSA	195	73.9
Confident in their capability to care for OSA patients	150	56.8
Confident in their skills to manage OSA patients on CPAP treatment	125	47.3

Spearman's correlation of the current study identified a positive (weak) correlation between knowledge scores and attitude scores (rho—0.151, p = 0.017) (Table 6).

Table 6. Correlation between knowledge and attitude scores, assessed by Spearman's correlation test.

	Spearman's Coefficient Value (Rho)	p-Value
Knowledge–Attitude	0.151	0.017 *

* Significant value.

4. Discussion

The proper management of sleep disorders, including OSA, could help prevent several chronic diseases. The role of PCPs is vital in diagnosing and referring patients to secondary care, as most cases require this step. Our survey assessed PCPs' knowledge and attitudes towards OSA and its referral patterns.

Our study results explored a wide variation in the knowledge questionnaire items, ranging from 36.0% to 81.8%, which is comparable to the studies performed by Corso et al. and Embarak et al. [24,25]. This result demonstrates that knowledge regarding OSA is inadequate and needs appropriate curriculum training. Our study outlined that the highest proportion of correct answers from PCPs was for the item related to snoring. This finding is in alignment with an Egyptian study conducted in 2020. In this study, the majority (79.7%) of the participants also agreed that most patients with OSA were snorers. The present study reported that the proportion of median (IQR) total knowledge scores of PCPs was 59.4 (33.3%). Recent studies conducted in Ecuador and Saudi Arabia also reported a similar finding, and their results found that the respondents' mean score was around 10 out of 18 [18,26]. However, some other studies have reported slightly higher knowledge mean scores among participants [14,24]. The most likely factors for the dissimilarities in the results could be the study settings and the inclusion of participants. Regarding referral patterns, PCPs most commonly referred suspected and diagnosed OSA cases to an ENT specialist; Devaraj et al. also found similar results [19].

Knowledge regarding the association between hypertension and OSA is essential for physicians. The present study revealed that only two-thirds of the PCPs answered correctly to the statement "OSA is associated with hypertension". Interestingly, a cross-sectional study conducted by Cherrez et al. found that a lower proportion (less than 50%) of the physicians responded with correct answers to the above statement [27]. The present study found that a lower proportion of the participants answered correctly to the statement, "Continuous positive airway pressure (CPAP) is the first line of therapy for severe OSA management". Similar to our findings, numerous recent surveys have explored a lower level of knowledge regarding this statement among their study participants [27–30]. Our study findings and studies from other countries indicate that PCPs have insufficient knowledge regarding OSA, which could decrease their ability to diagnose and refer patients to a specialist for necessary care. Regarding the identification of associated factors for the PCPs' knowledge of OSA, we did not find any significantly associated factors, except for regional distinctions.

Numerous existing texts suggest that self-confidence is an essential feature of a great physician, including PCPs [31–33]. This northern Saudi Arabian survey revealed that only a low proportion of the PCPs were confident in caring for OSA patients (56.8%), and the same was true regarding their ability to handle OSA patients on CPAP. Similar to this study's findings, another study by Chang et al. compared PCPs' attitudes toward OSA in three African regions, and they reported that their study participants had low confidence in caring for OSA patients [28]. However, an Italian study by Corso et al. noted that a higher proportion of their participants had confidence in the items mentioned. The possible variations in the study findings could be due to the differences between the respective study participants [24]. Both our study and the study by Chang et al. conducted the survey using the OSAKA questionnaire, whereas the latter survey was conducted among anesthesia specialists. Al-Khafaji et al. 2021, assessed the confidence of Middle Eastern and North African physicians of different specialties' in managing patients with OSA; they found that 72% of practitioners in internal medicine and 49% of practitioners in family medicine/general medicine were confident in managing patients with OSA [16]. However, most primary care physicians executed referrals for patients with suspected OSA to otorhinolaryngologists (72–83%) [14,28]. In addition, only 10% of PCPs used screening tools for OSA, and only 16% of PCPs used the latest clinical practice guidelines, according to Devaraj et al. in a 2020 study [14].

A positive attitude among healthcare workers is critical for patient care. The present study explored a positive correlation between knowledge and attitude, assessed by Spearman's correlation test (Spearman's rho = 0.151, $p = 0.014$). Similar to the present study's results, Al-Khafaji et al., in 2021, and Odeja et al., in 2019, also revealed the same findings [16,27].

5. Strengths and Weaknesses of the Present Study

The current survey is the first of its kind in the northern region of Saudi Arabia and was conducted recently. We also used a standard and validated data collection tool. However, cross-sectional and questionnaire-related survey biases, such as self-selection bias, could have influenced the results. Additionally, the study is limited to northern regions, and the findings may not be suitable for other regions of Saudi Arabia.

6. Conclusions

The present study explored inadequate knowledge of OSA among primary care physicians, and we also examined a positive correlation between knowledge and attitude among PCPs. Hence, improving PCPs' knowledge regarding OSA and the necessity for referral in this region arise recommended through the use of different training methods. Furthermore, the study findings highlight the need to include appropriate OSA programs and CME for PCPs, effective OSA education for undergraduates, and enhanced residency training with the provision of sleep medicine rotations, lectures, and workshops on OSA screening, diagnosis, and management.

Author Contributions: Conceptualization, A.N.A.-R., A.T., O.A. and A.D.; methodology, A.T., A.A., S.A., H.A., W.A. and F.A.; software, F.A., O.A. and A.D.; validation, A.N.A.-R., A.T., A.A., H.A. and A.D.; formal analysis, A.T. and W.A.; investigation, A.N.A.-R., A.A. and S.A.; resources, A.N.A.-R. and A.A.; data curation, S.A., H.A., W.A., F.A., O.A. and A.D.; writing—original draft preparation, A.N.A.-R., A.T., A.A., S.A. and H.A.; writing—review and editing, W.A., F.A., O.A. and A.D.; visualization, H.A., O.A. and A.D.; supervision, A.N.A.-R. and S.A.; project administration, F.A., O.A. and A.D.; funding acquisition, A.N.A.-R. All authors have read and agreed to the published version of the manuscript.

Funding: This research received no external funding.

Institutional Review Board Statement: The study was conducted in accordance with the Declaration of Helsinki and approved by the regional health affairs ethics committee (Qurrayat, Wide approval no. 120).

Informed Consent Statement: Informed consent was obtained from all subjects involved in the study.

Data Availability Statement: The raw SPSS data used in the present study is available upon request from the corresponding author.

Acknowledgments: The authors thank the primary care physicians who participated in the present study.

Conflicts of Interest: The authors declare no conflict of interest.

References

1. CDC. CDC—Data and Statistics—Sleep and Sleep Disorders. Available online: https://www.cdc.gov/sleep/data_statistics.html (accessed on 15 March 2022).
2. Almeneessier, A.S.; BaHammam, A.S. Sleep Medicine in Saudi Arabia. *J. Clin. Sleep Med.* **2017**, *13*, 641–645. [CrossRef]
3. Wali, S.O.; Abalkhail, B.; Krayem, A. Prevalence and risk factors of obstructive sleep apnea syndrome in a Saudi Arabian population. *Ann. Thorac Med.* **2017**, *12*, 88–94. [CrossRef]
4. Alsultan, A.; Al Sahlawi, M.; Agha, M. Prevalence of Obstructive Sleep Apnea Symptoms Among the Adult Population in Al-Ahsa, Saudi Arabia. *Cureus* **2022**, *14*, e31082. [CrossRef]
5. Alhejaili, F.; Hafez, A.; Wali, S.; Alshumrani, R.; Alzehairi, A.M.; Balkhyour, M.; Pandi-Perumal, S.R. Prevalence of Obstructive Sleep Apnea Among Saudi Pilots. *Nat. Sci. Sleep* **2021**, *13*, 537–545. [CrossRef]
6. Almeneessier, A.S.; Alangari, M.; Aldubayan, A.; Alsharidah, A.; Altaki, A.; Olaish, A.H.; Sabr, Y.S.; BaHammam, A.S. Prevalence of symptoms and risk of obstructive sleep apnea in Saudi pregnant women. *Ann. Thorac. Med.* **2020**, *15*, 163. [CrossRef]
7. Karna, B.; Sankari, A.; Tatikonda, G. Sleep disorder. In *StatPearls*; StatPearls Publishing: Treasure Island, FL, USA, 2022.
8. Medic, G.; Wille, M.; Hemels, M.E. Short- and long-term health consequences of sleep disruption. *Nat. Sci. Sleep* **2017**, *9*, 151–161. [CrossRef] [PubMed]
9. Benjafield, A.V.; Ayas, N.T.; Eastwood, P.R.; Heinzer, R.; Ip, M.S.M.; Morrell, M.J.; Nunez, C.M.; Patel, S.R.; Penzel, T.; Pépin, J.L.; et al. Estimation of the global prevalence and burden of obstructive sleep apnoea: A literature-based analysis. *Lancet Respir. Med.* **2019**, *7*, 687–698. [CrossRef]
10. Peppard, P.E.; Young, T.; Barnet, J.H.; Palta, M.; Hagen, E.W.; Hla, K.M. Increased prevalence of sleep-disordered breathing in adults. *Am. J. Epidemiol.* **2013**, *177*, 1006–1014. [CrossRef] [PubMed]
11. Senaratna, C.V.; Perret, J.L.; Lodge, C.J.; Lowe, A.J.; Campbell, B.E.; Matheson, M.C.; Hamilton, G.S.; Dharmage, S.C. Prevalence of obstructive sleep apnea in the general population: A systematic review. *Sleep Med. Rev.* **2017**, *34*, 70–81. [CrossRef] [PubMed]
12. Chung, S.A.; Jairam, S.; Hussain, M.R.; Shapiro, C.M. Knowledge of sleep apnea in a sample grouping of primary care physicians. *Sleep Breath* **2001**, *5*, 115–121. [CrossRef]
13. Thirunavukkarasu, A.; Almulhim, A.K.; Albalawi, F.A.; Alruwaili, Z.M.; Almajed, O.A.; Alruwaili, S.H.; Almugharriq, M.M.; Alruwaili, A.S.; Alkuwaykibi, M.K. Knowledge, Attitudes, and Practices towards Diabetic Retinopathy among Primary Care Physicians of Saudi Arabia: A Multicenter Cross-Sectional Study. *Healthcare* **2021**, *9*, 1697. [CrossRef] [PubMed]
14. Devaraj, N.K. Knowledge, attitude, and practice regarding obstructive sleep apnea among primary care physicians. *Sleep Breath* **2020**, *24*, 1581–1590. [CrossRef] [PubMed]
15. Miller, J.N.; Berger, A.M. Screening and assessment for obstructive sleep apnea in primary care. *Sleep Med. Rev.* **2016**, *29*, 41–51. [CrossRef] [PubMed]
16. Al-Khafaji, H.; Bilgay, I.B.; Tamim, H.; Hoteit, R.; Assaf, G. Knowledge and attitude of primary care physicians towards obstructive sleep apnea in the Middle East and North Africa region. *Sleep Breath* **2021**, *25*, 579–585. [CrossRef] [PubMed]
17. Ansari, S.; Hu, A. Knowledge and confidence in managing obstructive sleep apnea patients in Canadian otolaryngology—Head and neck surgery residents: A cross sectional survey. *J. Otolaryngol. Head Neck Surg.* **2020**, *49*, 21. [CrossRef] [PubMed]
18. Hodibi, M.; Aljubran, Z.; Sattar, A. Knowledge and attitude of primary health care physicians in Al-hasa towards obstructive sleep apnea. *Hypertension* **2020**, *77*, 114.
19. Devani, N.; Aslan, T.; Leske, F.; Mansell, S.K.; Morgan, S.; Mandal, S. Integrated diagnostic pathway for patients referred with suspected OSA: A model for collaboration across the primary-secondary care interface. *BMJ Open Respir. Res.* **2020**, *7*, e000743. [CrossRef]
20. Cochran, W.G. *Sampling Techniques*; John Wiley & Sons: Hoboken, NJ, USA, 1977.
21. Schotland, H.M.; Jeffe, D.B. Development of the obstructive sleep apnea knowledge and attitudes (OSAKA) questionnaire. *Sleep Med.* **2003**, *4*, 443–450. [CrossRef]
22. Thirunavukkarasu, A.; Al-Hazmi, A.H.; Dar, U.F.; Alruwaili, A.M.; Alsharari, S.D.; Alazmi, F.A.; Alruwaili, S.F.; Alarjan, A.M. Knowledge, attitude and practice towards bio-medical waste management among healthcare workers: A northern Saudi study. *PeerJ* **2022**, *10*, e13773. [CrossRef]

23. Asdaq, S.M.B.; Alshari, A.S.; Imran, M.; Sreeharsha, N.; Sultana, R. Knowledge, attitude and practices of healthcare professionals of Riyadh, Saudi Arabia towards COVID-19: A cross-sectional study. *Saudi J. Biol. Sci.* **2021**, *28*, 5275–5282. [CrossRef]
24. Corso, R.M.; Sorbello, M.; Buccioli, M.; Carretta, E.; Nanni, O.; Piraccini, E.; Merli, G.; Petrini, F.; Guarino, A.; Frova, G. Survey of Knowledge and Attitudes about Obstructive Sleep Apnoea Among Italian Anaesthetists. *Turk. J. Anaesthesiol. Reanim.* **2017**, *45*, 146–152. [CrossRef] [PubMed]
25. Embarak, S.; Zake, L.G.; Abd-El-Azem, W.; Sileem, A.E. Awareness of obstructive sleep apnea among critical care physicians in Sharkia Governorate, Egypt. *Egypt. J. Bronchol.* **2020**, *14*, 6. [CrossRef]
26. Chérrez-Ojeda, I.; Calderón, J.C.; Fernández García, A.; Jeffe, D.B.; Santoro, I.; Vanegas, E.; Cherrez, A.; Cano, J.; Betancourt, F.; Simancas-Racines, D. Obstructive sleep apnea knowledge and attitudes among recent medical graduates training in Ecuador. *Multidiscip. Respir. Med.* **2018**, *13*, 5. [CrossRef] [PubMed]
27. Cherrez Ojeda, I.; Jeffe, D.B.; Guerrero, T.; Mantilla, R.; Santoro, I.; Gabino, G.; Calderon, J.C.; Caballero, F.; Mori, J.; Cherrez, A. Attitudes and knowledge about obstructive sleep apnea among Latin American primary care physicians. *Sleep Med.* **2013**, *14*, 973–977. [CrossRef] [PubMed]
28. Chang, J.R.; Akemokwe, F.M.; Marangu, D.M.; Chisunkha, B.; Irekpita, E.; Obasikene, G.; Kagima, J.W.; Obonyo, C.O. Obstructive Sleep Apnea Awareness among Primary Care Physicians in Africa. *Ann. Am. Thorac Soc.* **2020**, *17*, 98–106. [CrossRef] [PubMed]
29. Simmons, M.; Sayre, J.; Schotland, H.; Jeffe, D. Obstructive sleep apnea knowledge among dentists and physicians. *J. Dent. Sleep Med.* **2021**, *8*. [CrossRef]
30. Alshehri, A.M.; Alshehri, M.S.; Alamri, O.M.; Alshehri, F.S.; Alshahrani, M.; Alflan, M.A.; Alshahrani, M.S. Knowledge, Awareness, and Attitudes Toward Obstructive Sleep Apnea among the Population of the Asir Region of Saudi Arabia in 2019. *Cureus* **2020**, *12*, e7254. [CrossRef]
31. Bendapudi, N.M.; Berry, L.L.; Frey, K.A.; Parish, J.T.; Rayburn, W.L. Patients' perspectives on ideal physician behaviors. *Mayo Clin. Proc.* **2006**, *81*, 338–344. [CrossRef]
32. Howard, M.; Langevin, J.; Bernard, C.; Tan, A.; Klein, D.; Slaven, M.; Barwich, D.; Elston, D.; Arora, N.; Heyland, D.K. Primary care clinicians' confidence, willingness participation and perceptions of roles in advance care planning discussions with patients: A multi-site survey. *Fam. Pract.* **2020**, *37*, 219–226. [CrossRef]
33. Owens, K.M.; Keller, S. Exploring workforce confidence and patient experiences: A quantitative analysis. *Patient Exp. J.* **2018**, *5*, 97–105. [CrossRef]

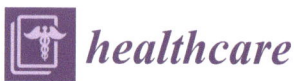

Article

The Impact of Mouth-Taping in Mouth-Breathers with Mild Obstructive Sleep Apnea: A Preliminary Study

Yi-Chieh Lee [1,2], Chun-Ting Lu [3], Wen-Nuan Cheng [4] and Hsueh-Yu Li [1,*]

[1] Department of Otolaryngology Head & Neck Surgery, Chang Gung Memorial Hospital at Linkou, 5 Fushing St., Taoyuan 333, Taiwan
[2] London School of Hygiene and Tropical Medicine, London WC1E 7HT, UK
[3] Department of Otolaryngology-Head and Neck Surgery, New Taipei Municipal Tucheng Hospital (Built and Operated by Chang Gung Medical Foundation), New Taipei City 236, Taiwan
[4] Department of Sports Sciences, University of Taipei, Taipei 100, Taiwan
* Correspondence: hyli38@cgmh.org.tw; Tel.: +886-3-3281200 (ext. 3966); Fax: +886-3-3979361

Abstract: Background: Many patients with obstructive sleep apnea (OSA) are mouth-breathers. Mouth-breathing not only narrows the upper airway, consequently worsening the severity of OSA, but also it affects compliance with nasal continuous positive airway pressure (CPAP) treatment. This study aimed to investigate changes in OSA by the use of mouth tape in mouth-breathers with mild OSA. Method: Mouth-breathers with mild OSA who met inclusion criteria and tolerated the sealing of the mouth were enrolled in the study. We used 3M silicone hypoallergenic tape was used to seal the mouths of the participants during sleep. The home sleep test (HST) used in this study was ApneaLink®. Subjects received both a baseline HST and an outcome HST to be used 1 week later while their mouths were taped. The changes between the baseline and the outcome HSTs were compared, and the factors that influenced the differences in the sleep-test parameters after the shift of the breathing route were analyzed. A "responder" was defined as a patient who experienced a reduction from the baseline snoring index of at least 50% under mouth-taping in the HST; otherwise, patients were considered as having a poor response. Results: A total of 20 patients with mild OSA were included. Following the taping of the mouth, a good response was found in 13 patients (65%). The median apnea/hypopnea index (AHI) decreased significantly, from 8.3 to 4.7 event/h (by 47%, $p = 0.0002$), especially in supine AHI (9.4 vs. 5.5 event/h, $p = 0.0001$). The median snoring index (SI) was also improved (by 47%, 303.8 vs. 121.1 event/h, $p = 0.0002$). Despite no significant difference in the mean saturation, improvements in the oxygen desaturation index (8.7 vs. 5.8, $p = 0.0003$) and the lowest saturation (82.5% vs. 87%, $p = 0.049$) were noted. The change in AHI was associated with baseline AHI ($r = -0.52$, $p = 0.02$), oxygen desaturation index (ODI) ($r = -0.54$, $p = 0.01$), and SI ($r = -0.47$, $p = 0.04$). The change in SI was strongly associated with baseline SI ($r = -0.77$, $p = 0.001$). Conclusions: Mouth-taping during sleep improved snoring and the severity of sleep apnea in mouth-breathers with mild OSA, with AHI and SI being reduced by about half. The higher the level of baseline AHI and SI, the greater the improvement was shown after mouth-taping. Mouth-taping could be an alternative treatment in patients with mild OSA before turning to CPAP therapy or surgical intervention.

Keywords: obstructive sleep apnea; snoring; mouth-taping; mouth-breathing

1. Introduction

Preferentially, people breathe through the nasal route for its physiological functions—heating, humidifying, and filtration—during the daytime and while sleeping. During the daytime, the resistance of the upper airway is similar in nasal-breathing and mouth-breathing [1,2]. During sleep, the resistance is lower in those breathing through the nasal route than in those breathing through the mouth [1,2]. Therefore, the fraction of mouth-breathing normally decreases during sleep. However, for patients with obstructive sleep apnea (OSA), open-mouth-breathing (OMB) is a common symptom during sleep. Mouth-breathing during sleep decreases the retropalatal and retroglossal areas via the posterior displacement of the soft palate and the inferior movement of the mandible, causing a reduction in the length of the upper-airway dilator muscles, which altogether aggravates the severity of OSA [3–7].

Continuous positive airway pressure (CPAP) is the treatment of choice for obstructive sleep apnea (OSA). However, poor adherence to CPAP therapy remains the major issue for OSA patients as nearly one-third of patients cannot tolerate CPAP use after 1 month [8,9]. Studies have shown that mouth-breathing is one reason for poor adherence [10]. Overall, OMB not only affects the severity of OSA [1,5] but also the compliance with nasal CPAP therapy [1,8,10].

Chronic nasal obstruction may lead to mouth-breathing due to decreased nasal flow. Although nasal obstruction is not alone in causing OSA [4], it is frequently associated with mouth-breathing during sleep. Therefore, treating nasal congestion consequently improves mouth-breathing, sleep quality, and compliance with nasal CPAP therapy [11]. The use of mouth tape is one way to maintain nasal-breathing during sleep. A previous pilot study has demonstrated the positive effect of the use of mouth tape against mild OSA (AHI 5, <15) by reducing the AHI and snoring index [12]. However, the previous study used a specially designed tape that limited its use because of low accessibility. In this study, we adopted a widely used 3M tape with advantages (easy to adhere, easy to remove, and non-allergenic) through a simple paste method to seal off the mouth. This tape made mouth-taping easy to perform, and the results are prone to be reproducible for scientific verification. This method can also be implemented easily as a first line of treatment before turning to mainstream therapies, such as CPAP, oral appliances, or surgery. The novelty of this study is that it is a proof of concept and technique—mouth-taping can improve snoring and sleep apnea in mouth-breathers with mild OSA.

The study aimed to investigate the impact of using 3M tape to seal the mouth in mouth-breathers with mild OSA and to explore the factors that influence the reduction of snoring during the shift of the breathing route.

2. Methods

2.1. Ethics Statement

The study was approved by the Institutional Review Board (IRB) of Chang Gung Memorial Hospital (IRB no. 202201088B0) accompanied by with waivers of the participants' consent. Linkou Chang Gung Memorial Hospital is the main branch of Chang Gung Memorial Hospital. The IRB of Chang Gung Memorial Foundation is the representative and is responsible for all branches of the Chang Gung Memorial Hospital in IRB review affairs.

2.2. Study Population

This retrospective study was conducted between 2020 and 2021 in Chang Gung Memorial Hospital, Linkou Medical Center, Taoyuan, Taiwan. Eligible candidates were diagnosed with adult OSA with a major complaint of snoring.

2.3. Study Design

The **inclusion criteria** included patients between the ages of 20 and 60 years, with a body mass index (BMI) of <30 kg/m^2, AHI < 15 event/h, symptoms of sleep-disordered breathing, witnessed mouth-breathing during sleep, and dryness of throat upon waking in the morning. The **exclusion criteria** were: significant retrognathia; an allergy to mouth tape; intolerance to the sealing of the mouth (the mouth tape was dislodged from the origin site by morning); comorbidity of severe medical diseases; hypertrophy of the palatine tonsil (grade III/IV); previous nose, palate, or tongue surgery; and shift workers. For patients with nasal obstruction, medication and nasal spray were used to ameliorate clinical symptoms and facilitate mouth-taping. Since all subjects visited our clinic for the improvement of snoring, the response was therefore based on the change in snoring index. A **"responder"** was defined as a patient who experienced a reduction from the baseline snoring index of at least 50% under mouth tape in a home sleep test; otherwise, patients were considered as having a poor response.

2.4. Home Sleep Test (HST)

Because of the COVID-19 pandemic, we decided to shift away from in-lab sleep tests to HST in some of our sleep-disordered-breathing patients out of a concern for safety and to avoid a delayed diagnosis of OSA. For those patients who had a comorbidity with insomnia, other sleep disorders, or major medical diseases, standard polysomnography was arranged as usual. The HST used in this study was ApneaLink® (ResMed, Sydney, Australia), which is an ambulatory sleep monitor that can detect OSA with acceptable reliability [13,14]. Parameters were measured and analyzed automatically, and then they were reviewed and rescored by an experienced sleep specialist. Reports with incomplete data, such as insufficient recording time (<4 h), a signal that was too weak/sensor loss, or a chaotic signal were excluded, and those patients received new home sleep tests. Subjects received both a baseline HST and an outcome HST to be administered 1 week later under mouth-taping.

2.5. Mouth-Taping

The mouth tape used in the study was 3M silicone hypoallergenic tape (1 inch in length). The tape was trimmed to measure 4 cm in length and placed on the philtrum, spanning the upper and lower lips, so as to seal the mouth during sleep. The nocturnal change in airflow during mouth-breathing vs. nasal-breathing is demonstrated in Figure 1.

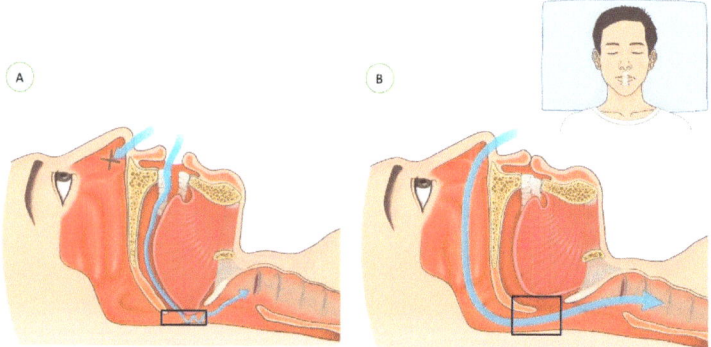

Figure 1. Figures demonstrating the breathing routes of (**A**) mouth-breathing and (**B**) nasal-breathing after mouth-taping.

2.6. Data Collection

Basic demographic information (age, sex, and body mass index) was obtained. The variables of the HST included the apnea/hypopnea index (AHI, the sum of AI and HI per hour); the apnea index (AI, decrease in airflow by 90% of baseline for at least 10 s); the hypopnea index (HI, decrease in airflow by 30% to 90% of baseline in addition to a $\geq$3% reduction of oxygen saturation for at least 10 s per hour) [13]; the supine AHI (AHI of patients in a supine position); the non-supine AHI (AHI of patients in a non-supine position); the mean saturation (the mean saturation during sleep); the lowest saturation (the lowest saturation during sleep) [15]; the 90% saturation percentage (the percentage of total time with an oxygen saturation level lower than 90%); the oxygen desaturation index (ODI, the average number of desaturation events per hour) [16]; and the snoring index (SI, the number of snoring events per hour).

2.7. Statistical Analysis

Statistical analysis was conducted using STATA v. 15 (StataCorp LLC, College Station, TX, USA). Data are presented as the median with the interquartile range (IQR, 25th–75th percentile) or number (percentage, %). Wilcoxon signed-rank tests were used to compare the baseline and outcome HST data, and Chi-square tests were used for comparing the categorical data between the groups. Spearman rank-order correlation analysis was used to evaluate the relationships between variables. A p-value < 0.05 was regarded as statistically significant.

3. Results

A total of 20 patients met the inclusion criteria and were included for further analysis. Table 1 summarizes the distribution of the baseline characteristics. The study population consisted of 19 men (95.0%) and 1 woman (5.0%) with a median age of 38 years (IQR: 30–43 years old). The median BMI was 24.5 kg/m^2 (IQR: 23.6–26.0 kg/m^2). Median AHI values before the use of the mouth tape were 8.3 (IQR: 6.2–12.9) events per hour.

Table 1. Demographic information.

	n (%) or Median (IQR)
Age (in years)	38 (30–43)
Sex (male/female)	19 (95.0%)/1 (5.0%)
Height (cm)	175 (170.9–177.25)
Weight (kg)	74 (67.7–79.5)
BMI (kg/m^2)	24.5 (23.6–26.0)

A comparison of the HST data from before and after the use of the mouth tape is shown in Table 2. The severity of OSA decreased in all participants after the mouth tape was used. Specifically, a significant reduction of values was seen in the AHI (p value = 0.0002), the AI (p value = 0.002), and the HI (0.003) (see Figure 2). The individual SI improved significantly after mouth-taping (see Figure 3). Moreover, most of the participants experienced worse symptoms in the supine position (median AHI: 9.4, IQR: 7.3–15.7) than in the non-supine position (median AHI: 3.2, IQR: 0.1–5.0). Mouth-tape use predominantly improved the OSA symptoms in the supine position, with a reduction of the median AHI from 9.4 to 5.5 events per hour (p value = 0.0001).

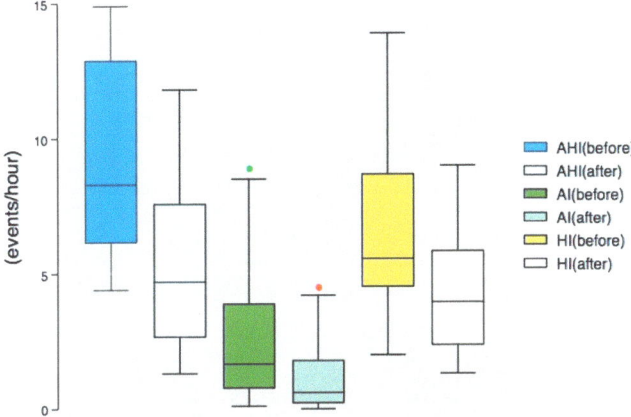

Figure 2. Box graph of apnea/hypopnea index (AHI), apnea index (AI), and hypopnea index (HI) before and after mouth-taping. (The green and red dots represent outliners of each parameter).

Table 2. HST data from before and after mouth-taping.

HST Parameters	Mouth-Breathing		Nasal-Breathing		Changes (Percentage %) †		p-Value
	Median	IQR	Median	IQR	Median	IQR	
AHI (event/h)	8.3	6.2–12.9	4.7	2.7–7.6	−47%	−59%~−23%	0.0002
AI (event/h)	1.7	0.8–3.9	0.6	0.2–1.8	−51%	−76%~−18%	0.002
HI (event/h)	5.6	4.5–8.7	4	2.4–5.9	−44%	−56%~−14%	0.003
Supine AHI (event/h)	9.4	7.3–15.7	5.5	3.8–8.9	−41%	−54%~−41%	0.0001
Non-supine AHI (event/h)	3.2	0.1–5.0	0.6	0.1–2.2	−55%	−95%~−44%	0.03
Mean saturation (%)	95	94.5–95.5	95	94.5–96	0%	−1%~1%	0.9
Lowest saturation (%)	82.5	80.5–88	87	84–89.5	2%	−1%~8%	0.049
90% saturation (%)	1	0–2.5	0	0–1	−67%	−100%~0%	0.12
ODI (event/h)	8.7	6.6–12.8	5.8	3.3–8.1	−36%	−58%~−20%	0.0003
Snoring index (event/h)	303.8	137.8–348.3	121.1	41.8–168.4	−47%	−59%~−23%	0.0002

HST: home sleep test, AHI: apnea/hypopnea index; AI: apnea index; HI: hypopnea index; ODI: oxygen desaturation index; IQR: interquartile range. † changes (percentage %) = (value of nasal-breathing − value of mouth-breathing)/value of mouth-breathing.

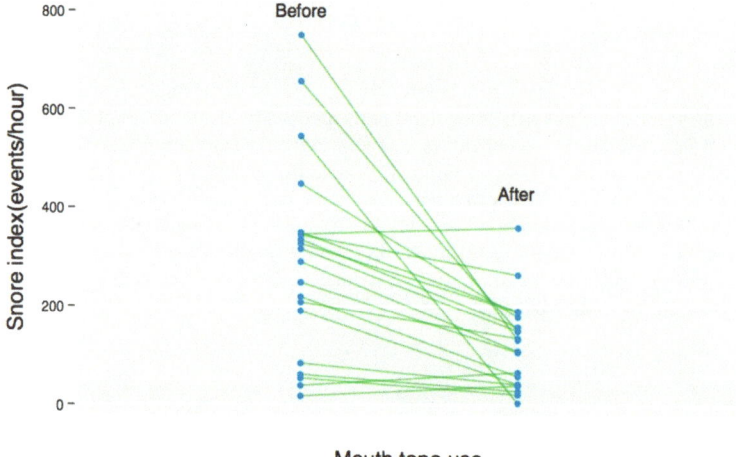

Figure 3. Individual change in snoring index (SI) before and after mouth-taping.

An association between the use of mouth tape and a change in the mean saturation and 90% saturation during sleep was not found in the study. However, significant improvements in ODI (*p* value = 0.0003) and SI (*p* value = 0.0002) were shown, from 8.7 to 5.8 and 303.8 to 121.1, respectively. No significant factors (including age, sex, BMI, and all sleep parameters) affecting response (>50% reduction from baseline snoring index) of the use of mouth tape were found in the analysis. The correlations between variables contributing to the change in the AHI and SI were also examined. A statistically significant correlation of change in AHI was seen in the baseline AHI (r = −0.52, *p* value =0.02), the baseline oxygen desaturation index (ODI) (r = −0.54, *p* value =0.01), and the baseline SI (ρ = −0.47, *p* value = 0.04). Furthermore, a change in SI was associated with a baseline SI (r = −0.77, *p* value =0.001) (see Figure 4).

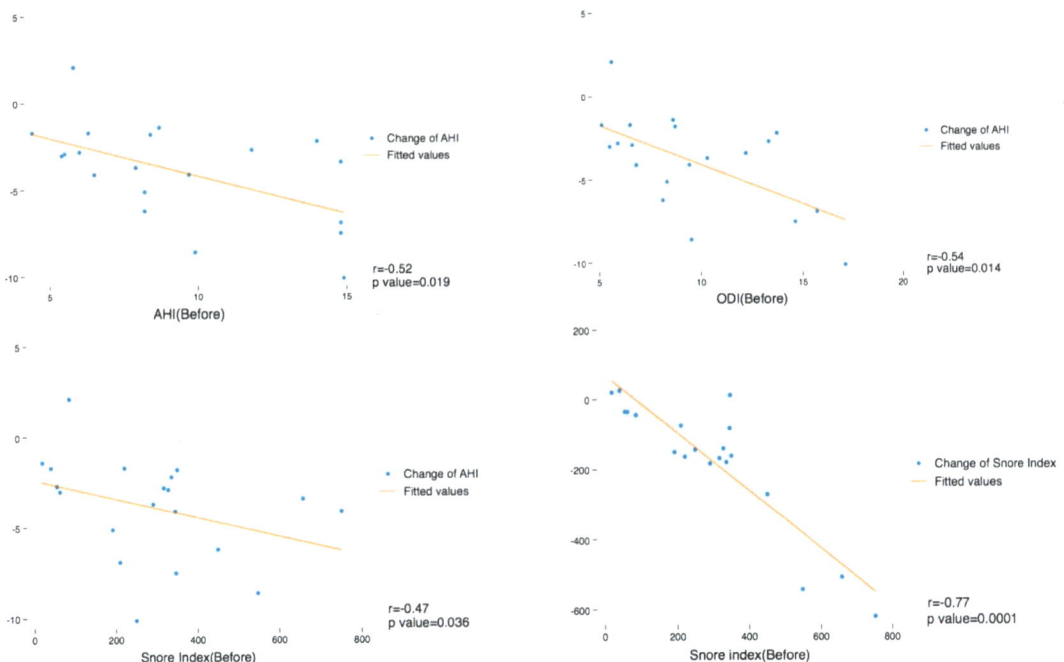

Figure 4. Correlation tests between variables (including the change of AHI from baseline AHI, ODI, and snoring index, and the change in snoring index from baseline snoring index).

4. Discussion

Studies have shown an association between OMB and OSA [1,17]. OMB elongates and narrows the upper airway, which negatively affects the severity of OSA [6]. Therefore, a higher percentage of mouth-breathers is found among people with OSA. Humans preferentially breathe through the nasal route during the daytime and while sleeping for the benefit of physiological functions. However, during sleep, people might have OMB resulting from chronic nasal obstruction or habitual mouth-breathing [3]. For people with nasal obstruction, medication and nasal spray were given before the use of mouth tape. In the study, we evaluated the potential benefits of using mouth tape in treating mild OSA patients with open-mouth-breathing (OMB). The study only enrolled patients who tolerated the use of mouth tape during sleep. The hypothesis is that taping the mouth in these patients during sleep may improve their OSA by causing them to switch from oral- to nasal-breathing.

The results showed improvements in most of the parameters in the sleep tests. There was a significant decrease ($p = 0.0002$) in AHI after the use of mouth tape. The level of the AHI was even lowered to the normal range in some participants.

In the study, most (75%) of the participants had positional sleep apnea [18,19]. The supine AHI experienced a significant reduction after the use of mouth tape (p-value: 0.0001). In a previous study, positional sleep apnea was demonstrated as being more common in mild OSA patients [19], and the obstruction site was more likely in the soft palate [20]. Lee et al. also demonstrated significant changes in the retropalatal space between the closed-mouth and the open-mouth positions due to the posterior displacement of the soft palate when the mouth is open [1]. More-elongated and narrower upper-airway spaces were also found in patients with OSA using 3D multidetector computed tomography (3D MDCT) [6]. We can infer that, after the treatment of any nasal obstruction and the switch to nasal-breathing via the taping of the mouth, the retropalatal space might be widened and therefore improve snoring and the severity of OSA. Since ODI and AHI have a good concordance, a significant reduction of ODI after mouth-taping is also conceivable [21].

No significant factor affecting the effectiveness of the use of mouth tape was seen in the analysis. However, in positional sleep apnea patients ($n = 15$), 11 (73.3%) of them were classified as responders. In comparison, only 2 (40%) out of the 5 non-positional sleep apnea patients were responders. Although the results did not show a statistical significance, that could be attributable to the small sample size as the percentage difference (33.3%) was substantial. A study with a larger sample size could be performed to investigate the effectiveness.

A statistically significant negative correlation was observed between the change of the AHI with the baseline AHI, ODI, and SI. For patients with a higher level of baseline AHI, ODI, and SI, the effectiveness of mouth-taping was greater. The improvement of the AHI was greater in the more severe cases of mild OSA, but not in the moderate or severe cases of OSA (AHI > 15). Mouth-taping is not recommended for moderate or severe OSA patients because it may impose dangers rather than benefits in these patients. Besides, a strong negative correlation between the change in SI and the baseline SI was found in the analysis, which could be a good predictor of the effectiveness of mouth-taping treatment.

In recent years, oral appliances such as mouth tape and oral shield devices have been invented and have been shown to be effective in clinical use [22]. Foellner et al. [23] showed the positive effect of using an oral shield device concomitantly with nasal CPAP. Huang et al. [12] also demonstrated the promising result of using novel oral patches for treating mild OSA. However, the device and the patch are of limited use due to their accessibility. The 3M mouth tape is already a product on the market, and it is prevalent and accessible. Moreover, the product is affordable and user-friendly. Our study highlights the utility of 3M mouth tape as an easy and inexpensive tool to mitigate the severity of OSA in selective patients.

There are some limitations to this study. First, the study has a small sample size without a control group, and no comparison could be made to determine whether there was a placebo effect. Second, this is a retrospective study with a short follow-up period, and no long-term effect was evaluated. Besides, the home sleep test used in the study may underestimate the severity of OSA. Also, the low proportion of women is another drawback. Finally, the follow-up period is short, and there could possibly be an issue of low adherence to mouth-taping in the long term. For further research, prospective studies with larger sample sizes and control groups can be done to assess the efficacy of the mouth tape.

5. Conclusions

Our study provided a simple and effective treatment modality using 3M mouth tape for mild OSA patients with open-mouth-breathing. The AHI and SI were reduced by nearly half after mouth-taping during sleep; the more severe the baseline AHI and SI, the greater the improvement after mouth-taping. For mild OSA mouth-breathers, mouth-taping could be an alternative treatment before CPAP therapy or surgical intervention are tried.

Author Contributions: Conceptualization, H.-Y.L.; methodology, H.-Y.L. and W.-N.C.; software, Y.-C.L.; validation, C.-T.L. and Y.-C.L.; formal analysis, Y.-C.L.; investigation, H.-Y.L.; resources C.-T.L.; data curation, C.-T.L.; writing—original draft preparation, Y.-C.L.; writing—review and editing, H.-Y.L.; visualization, H.-Y.L. and W.-N.C.; supervision, H.-Y.L.; project administration, H.-Y.L. All authors have read and agreed to the published version of the manuscript.

Funding: This research received no external funding.

Institutional Review Board Statement: The study was approved by the Institutional Review Board (IRB) of Chang Gung Memorial Hospital (IRB no. 202201088B0).

Informed Consent Statement: Informed consents were waived.

Data Availability Statement: The data is not publicly available due to the regulation of our institution and the protection of patients' privacy, particularly in the small sample size group. However, the data presented in the study is available on request from the corresponding author for further research.

Acknowledgments: The authors would like to express our gratitude to Yen-Ting Chiang for editing the manuscript. The authors also wish to thank Nan-Chen Huang for the original illustrations in the popular science book, *HY Li. Deep sleep every night* (in Chinese), Medicalnews/Walkers Cultural Co., Ltd. Ark Couture Publishing House.

Conflicts of Interest: The named authors have no conflicts of interest, financial or otherwise.

References

1. Lee, S.H.; Choi, J.H.; Shin, C.; Lee, H.M.; Kwon, S.Y.; Lee, S.H. How does open-mouth breathing influence upper airway anatomy? *Laryngoscope* **2007**, *117*, 1102–1106. [CrossRef] [PubMed]
2. Georgalas, C. The role of the nose in snoring and obstructive sleep apnoea: An update. *Eur. Arch. Otorhinolaryngol.* **2011**, *268*, 1365–1373. [CrossRef] [PubMed]
3. Warren, D.W.; Hairfield, W.M.; Seaton, D.; Morr, K.E.; Smith, L.R. The relationship between nasal airway size and nasal-oral breathing. *Am. J. Orthod. Dentofacial. Orthop.* **1988**, *93*, 289–293. [CrossRef]
4. Meurice, J.C.; Marc, I.; Carrier, G.; Sériès, F. Effects of mouth opening on upper airway collapsibility in normal sleeping subjects. *Am. I Respir. Crit. Care Med.* **1996**, *153*. [CrossRef]
5. Koutsourelakis, I.; Vagiakis, E.; Roussos, C.; Zakynthinos, S. Obstructive sleep apnoea and oral breathing in patients free of nasal obstruction. *Eur. Respir. J.* **2006**, *28*, 1222–1228. [CrossRef]
6. Kim, E.J.; Choi, J.H.; Kim, K.W.; Kim, T.H.; Lee, S.H.; Lee, H.M.; Shin, C.; Lee, K.Y.; Lee, S.H. The impacts of open-mouth breathing on upper airway space in obstructive sleep apnea: 3-D MDCT analysis. *Eur. Arch. Otorhinolaryngol.* **2011**, *268*, 533–539. [CrossRef]
7. Harari, D.; Redlich, M.; Miri, S.; Hamud, T.; Gross, M. The effect of mouth breathing versus nasal breathing on dentofacial and craniofacial development in orthodontic patients. *Laryngoscope* **2010**, *120*, 2089–2093. [CrossRef]
8. Bachour, A.; Maasilta, P. Mouth breathing compromises adherence to nasal continuous positive airway pressure therapy. *Chest* **2004**, *126*, 1248–1254. [CrossRef]
9. Poulet, C.; Veale, D.; Arnol, N.; Lévy, P.; Pepin, J.L.; Tyrrell, J. Psychological variables as predictors of adherence to treatment by continuous positive airway pressure. *Sleep Med.* **2009**, *10*, 993–999. [CrossRef]
10. Madeiro, F.; Andrade, R.G.S.; Piccin, V.S.; Pinheiro, G.D.L.; Moriya, H.T.; Genta, P.R.; Lorenzi-Filho, G. Transmission of Oral Pressure Compromises Oronasal CPAP Efficacy in the Treatment of OSA. *Chest* **2019**, *156*, 1187–1194. [CrossRef]
11. Bachour, A.; Hurmerinta, K.; Maasilta, P. Mouth closing device (chinstrap) reduces mouth leak during nasal CPAP. *Sleep Med.* **2004**, *5*, 261–267. [CrossRef] [PubMed]
12. Huang, T.W.; Young, T.H. Novel porous oral patches for patients with mild obstructive sleep apnea and mouth breathing: A pilot study. *Otolaryngol. Head Neck Surg.* **2015**, *152*, 369–373. [CrossRef] [PubMed]
13. Erman, M.K.; Stewart, D.; Einhorn, D.; Gordon, N.; Casal, E. Validation of the ApneaLink for the Screening of Sleep Apnea: A Novel and Simple Single-Channel Recording Device. *J. Clin. Sleep Med.* **2007**, *03*, 387–392. [CrossRef]
14. Cho, J.H.; Kim, H.J. Validation of ApneaLink Plus for the diagnosis of sleep apnea. *Sleep Breath* **2017**, *21*, 799–807. [CrossRef]
15. Marchi, N.A.; Ramponi, C.; Hirotsu, C.; Haba-Rubio, J.; Lutti, A.; Preisig, M.; Marques-Vidal, P.; Vollenweider, P.; Kherif, F.; Heinzer, R.; et al. Mean Oxygen Saturation during Sleep Is Related to Specific Brain Atrophy Pattern. *Ann. Neurol.* **2020**, *87*, 921–930. [CrossRef]
16. Temirbekov, D.; Gunes, S.; Yazici, Z.M.; Sayin, I. The Ignored Parameter in the Diagnosis of Obstructive Sleep Apnea Syndrome: The Oxygen Desaturation Index. *Turk Arch. Otorhinolaryngol.* **2018**, *56*, 1–6. [CrossRef]
17. Hsu, Y.B.; Lan, M.Y.; Huang, Y.C.; Kao, M.C.; Lan, M.C. Association Between Breathing Route, Oxygen Desaturation, and Upper Airway Morphology. *Laryngoscope* **2021**, *131*, E659–E664. [CrossRef]
18. Mador, M.J.; Kufel, T.J.; Magalang, U.J.; Rajesh, S.K.; Watwe, V.; Grant, B.J. Prevalence of Positional Sleep Apnea in Patients Undergoing Polysomnography. *Chest* **2005**, *128*, 2130–2137. [CrossRef]
19. Richard, W.; Kox, D.; den Herder, C.; Laman, M.; van Tinteren, H.; de Vries, N. The role of sleep position in obstructive sleep apnea syndrome. *Eur. Arch. Otorhinolaryngol.* **2006**, *263*, 946–950. [CrossRef]
20. Sunwoo, W.S.; Hong, S.L.; Kim, S.W.; Park, S.J.; Han, D.H.; Kim, J.W.; Lee, C.H.; Rhee, C.S. Association between Positional Dependency and Obstruction Site in Obstructive Sleep Apnea Syndrome. *Clin. Exp. Otorhinolaryngol.* **2012**, *5*, 218–221. [CrossRef]
21. Varghese, L.; Rebekah, G.; N., P.; Oliver, A.; Kurien, R. Oxygen desaturation index as alternative parameter in screening patients with severe obstructive sleep apnea. *Sleep Sci.* **2022**, *15*, 224–228. [CrossRef] [PubMed]
22. Jau, J.Y.; Kuo, T.B.J.; Li, L.P.H.; Chen, T.Y.; Lai, C.T.; Huang, P.H.; Yang, C.C.H. Mouth puffing phenomena of patients with obstructive sleep apnea when mouth-taped: Device's efficacy confirmed with physical video observation. *Sleep Breath* **2022**. [CrossRef] [PubMed]
23. Foellner, S.; Guth, P.; Jorde, I.; Lucke, E.; Ganzert, C.; Stegemann-Koniszewski, S.; Schreiber, J. Prevention of leakage due to mouth opening through applying an oral shield device (Sominpax) during nasal CPAP therapy of patients with obstructive sleep apnea. *Sleep Med.* **2020**, *66*, 168–173. [CrossRef] [PubMed]

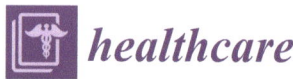

Article

Sleep Disorders and Mental Stress of Healthcare Workers during the Two First Waves of COVID-19 Pandemic: Separate Analysis for Primary Care

Athanasia Pataka [1,2,*], Seraphim Kotoulas [1,2], Asterios Tzinas [1,2], Nectaria Kasnaki [2], Evdokia Sourla [1,2], Evangelos Chatzopoulos [1,2], Ioanna Grigoriou [2] and Paraskevi Argyropoulou [1]

[1] Medical School, Aristotle University of Thessaloniki, 54124 Thessaloniki, Greece; akiskotoulas@hotmail.com (S.K.); stergiostzinas@hotmail.com (A.T.); evisou@yahoo.gr (E.S.); vaggchatz@hotmail.com (E.C.); pargyrop@auth.gr (P.A.)
[2] Respiratory Failure Unit, G. Papanikolaou Hospital, 57010 Thessaloniki, Greece; kasnakinek@gmail.com (N.K.); ioagrig@hotmail.com (I.G.)
* Correspondence: patakath@yahoo.gr

Abstract: Background: During the recent pandemic, Healthcare Professionals (HCPs) presented a significant prevalence of psychological health problems and sleep disturbances. The aim of this study was to assess the impact of COVID-19 on HCPs' sleep and mental stress with a separate analysis for primary care HCPs. Methods: A cross-sectional observational study with an online anonymized, self-reported questionnaire was conducted in May 2020 (1st wave) and repeated in December 2020 (2nd wave). Patient health questionnaire-4 (PHQ-4), dimensions of anger reactions-5 (DAR-5) scale, 3-item UCLA loneliness scale (LS) and sleep condition indicator (SCI) were used. Results: Overall, 574 participants were included from the 1st wave, 514 from the 2nd and 469 were followed during both. Anxiety and depression were significantly higher during the 2nd wave vs. the 1st (32.8% vs. 12.7%, $p < 0.001$ and 37.7% vs. 15.8%, $p < 0.001$). During the 2nd wave, HCPs scored significantly higher in DAR-5 (9.23 ± 3.82 vs. 7.3 ± 3.3, $p < 0.001$) and LS (5.88 ± 1.90 vs. 4.9 ± 1.9, $p < 0.001$) with worse sleep quality SCI (23.7 ± 6.6 vs. 25.4 ± 3.2, $p < 0.001$). This was more evident in primary care HCPs. Significant correlations were found between SCI and PHQ4, DAR5 and LS. Conclusion: There is a need to support HCPs' mental health and sleep, especially in those working in primary care.

Keywords: sleep disorders; COVID 19; waves; primary care; sleep condition indicator; anger; anxiety; depression; PHQ4; DAR-5; loneliness

1. Introduction

In December 2019, a novel coronavirus was identified (SARS-CoV-2) leading to a global pandemic and subsequently increasing the amount of pressure on Healthcare Professionals (HCPs). HCPs were exposed to situations outside their ordinary work and experienced high levels of stress and irregular schedules with frequent and long work shifts [1–3]. During the previous epidemics, such as H1N1, SARS and MERS, HCPs reported significant levels of physiological distress and sleep disorders and it has been shown that disturbed sleep is closely associated with anxiety, depression and post-traumatic stress [4–6]. During the recent pandemic, HCPs presented a significant prevalence of psychological health problems, burnout and sleep disturbances, especially insomnia [7–15]. Sleep disorders are a common problem also reported in the general population during the pandemic with prevalence similar or lower than that of HCPs. However, significant variations were observed in the literature with estimates for sleep problems among different populations ranging from 8% to 91% [16]. Patients infected from SARS-COV-2 appeared to be the most affected group with a prevalence reaching 75% [16]. Furthermore, in a recent systematic review with a meta-analysis, the rates of sleep problems were found to be comparable in both HCPs and the general population (i.e., 36% in HCPs vs. 32% in the general population) [16]. Despite the variation between different systematic reviews and meta-analysis, the pooled prevalence of sleep disorders in HCPs ranged from 36% to 45% [9,16,17].

HCPs are considered as pivotal to COVID 19 crisis management, playing a major role in screening and treating patients, especially HCPs working in primary care. Furthermore, at the beginning of the COVID 19 pandemic, the failure of providing essential care protective equipment, the rapid transmission of the disease and the lack of a definite treatment increased the feeling of insecurity, powerlessness and frustration which further increased psychological and mental health problems. Increased pressure during work results in an increased risk of adverse mental health outcomes and also sleep disorders [11–20]. Lifestyle factors such as smoking and alcohol use, the use of substances and the pre-existence of mental health disorders may influence the development of subsequent mental health conditions and sleep disorders in HCPs [21–23].

During the pandemic, the role of primary care, and primary care HCPs became more important as primary care centers were the first point of contact for patients suspected of COVID-19; additionally, the majority of hospitals were transformed into COVID 19 pandemic facilities. Primary care HCPs served in the diagnosis and treatment of suspicious or diagnosed COVID 19 cases in the hospitals, especially in the emergency departments. This led to an increase in the workload but also in the risk of primary care HCPs' exposure to COVID 19. The effect of the pandemic on the mental health and sleep of frontline HCPs has been proven to be significantly worse compared with non-frontline HCPs [24].

As the pandemic evolves, its effects on the mental health of HCPs may change. Notably, the majority of studies so far have been web-based and several of them were performed during 2020, i.e., before the initiation of vaccination [9–11,25,26]. Most of the existing research examines the impact of COVID-19 on sleep using cross-sectional surveys with questions addressing possible changes in sleep and an evaluation of changes from one time point to another (between different waves of the pandemic or before and after different lock downs) [27,28].

We hypothesized that, after experiencing the first COVID-19 wave, HCPs' level of sleep quality together with psychological distress, such as anxiety and depression, anger and loneliness, further deteriorated, especially in primary care HCPs more exposed to COVID 19. We aimed to compare the same groups of HCPs during the two first consecutive waves and to evaluate if demographic and social factors, exposure to COVID 19 and psychological distress affected sleep quality with a separate analysis for primary care HCPs.

2. Methods

This was a cross-sectional time-series study (https://dam.ukdataservice.ac.uk/media/455362/changeovertime.pdf (last accessed 8 July 2022)). The protocol was approved by the institutional review board of G Papanikolaou General Hospital, Exohi, Thessaloniki, Greece (N 876, Approval Date 20 May 2020), and all the participants provided their written electronic consent that was included in the online questionnaire before the initiation of enrolment. An information sheet with detailed explanations of the research purpose was included in the survey. For several questions, the participants were not able to continue to the next question of the survey unless they had provided a response. The participants were informed about the anonymization of the data and no incentives were offered. A pilot study was conducted from a sample of 30 HCPs working in G Papanikolaou Hospital before the initiation of data collection in both waves and these results were excluded from the survey.

The questionnaire of the study was sent to all employees of the hospitals and healthcare centers (physicians, nurses, physiotherapists, etc.) of both the public and private sector in the province of Thessaloniki, Greece, via emails delivered from the local medical and nurses associations during the first two epidemic waves of COVID-19; the first during May 2020 and the second during December 2020. The questionnaire included questions about the baseline characteristics of the participants (age, gender, marital status, children, education, occupation, job location, specialty, work in an intensive care unit (ICU) and with COVID patients), as well as alcohol consumption, smoking habits assessed by the Heaviness of Smoking Index (HSI) [29], anxiety and depression using the patient health questionnaire-4 (PHQ-4) [30], anger using the dimensions of anger reactions-5 (DAR-5) scale [31], loneliness using the 3-item UCLA loneliness scale [32], and sleep related disorders using the sleep condition indicator (SCI) [33]. During the follow up of the HCPs (second wave), the questionnaire included a question asking the participants to declare whether they had completed the questionnaire previously. From this question and by crosschecking with the demographics of the participants, we managed to maintain the same groups of HCPs that were followed up during both waves and measured the variables in the same respondents over time.

The HSI is a questionnaire that evaluates nicotine dependence by using only the following two items: the time to first cigarette in the morning and the number of cigarettes per day. Scores ranging from 0 to 2 indicate low addiction, from 3 to 4 moderate addiction and from 5 to 6 high addiction [29].

The PHQ4 [30] is a brief screening scale for the evaluation of anxiety and depression consisting of 4 questions rated from 0 to 3. The total score of PHQ4 is determined by the addition of each of the 4 questions together with scores from 0–2 rated as normal, 3–5 as mild, 6–8 as moderate and 9–12 as severe. If the total score of the first two questions is ≥ 3, anxiety is suggested, whereas if the total score of the last two questions is ≥ 3, depression is suggested [30].

The DAR-5 [31] is a 5-item self-report five-point Likert scale, ranging from 1–5, which is used for the assessment of anger intensity, duration, frequency and impact on social functioning over a 4-week period. The total score ranges from 5 to 25 with higher scores indicating worse symptomatology. A cut-off score of above 12 is indicative of functional impairment and psychological distress related to anger [31].

The UCLA loneliness scale comprises of three questions that evaluate three dimensions of loneliness (relational and social connectedness and self-assessed isolation). The scores for each question are added together with a range of scores from 3 to 9; with individuals with scores of 6–9 characterized as "lonely" [32].

The SCI [33] is an eight-item scale, based upon DSM-5 insomnia criteria, comprising two items evaluating sleep continuity, two items evaluating sleep satisfaction or dissatisfaction, two items evaluating the severity of the sleep disorder (nights per week; duration of problem) and two evaluating the daytime consequences of poor sleep (effects on mood, energy or relationships, concentration, daytime performance). Each item is scored on a five-point scale (0–4), with lower scores (ranging from 0 to 2) reflecting DSM-5 threshold criteria for insomnia disorder. Total SCI scores ranged from 0 to 32, with higher values indicating better sleep. An SCI score of ≤ 16 was found to be indicative of possible insomnia disorder [33,34].

3. Statistical Analysis

Statistical analysis was performed using SPSS (version-20 IBM-SPSS-statistical-software, Armonk, NY, USA). Continuous variables were presented as mean ± SD and categorical variables as number (%). $p < 0.05$ was accepted as statistically significant. The normality of continuous data was assessed using the Kolmogorov–Smirnov test. For the detection of statistically significant differences between the whole population of responders of the two waves, independent-samples-T-test for parametric and the Mann–Whitney-U-test for non-parametric variables were used. Paired t-test or McNemar's test were used to compare the same HCPs that were followed up during both the first and second waves for parametric and non-parametric variables, respectively. A chi-square was used for the detection of significant differences between the two waves in categorical variables. Regression analyses were performed to evaluate the association of predictive factors with changes in sleep quality across the two time points, whereas Pearson's Correlation was used to explore the associations of different of factors (SCI, PHQ4, DAR5, LS) in the two different waves. Variables including age, gender, employment status (working in primary care or not, working in the private sector), depression, anxiety, anger and loneliness were included. Associations between different risk factors and poor sleep quality, assessed by SCI cut off 16, were determined with binary logistic regression analysis. The identified covariates were presented in terms of correlation coefficient (r or R2). Additionally, a separate analysis was performed only for primary care HCPs. G*Power software was used to calculate the sample size showing that a sample size of 248 would be required for an expected effect size of d = 0.55, an alpha of 5%, and beta of 20% for two groups with an allocation ratio of 1.8 when performing Mann–Whitney U tests.

4. Results

Five hundred and seventy-four participants answered the questionnaire during the first wave, 514 during the second wave and 469 were followed during both the waves. The socio-demographic characteristics of the participants of the two groups were comparable, apart from the absence of physiotherapists among the participants from the second wave (Table 1). It was also evident that during the second wave, the participants had been treating COVID-19 patients more often than in the first ($p < 0.001$). According to the answers of the PHQ-4 questionnaire, HCPs presented significantly worse mental status during the second wave with more anxiety and depression symptoms (Table 1). Additionally, the participants felt angrier and lonelier compared to the first wave. They scored significantly higher in the DAR-5 and the UCLA loneliness scale (Table 1).

Table 1. Differences between socio-demographic characteristics, mental health indices and sleep quality of al the responders of the 1st and of the 2nd wave. (Mean ± s.d.).

	Wave 1 n = 574	Wave 2 n = 514	p
Age, years	45.5±11	45.1±8.2	0.4
Gender (males%)	47.4%	45.3%	0.39
Married	63.4%	64.2%	0.61
Children	33.6%	36.8%	0.4
Smoking	32.9%	33.1%	0.3
Physician	79.2%	81.8%	0.75
Pathological specialty	58.2%	59.0%	
Surgical specialty	32.7%	30.9%	0.87
Laboratory specialty	9.2%	10.1%	
Nurse	8.9%	10.7%	0.41
Physiotherapist	3.3%	0.0%	0.001
Work in ICU	9.9%	11.5%	0.22
Treating COVID 19 patients	19.3%	46.4%	<0.001
HSI	2.44 ± 1.7	2.41 ± 1.6	0.8
DAR5	7.7 ± 2.6	9.1 ± 3.6	<0.001
DAR-5 > 12	8.5%	22.4%	<0.001
LS	5.01 ± 1.6	5.9 ± 1.6	<0.001
LS > 6	35.4%	51.3%	<0.001
SCI	26.4 ± 5.7	23.4 ± 6.2	<0.001
SCI < 16	6.7%	19.7%	<0.001

Table 1. Cont.

	Wave 1 n = 574	Wave 2 n = 514	p
PHQ4	2.8 ± 2.3	4.5 ± 1.3	<0.001
Normal (0–2)	48.4%	26.9%	<0.001
Mild (3–5)	39.9%	41.0%	
Moderate (6–8)	9.6%	20.1%	
Severe (9–12)	2.1%	12.0%	
PHQ4 Anxiety	1.34 ± 1.21	2.2 ± 1.9	<0.001
PHQ4: Anxiety > 3	13.1%	33.1%	<0.001
PHQ4 Depression	1.53 ± 1.30	2.41 ± 2.1	<0.001
PHQ4: Depression > 3	16.9%	38.2%	<0.001

s.d. = standard deviation, ICU = Intensive Care Unit, HSI = Heaviness of Smoking Index, PHQ4 = patient health questionnaire-4, DAR-5 = Dimensions of Anger Reactions-5, LS = UCLA Loneliness Scale, SCI = Sleep Condition Indicator; Independent-samples-t-test for parametric and the Mann–Whitney-U-test for non-parametric variables were used for continuous variables; Chi-square was used for categorical variables.

When the mental health variables and sleep quality of the 469 respondents that were followed up during both first and second waves were compared, worse outcomes were found in all parameters. Sleep quality, anxiety, depression, anger and loneliness were significantly worse during the second wave of the pandemic (Table 2).

Table 2. Differences between socio-demographic characteristics, mental health indices and sleep quality of the responders that were followed up during both first and second waves (Mean ± s.d.).

	Wave 1 n = 469	Wave 2 n = 469	p
Work in ICU	9.2%	12.8%	0.08
Treating COVID 19 patients	21.%	48.6%	<0.001
HSI	2.3 ± 1.8	2.4 ± 1.7	0.78
DAR5	7.3 ± 3.3	9.2 ± 3.8	<0.001
DAR-5 > 12	7.6%	22.0%	<0.001
LS	4.9 ± 1.6	5.9 ± 1.9	<0.001
LS>6	34.1%	54.3%	<0.001
SCI	25.4 ± 3.2	23.7 ± 6.6	<0.001
SCI<16	6.1%	18.6%	<0.001
PHQ4	2.7 ± 3.4	4.4 ± 2.9	<0.001
Normal (0–2)	49.1%	26.2%	<0.001
Mild (3–5)	40.1%	42.0%	
Moderate (6–8)	8.9%	20.3%	
Severe (9–12)	1.9%	11.5%	
PHQ4 Anxiety	1.29 ± 1.26	2.08 ± 1.58	<0.001
PHQ4: Anxiety > 3	12.7%	32.8%	<0.001
PHQ4 Depression	1.47 ± 1.2	2.38 ± 1.60	<0.001
PHQ4: Depression > 3	15.8%	37.7%	<0.001

s.d. = standard deviation, ICU = Intensive Care Unit, HSI = Heaviness of Smoking Index, PHQ4 = patient health questionnaire-4, DAR-5 = Dimensions of Anger Reactions-5, LS = UCLA Loneliness Scale, SCI = Sleep Condition Indicator; Paired t-test or McNemar's test were used for parametric and non-parametric variables, respectively. Chi-square was used for categorical variables.

During the second wave, the participants presented significantly worse sleep quantity ($p < 0.001$) and quality ($p < 0.001$) with more awakenings compared with the first wave with 46.8% reporting that they experienced problems with their sleep $2 \geq$ nights per week (Table 3). Additionally, 16.3% of HCPs, compared with 5.7% in the first wave, thought that poor sleep affected their mood, energy or relationships during the past month, whereas 11.7% vs. 5.5% thought that poor sleep affected their productivity, concentration and ability to stay awake (Table 3). Almost 11% of HCPs during the second wave believed that poor sleep caused trouble to them in general, compared with 4.3% in the first (Table 3). During the second wave, a significantly lower total score in the SCI (23.7 ± 6.6 vs. 25.4 ± 3.2, $p < 0.001$) was found, a fact that meant more frequent insomnia symptoms with a SCI cut off 16 (18.6% vs. 6.1%, $p < 0.001$) (Table 2).

Table 3. Comparison of sleep-related variables of participants followed up during the 1st and 2nd wave.

		1st Lockdown ($n = 469$)	2nd Lockdown ($n = 469$)	p (Value)
What is the quality of your sleep during the pandemic compared to before that?	Worse	15.7%	32.8%	<0.001
	The same	71.1%	62.7%	
	Better	13.2%	4.5%	
The last 2–3 weeks how much of a problem were any episodes of awakening during your sleep?	No problem at all	43.2%	35.8%	<0.001
	Small problem	39.9%	37.7%	
	Moderate problem	15.7%	22.6%	
	Great problem	1.2%	3.8%	
Do you use sleeping pills?	I do not use	93.0%	92.3%	0.67
	I was using them before the lockdown	4.9%	4.7%	
	I started using them during the lockdown	2.1%	3.0%	
SCI: How long does it take you to fall asleep?	> 60 min (0)	4.9%	6.0%	<0.001
	46–60 min (1)	0.0%	13.9%	
	31–45 min (2)	0.0%	2.3%	
	16–30 min (3)	40.4%	31.8%	
	0–15 min (4)	54.7%	46.1%)	
SCI: If you then wake up during the night ... how long are you awake for in total? (add up all the awakenings)	> 60 min (0)	2.6%	5.8%	<0.001
	46–60 min (1)	7.7%	0.0%	
	31–45 min (2)	0.0%	10.0%	
	16–30 min (3)	12.9%	16.0%	
	0–15 min (4)	76.8%	68.2%	
SCI: How many nights a week do you have a problem with your sleep?	5–7 nights (0)	5.9%	10.7%	0.002
	4 nights (1)	6.4%	8.1%	
	3 nights (2)	8.9%	12.4%	
	2 nights (3)	13.9%	15.6%	
	0–1 nights (4)	64.8%	53.3%	

Table 3. Cont.

		1st Lockdown (n = 469)	2nd Lockdown (n = 469)	p (Value)
SCI: How would you rate your sleep quality?	Very poor (0)	0.3%	0.4%	<0.001
	Poor (1)	6.3%	0.0%	
	Average (2)	24.6%	17.3%	
	Good (3)	0.0%	28.8%	
	Very good (4)	68.8%	53.5%	
SCI: Thinking about the past month, to what extent has poor sleep affected your mood, energy, or relationships?	Very much (0)	1.2%	2.6%	<0.001
	Much (1)	4.5%	13.7%	
	Somewhat (2)	17.6%	25.1%	
	A little (3)	20.7%	19.8%	
	Not at all (4)	56.0%	38.8%	
SCI: Thinking about the past month, to what extent has poor sleep affected your concentration, productivity, or ability to stay awake?	Very much (0)	0.5%	2.3%	<0.001
	Much (1)	5.0%	9.4%	
	Somewhat (2)	16.3%	25.5%	
	A little (3)	18.0%	21.4%	
	Not at all (4)	60.2%	41.3%	
SCI: Thinking about the past month, to what extent has poor sleep troubled you in general?	Very much (0)	0.7%	1.8%	<0.001
	Much (1)	3.6%	9.1%	
	Somewhat (2)	12.2%	26.2%	
	A little (3)	18.7%	20.9%	
	Not at all (4)	64.8%	42.1%	
SCI: How long have you had a problem with your sleep?	>12 months (0)	10.3%	11.3%	<0.001
	7–12 months (1)	1.2%	5.6%	
	3–6 months (2)	2.8%	4.9%	
	1–2 months (3)	11.1%	11.5%	
	<1 month/I do not have a problem (4)	74.6%	66.7%	

s.d. = standard deviation, SCI = sleep condition indicator; Chi-square was used for categorical variables.

In a separate analysis of primary care HCPs, there were statistically significant differences between them and all the other HCPs, as they were younger, mostly female, and experienced a worse quality of sleep, more anxiety, anger and loneliness (Table 4). These differences were more evident during the first wave of the pandemic. During the second wave, no significant differences were observed between the groups of HCPs, with similar scores in SCI, PHQ4, DAR5 and LS. However, when the sleep quality, depression, anxiety, anger and loneliness of each group of HCPs, i.e., primary care HCPs or all the others, were compared between the two waves, significant aggravation was found in almost all variables and in both groups (Table 4).

In the regression analysis, the predictors that mostly affected sleep quality during the first wave were being a primary care HCP, being married and psychological distress assessed by PHQ4. However, during the second wave, the most important factors were again psychological distress, anger and loneliness, but not marital status and being a primary care HCP. Parenthood did not associate with sleep quality as assessed with SCI. Treating COVID patients did not have a significant effect on the quality of sleep of HCPs. In the separate analysis of primary HCPs, the most significant factor that affected sleep quality during the first wave was PHQ4, and during the second wave additionally DAR5 and loneliness (Table 5). Treating COVID 19 patients, parenthood and marital status were not associated with the sleep quality of primary care HCPs in the regression analysis during both waves.

Table 4. Comparison between primary care HCPs with all the others participants during the 1st and 2nd wave.

	Primary Care HCP 1st Wave $n = 236$	All the Others 1st Wave $n = 233$	p	Primary Care HCP 2nd Wave $n = 236$	All the Others 2nd Wave $n = 233$	p
Age	43.4 ± 11.1	47 ± 12.8	0.003	43.4 ± 11.1	47 ± 12.8	0.003
Gender (male%)	38.5%	49.3%	0.01	38.5%	49.3%	0.01
Married	59.7%	72.1%	0.004	59.7%	72.1%	0.004
HSI	2.2 ± 1.6	2.6 ± 1.7	0.07	2.3 ± 1.6	2.3 ± 1.7	0.8
SCITOTAL	25.4 ± 6.2 **	27.4 ± 5.2 *	0.001	23 ± 6.6 **	24.3 ± 6.4 *	0.1
SCI < 16	11.5% $	5.1% ***	0.02	20.6% $	14.3% ***	0.15
PHQ4TOTAL	3.15 ± 2.3 *	2.5 ± 2.2 *	0.001	4.65 ± 3 *	4.1 ± 2.8 *	0.07
PHQ4-anxiety ≥ 3	14.8% *	9.3% *	0.05	36% *	29.3% *	0.15
PHQ4-depression ≥ 3	17.8%*	14.9% *	0.4	40.6% *	34.2% *	0.19
DAR5TOTAL	8 ± 2.6 *	7.2 ± 2.5 *	0.001	9.3 ± 3.9 *	8.8 ± 3.3 *	0.18
DAR5≥12	9.7%*	6.7%*	0.2	23.5% *	17.3% *	0.12
LONELINESTOTAL	5.2 ± 1.7 *	4.8 ± 1.6 *	0.009	5.9 ± 1.9 *	5.7 ± 1.85 *	0.5
LS > 6	38.4% ***	29.9% *	0.04	53.4% ***	52.7% *	0.9

HIS = Heaviness of Smoking Index, PHQ4 = patient health questionnaire-4, DAR-5 = Dimensions of Anger Reactions-5, LS = UCLA Loneliness Scale, SCI = Sleep Condition Indicator; Independent-samples-T-test for parametric and the Mann–Whitney-U-test for non parametric continuous variables were used to compare between the different groups of HCPs; Paired t-test or McNemar's test were used for parametric and non-parametric variables, respectively in order to compare the same group during the two waves; Chi-square was used for categorical variables * comparison between 1st and 2nd wave $p < 0.001$ ** $p = 0.002$ *** $p = 0.003$, $ $p = 0.05$.

Table 5. Multiple regression analysis examining the association between sleep quality and characteristics of the population of HCPs and separately of primary care HCPs followed during the 1st and the 2nd waves.

	All Population ($n = 469$)					
Variables	Standardized β	t	p	R	R2	Adjusted R2
SCI 1st				0.58	0.34	0.32
age	−0.057	−1.25	0.2			
gender	−0.04	−0.85	0.4			
MARRIED	0.12	2.12	0.03			
Primary care HCP	0.092	2.045	0.04			
PHQ4	−0.49	−8.42	<0.001			
DAR5	−0.096	−1.75	0.08			
LONELINESS	−0.13	0.257	0.8			
Treating COVID patients	−0.057	−1.31	0.2			
SCI 2nd				0.616	0.38	0.36

Table 5. Cont.

Variables	Standardized β	t	p	R	R2	Adjusted R2
All Population (n = 4 69)						
age	0.11	1.29	0.2			
gender	−0.019	−0.228	0.8			
Married	−0.04	−0.67	0.5			
Primary care HCP	0.013	0.27	0.19			
PHQ4	−0.33	−4.9	<0.001			
DAR5	−0.17	−2.8	0.005			
LONELINESS	−0.23	−4.05	<0.001			
Treating COVID patients	−0.06	−1.16	0.25			
Only primary care (n = 236)						
SCI 1st				0.62	0.38	0.36
age	−0.04	−0.04	0.5			
gender	−0.03	−0.59	0.6			
PHQ4	−0.55	−6.85	<0.001			
DAR5	−0.065	−0.37	0.7			
LONELINESS	0.07	0.97	0.6			
Treating COVID patients	−0.08	−1.23	0.2			
SCI 2nd				0.59	0.35	0.32
age	−0.09	−1.13	0.3			
gender	−0.07	0.88	0.42			
PHQ4	−0.24	−2.34	0.02			
DAR5	−0.23	−2.5	0.015			
LONELINESS	−0.3	−3.6	<0.001			
Treating COVID patients	0.04	0.49	0.6			

PHQ4 = patient health questionnaire-4, DAR-5 = Dimensions of Anger Reactions-5, LS = UCLA Loneliness Scale, SCI = Sleep Condition Indicator.

In a separate gender analysis, the multiple regression analysis (age, primary care or not, PHQ4, DAR5, LS, HIS) revealed that apart from PHQ4, treating COVID patients (β = −0.175, t = −2.7, p = 0.008) and DAR5 (β = −0.16, t = −2.04, p = 0.04) were significantly associated with sleep quality (SCI) in men but only during the first wave. During the second wave in men, and in both waves in women, the associations did not differ from the analysis for both genders together (Table 5). The only factor associated with SCI cut off 16 was PHQ4 in men (OR: 1.94, 95% Confidential Interval 1.13–3.31, p = 0.015), but not women (OR: 1.6, 95% Confidential Interval 0.64–4.01, p = 0.21) and only during the first wave.

In the further analysis of psychological distress assessed by the PHQ4, marital status and parenthood did not associate with anxiety and depression. PHQ4 significantly associated with SCI, DAR5, Loneliness (p < 0.001) and female gender (p < 0.04) in both waves. Significant negative correlations were found between SCI and PHQ4, DAR5 and LS for all the participants in both waves and also in the separate analysis for primary care HCPs (Table 6).

Table 6. Correlation of sleep quality with mood changes, anger and loneliness during the two waves. Analysis of all participants and separately for primary care.

	PHQ4	p	DAR5	p	LS	p	HSI	p
	All Participants (n = 469)							
SCI 1st	−0.61	<0.001	−0.395	<0.001	−0.28	<0.001	−0.2	0.15
SCI 2nd	−0.46	<0.001	−0.45	<0.001	−0.45	<0.001	0.19	0.2
	Only Primary Care (n = 236)							
SCI 1st	−0.55	<0.001	−0.38	<0.001	−0.31	<0.001	−0.115	0.2
SCI 2nd	−0.56	<0.001	−0.49	<0.001	−0.47	<0.001	0.08	0.47

PHQ4 = patient health questionnaire-4, DAR-5 = Dimensions of Anger Reactions-5, LS = UCLA Loneliness Scale, SCI = Sleep Condition Indicator, HSI = Heaviness of Smoking Index.

5. Discussion

To the best of our knowledge, this is the first study that attempted to demonstrate the changes in sleep quality, mental distress, anger and loneliness in Greek HCPs in relation to the evolving COVID-19 pandemic. To date, no longitudinal studies evaluating these factors on HCPs and especially primary care HCPs have been conducted in northern Greece. Our results indicate that the sleep quality of all HCPs significantly worsened during the pandemic, together with the levels of anxiety, depression, anger and loneliness. Primary care HCPs were more significantly affected in both waves.

There is a bidirectional relationship between psychological distress and sleep quality. Anxiety and stress affect sleep quality by being the main precipitating factors for the development of sleep dysfunction and, on the other hand, sleep quality is an important factor for the regulation of stable emotional control [35–38]. In a meta-analysis evaluating the psychological and mental impact of COVID 19 on medical staff and the general population, the prevalence of anxiety was found to be rather similar between these groups (26% and 32%, respectively) [37]. The COVID-19 pandemic is the most recent global public health event after SARS and Middle East Respiratory Syndrome (MERS). There is evidence that HCPs suffered from emotional distress and psychiatric morbidity during all these previous outbreaks with prevalence reaching almost 50% [39,40].

During the early stage of the COVID-19 pandemic, anxiety symptoms were reported in 28.8% and depressive symptoms in 16.5% of the general population in China [41]. On the other hand, among HCPs the incidence of anxiety and depression was reported to be around 44% and 50%, respectively [42,43]. In our study, HCPs were found to have a significantly worse mental status during the second wave compared to the first, with anxiety symptoms reported in 32.8% and depression in 37.7% of the participants. This was more evident in primary care HCPs compared with the other groups of HCPs with 23.8% reporting symptoms of anxiety and 27.5% of depression. Anxiety symptoms were also found to be more frequent than depression in other studies [43]. The application of different tools to assess mental health, and using different cutoff points, may have contributed to the heterogeneity of results between different studies. Mild symptoms of fear and stress are considered a normal reaction to a newly recognized condition such as the COVID 19 pandemic. It seems that most HCPs experienced mild symptoms of both depression and anxiety, as in our study, while more severe symptoms were reported less frequently [9,43].

Considerable evidence, especially in the form of cross-sectional studies and systematic reviews, has demonstrated the significant impact of COVID 19 on psychological and mental health outcomes and sleep disorders [35–43]. However, until now, limited published studies were available evaluating the changes in the mental health of HCPs during the course of the pandemic and more specifically comparing the differences over the different waves. Similar to our findings, other studies [44] also reported higher odds of psychological distress, such as depression and anxiety, among those HCPs who were involved with the treatment of patients suffering from COVID19. Additionally, a longitudinal study that was carried out in Japan and evaluated four waves of the pandemic showed that even when the cases of COVID 19 were low, HCPs continuously experienced high psychological distress [45]. Our results indicate that the levels of anxiety, depression, anger and loneliness together with the worsening of sleep quality increased during the course of the pandemic. Several factors may influence mental health outcomes. Specifically, in our study, negative correlations were observed between psychological distress, anger, loneliness and sleep problems, especially in primary care HCPs, which makes more evident the importance of implementing strategies to improve the work environment and support HCPs.

The existing literature reported that the prevalence of psychological symptoms in HCPs during the COVID-19 pandemic was higher than in the previous epidemics [44–51]. We found that during the second wave, the participants felt angrier and lonelier compared to the first, with 22% presenting clinically significant anger and 54.3% indicating significant loneliness. This may have a negative impact on the provision of health services [52]. A survey evaluating the impact of COVID-19 on mental health and its associated factors among HCPs across 31 countries showed that more psychological consequences were found in the HCPs with less social support possibly because they did not have the opportunity to express their feelings [50]. This is in accordance with our study as loneliness was found to be an important factor affecting sleep quality especially during the second wave in the total population and separately in primary HCPs.

Stress is a well-known cause of sleep disturbances in HCPs [44–51] and possibly due to that, the prevalence of sleep disturbances in COVID-19 medical staff was higher than in other community groups [53]. In Wuhan, HCPs experienced high levels of depression anxiety, anger, fear and stress, due to the possibility of infection, the direct exposure to disease and excessive work pressure [51]. In addition, it was found that 39.2% of HCPs in China suffered from sleep disturbances during the pandemic [43]. In our study, a strong correlation was found between sleep quality (SCI) and mental health (PHQ4), even in the separate analysis of depression and anxiety, further verifying this important bidirectional relationship. This was even more evident in the separate analysis of primary care HCPs.

It was found that consultants and physicians with greater responsibility for treating COVID-19 patients developed sleep disturbance more frequently [19,50,54,55]. A systematic review and meta-analysis revealed that almost 35% of HCPs suffered from sleep disturbances, with those working at the front line against COVID-19 being more vulnerable. Increased stress in the workplace due to exposure to COVID 19 increased sleep problems in HCPs and especially nurses and physicians [56]. In our analysis, primary care HCPs presented worse sleep quality that was aggravated during the evolution of the pandemic in the second wave with 20.6% reporting symptoms of insomnia. During that time, almost 50% of HCPs that responded were providing treatment to COVID 19 patients.

On the other hand, a study during the early outbreak of COVID-19 in Hubei Province [57] demonstrated that the sleep problems (PSQI scores) of both frontline and non-frontline workers did not differ significantly; however frontline HCPs were more susceptible to more severe sleep disturbances (PSQI > 10). In that study, binary logistic regression analysis revealed associations between medical occupation, parenthood, anxiety and depression with poor sleep quality. In our study, the most significant associations were between being primary care HCP and psychological distress (PHQ4) during the first wave and between psychological distress, anger and loneliness during the second wave with poor sleep quality.

Other factors that may contribute to sleep problems in HCPs are being female [58–60], aged 41–45 years [51,60], caring for children [57,58] and being single [60]. Importantly, in our study female gender did not show an independent effect on SCI as well as parenthood and marital status. In previous studies, female sex was associated with poor sleep quality, increased anxiety and stress compared with men [61,62], and this also applied for HCPs during COVID-19 pandemic [52,56,63]. Additionally, it was found that sleep disturbances among HCPs positively related to increased age and this could be attributed to increased fatigue from work during the years, physical problems and increased need for rest and sleep with older age [56,63]. In our study, age did not affect the results probably because most of the HCPs were of the same age range (40–50 years old).

The majority of studies so far quantified sleep habits with the use of self-reported questionnaires such as the Pittsburgh Sleep Quality Index (PSQI), Athens Insomnia Scale (AIS), Insomnia Severity Index (ISI), and some also used questionnaires designed by the researchers [64]. The selection of the questionnaire may have a significant impact on the results and may possibly explain the heterogeneity of prevalence rates of sleep disorders across different studies [9,16]. For example, with the administration of PSQI, higher rates of sleep disturbances were demonstrated compared with AIS and ISI; this could be attributed to the fact that the PSQI evaluates sleep quality in general assessing a broad range of sleep disorders such as snoring, sleep medications and nightmares, whereas AIS and ISI are more specific to insomnia symptoms [16]. Based on scores such as the PSQI, the prevalence of poor sleep quality in HCPs ranged between 18.4 to 84.7% [16,43,55,61,64–68]. A study showed that HCPs' sleep quality worsened after one-month during the early COVID-19 pandemic, with the percentage of HCPs presenting PSQI > 5 increasing from 62% to 69.3% [68]. In a rather recent study evaluating Italian pediatric HCPs, the median PSQI value was 8.0 (5.0–10.0) with 68.6% of the participants having a score higher than 5 indicating sleep disturbance, 20.0% of 11–16 indicating poor sleep quality and 2.3% more than 16 indicating very poor sleep quality [69]. In our study, we used the SCI for the assessment of sleep disorders with a cut off of 16 being indicative of insomnia disorder. During the progression of the pandemic, 18.6% of HCPs had a SCI score ≤ 16 which is indicative of a possible insomnia disorder. The deterioration of insomnia was evident in both primary care and non-primary care HCPs during the second wave pandemic with 20.6% of primary care HCPs and 14.3% of all the other HCPs having SCI score ≤ 16.

Insomnia was the most frequent sleep disorder found in other studies with a prevalence ranging from 23.6% to 68% when assessed by ISI scores, with ISI ≥ 15 indicating moderate-to-severe insomnia in 7–15% [70]. Other studies using AIS with a cut-off of 6 found that 68% of physicians and 53% of nurses suffered from insomnia [69–72]. Apart for insomnia, other sleep disorders such as nightmares, sleep terrors and sleepwalking were more frequently reported in HCPs [66]. Furthermore, a study that evaluated HCPs insomnia using wearable sleep oximeters found a high rate of co-morbid moderate to severe sleep apnea in HCPs with insomnia being attributable to stress reaching up to 38.5% [73].

The main strength of our study lies on the cross-sectional time-series design to study differences in sleep quality and mental health symptoms among the same groups of HCPs during two consecutive waves of the pandemic. However, our study has some limitations. It was based on an online questionnaire that cannot guarantee the accuracy of all the information provided from the participants. Additionally, it was very difficult to overcome the selection bias as the study was based on an online survey and the sampling from each facility might not be representative. Unfortunately, the majority of the participants of our study were physicians, and this could be the reason that we did not find any significant differences between different types of HCPs, especially in nurses so we cannot make safe conclusions and comparisons between different groups of HCPs. Unfortunately, the existence of previous history of anxiety and/or depression before the pandemic was not evaluated and this could have affected our results. However, the significant deterioration of these symptoms over the pandemic is an important finding even in the absence of data of a possible prior disorder.

The relationship between COVID-19- related sleep disturbance and stress is bidirectional. Poor sleep may lead to daytime sleepiness, fatigue and impaired daytime performance resulting in work errors further worsening the psychological condition of HCPs. During a crisis such as COVID-19, the good quality of sleep of HCPs becomes of essence as poor sleep or sleep deprivation may reduce work efficiency by impairing cognitive functioning and decision-making processes, increasing the risk of medical errors and poor patient outcomes. In addition to poor patient outcomes, reduced sleep quality has been related to decreased personal satisfaction, adverse mental health and increased burnout and may also be associated with increased morbidity, risk for obesity, diabetes and cardiovascular complications such as heart attack and stroke [23]. Stress and depression have been linked with increased likelihood of impaired professional behavior [39,53]. The psychological impact of the pandemic is more evident in frontline HCPs, but it is also felt by HCPs of other specialties [9,16,69]. Sadly, the emotional impact of the pandemic has led to suicides among HCPs [66]; something that is very alerting as compared with the general population physicians are at an increased risk of committing suicide [74].

As sleep disorders, especially insomnia, have been related in the development of mood changes, and vice versa [36,59,75], a position paper referring to the protection of HCPs during the COVID-19 pandemic emphasized that apart from personal protective equipment and food, psychological and family support are also important [76]. The European Academy for Cognitive-Behavioral Treatment of Insomnia (the European CBT-I Academy) provided some recommendations addressing the sleep problems of HCPs who experienced an increased work burden during the COVID-19 pandemic. Practical recommendations such as expressing concerns to family members, relaxing by exercising with yoga or reading, were some of the methods proposed for dealing with sleep disorders at home [77].

6. Conclusions

Our study emphasized the need for supporting HCPs' mental health and sleep, especially in those treating COVID patients and working in the primary care. Poor sleep is associated with a higher risk of developing mental illness such as generalized anxiety and depressive symptoms especially during a pandemic. Improving the sleep of HCPs is essential during the COVID-19 pandemic. The national health systems should implement effective strategies for the early identification of various risk factors and accurate recognition of sleep disorders and mental distress. The provision of effective management strategies in a timely manner is essential for the protection of HCPs and also of their patients [74–76]. Reasonable working schedules that allow the appropriate recovery of HCPs and relaxation techniques such as mindfulness and emotional support are essential [78]. On the other hand, there is still no longitudinal investigation assessing the duration and intensity of sleep disorders and psychological distress in medical staff. It is very important to evaluate the long-term effects of the pandemic and the effectiveness of the implemented supporting strategies. Additionally, it is necessary to assess the different outcome measures across different time points, the effect of vaccination or of other possible treatments for COVID 19, as the impact of the pandemic on mental health and sleep may change over time.

Author Contributions: Conceptualization, A.P., S.K. and P.A.; Methodology, A.T., N.K. and E.S.; Software, S.K. and A.T.; Validation, A.T., E.S. and I.G.; Formal Analysis, A.P. and S.K.; Investigation, A.T., N.K., E.C. and I.G.; Data Curation, S.K., N.K., E.S. and E.C.; Writing—Original Draft Preparation, A.P., S.K. and E.S.; Writing—Review and Editing, P.A., E.C. and N.K.; Supervision, A.P. and P.A. All authors have read and agreed to the published version of the manuscript.

Funding: This research received no external funding.

Institutional Review Board Statement: The protocol was approved by the institutional review board of G Papanikolaou General Hospital, Exohi, Thessaloniki, Greece (N 876, Approval Date 20 May 2020).

Informed Consent Statement: Informed consent was obtained from all subjects involved in the study.

Data Availability Statement: The data presented in this study are available on request from the corresponding author. The data are not publicly available due to institutional ethics policy.

Conflicts of Interest: The authors declare no conflict of interest.

References

1. Adams, J.G.; Walls, R.M. Supporting the Health Care Workforce During the COVID-19 Global Epidemic. *JAMA* **2020**, *323*, 1439–1440. [CrossRef] [PubMed]
2. Shanafelt, T.; Ripp, J.; Trockel, M. Understanding and Addressing Sources of Anxiety Among Health Care Professionals During the COVID-19 Pandemic. *JAMA* **2020**, *323*, 2133–2134. [CrossRef] [PubMed]
3. El-Hage, W.; Hingray, C.; Lemogne, C.; Yrondi, A.; Brunault, P.; Bienvenu, T.; Etain, B.; Paquet, C.; Gohier, B.; Bennabi, D.; et al. Health professionals facing the coronavirus disease 2019 (COVID-19) pandemic: What are the mental health risks? *Encephale* **2020**, *46*, 73–80. [CrossRef] [PubMed]
4. Ji, D.; Ji, Y.J.; Duan, X.Z.; Li, W.G.; Sun, Z.Q.; Song, X.A.; Meng, Y.H.; Tang, H.M.; Chu, F.; Niu, X.X.; et al. Prevalence of psychological symptoms among Ebola survivors and healthcare workers during the 2014–2015 Ebola outbreak in Sierra Leone: A cross-sectional study. *Oncotarget* **2017**, *8*, 12784–12791. [CrossRef] [PubMed]
5. Lin, C.Y.; Peng, Y.C.; Wu, Y.H.; Chang, J.; Chan, C.H.; Yang, D.Y. The psychological effect of severe acute respiratory syndrome on emergency department staff. *Emerg. Med. J.* **2007**, *24*, 12–17. [CrossRef]
6. Mohammed, A.; Sheikh, T.L.; Gidado, S.; Poggensee, G.; Nguku, P.; Olayinka, A.; Ohuabunwo, C.; Waziri, N.; Shuaib, F.; Adeyemi, J.; et al. An evaluation of psychological distress andsocial support of survivors and contacts of Ebola virus disease infection and theirrelatives in Lagos, Nigeria: A cross sectional study—2014. *BMC Public Health* **2015**, *15*, 824. [CrossRef]
7. Krishnamoorthy, Y.; Nagarajan, R.; Saya, G.K.; Menon, V. Prevalence of psychological morbidities among general population, healthcare workers and COVID-19 patients amidst the COVID-19 pandemic: A systematic review and meta-analysis. *Psychiatry Res.* **2020**, *293*, 113382. [CrossRef]
8. Giorgi, G.; Lecca, L.I.; Alessio, F.; Finstad, G.L.; Bondanini, G.; Lulli, L.G.; Arcangeli, G.; Mucci, N. COVID-19-Related Mental Health Effects in theWorkplace: A Narrative Review. *Int. J. Environ. Res. Public Health* **2020**, *17*, 7857. [CrossRef] [PubMed]
9. Pappa, S.; Ntella, V.; Giannakas, T.; Giannakoulis, V.G.; Papoutsi, E.; Katsaounou, P. Prevalence of depression, anxiety, and insomnia among healthcare workers during the COVID-19 pandemic: A systematic review and meta-analysis. *Brain Behav. Immun.* **2020**, *88*, 901–907. [CrossRef]
10. Vanhaecht, K.; Seys, D.; Bruyneel, L.; Cox, B.; Kaesemans, G.; Cloet, M.; Broeck, K.V.D.; Cools, O.; DeWitte, A.; Lowet, K.; et al. COVID-19 is having a destructive impact on health-care workers' mental well-being. *Int. J. Qual. Health Care* **2021**, *33*, mzaa158. [CrossRef] [PubMed]
11. Marvaldi, M.; Mallet, J.; Dubertret, C.; Moro, M.R.; Guessoum, S.B. Anxiety, depression, trauma-related, and sleep disorders among healthcare workers during the COVID-19 pandemic: A systematic review and meta-analysis. *Neurosci. Biobehav. Rev.* **2021**, *126*, 252–264. [CrossRef] [PubMed]
12. Young, K.P.; Kolcz, D.L.; O'Sullivan, D.M.; Ferrand, J.; Fried, J.; Robinson, K. Health Care Workers' Mental Health and Quality of Life During COVID-19: Results from a Mid-Pandemic, National Survey. *Psychiatr. Serv.* **2021**, *72*, 122–128. [CrossRef] [PubMed]
13. Serrano-Ripoll, M.J.; Meneses-Echavez, J.F.; Ricci-Cabello, I.; Fraile-Navarro, D.; Fiol-de Roque, M.A.; Pastor-Moreno, G.; Castro, A.; Ruiz-Pérez, I.; Zamanillo Campos, R.; Gonçalves-Bradley, D.C. Impact of viral epidemic outbreaks on mental health ofhealthcare workers: A rapid systematic review and meta-analysis. *J. Affect. Disord.* **2020**, *277*, 347–357. [CrossRef] [PubMed]
14. Ibar, C.; Fortuna, F.; Gonzalez, D.; Jamardo, J.; Jacobsen, D.; Pugliese, L.; Giraudo, L.; Ceres, V.; Mendoza, C.; Repetto, E.M.; et al. Evaluation of stress, burnout and hair cortisol levels in health workers at a University Hospital during COVID-19 pandemic. *Psychoneuroendocrinology* **2021**, *128*, 105213. [CrossRef] [PubMed]
15. Barello, S.; Palamenghi, L.; Graffigna, G. Stressors and Resources for Healthcare Professionals During the COVID-19 Pandemic: Lesson Learned from Italy. *Front. Psychol.* **2020**, *11*, 2179. [CrossRef] [PubMed]
16. Jahrami, H.; BaHammam, A.S.; Bragazzi, N.L.; Saif, Z.; Faris, M.A.; Vitiello, M.V. Sleep problems during the COVID-19 pandemic by population: A systematic review and meta—Analysis. *J. Clin. Sleep Med.* **2021**, *17*, 299–313. [CrossRef] [PubMed]
17. Xia, L.; Chen, C.; Liu, Z.; Luo, X.; Guo, C.; Liu, Z.; Zhang, K.; Liu, H. Prevalence of sleep disturbances and sleep quality in Chinese healthcare workers during the COVID-19 pandemic: A systematic review and meta-analysis. *Front. Psychiatr.* **2021**, *12*, 646342. [CrossRef] [PubMed]
18. Spoorthy, M.S.; Pratapa, S.K.; Mahant, S. Mental health problems faced by healthcare workers due to the COVID-19 pandemic-a review. *Asian J. Psychiatr.* **2020**, *51*, 102119. [CrossRef] [PubMed]
19. Giardino, D.L.; Huck-Iriart, C.; Riddick, M.; Garay, A. The endless quarantine: The impact of the COVID-19 outbreak on healthcare workers after three months of mandatory social isolation in Argentina. *Sleep Med.* **2020**, *76*, 16–25. [CrossRef] [PubMed]
20. Ballesio, A.; Lombardo, C.; Lucidi, F.; Violani, C. Caring for the carers: Advice for dealing with sleep problems of hospital staff during the COVID-19 outbreak. *J. Sleep Res.* **2020**, *30*, 13096. [CrossRef]
21. Nguyen, L.H.; Drew, D.A.; Graham, M.S.; Joshi, A.D.; Guo, C.G.; Ma, W.; Mehta, R.S.; Warner, E.T.; Sikavi, D.R.; Lo, C.L.; et al. Risk of COVID-19 among front-line health-care workers and the general community: A prospective cohort study. *Lancet Public Health* **2020**, *5*, 475–483. [CrossRef]
22. Li, L.; Wu, C.; Gan, Y.; Qu, X.; Lu, Z. Insomnia and the risk of depression: A meta-analysis of prospective cohort studies. *BMC Psychiatr.* **2016**, *16*, 375. [CrossRef] [PubMed]
23. Wu, K.; Wei, X. Analysis of psychological and sleep status and exercise rehabilitation of front-line clinical staff in the fight against COVID-19 in China. *Med. Sci. Monit. Basic Res.* **2020**, *26*, 924085. [CrossRef] [PubMed]

24. Kang, L.; Li, Y.; Hu, S.; Chen, M.; Yang, C.; Yang, B.X.; Wang, Y.; Hu, J.; Lai, J.; Ma, X.; et al. The mental health of medical workers in Wuhan, China dealing with the 2019 novel coronavirus. *Lancet Psychiatry* **2020**, *7*, 14. [CrossRef]
25. Fiest, K.M.; Leigh, J.P.; Krewulak, K.D.; Plotnikoff, K.M.; Kemp, L.G.; Ng-Kamstra, J.; Stelfox, H.T. Experiences and management of physician psychological symptoms during infectious disease outbreaks: A rapid review. *BMC Psychiatry* **2021**, *21*, 91. [CrossRef]
26. Phiri, P.; Ramakrishnan, R.; Rathod, S.; Elliot, K.; Thayanandan, T.; Sandle, N.; Haque, N.; Chau, S.W.; Wong, O.W.; Chan, S.S.; et al. An evaluation of the mental health impact of SARS-CoV-2 on patients, general public and healthcare professionals: A systematic review and meta-analysis. *EClinicalMedicine* **2021**, *34*, 100806. [CrossRef] [PubMed]
27. Pérez-Carbonell, L.; Meurling, I.J.; Wassermann, D.; Gnoni, V.; Leschziner, G.; Weighall, A.; Ellis, J.; Durrant, S.; Hare, A.; Steier, J.; et al. Impact of the novel coronavirus (COVID-19) pandemic on sleep. *J. Thorac. Dis.* **2020**, *12*, 163–175. [CrossRef]
28. Cellini, N.; Canale, N.; Mioni, G.; Costa, S. Changes in sleep pattern, sense of time and digital media use during COVID-19 lockdown in Italy. *J. Sleep Res.* **2020**, *29*, 13074. [CrossRef]
29. Heatherton, T.F.; Kozlowski, L.T.; Frecker, R.C.; Rickert, W.; Robinson, J. Measuring the heaviness of smoking: Using self-reported time to the first cigarette of the day and number of cigarettes smoked per day. *Br. J. Addict.* **1989**, *84*, 791–799. [CrossRef] [PubMed]
30. Kroenke, K.; Spitzer, R.L.; Williams, J.B.; Löwe, B. An ultra-brief screening scale for anxiety and depression: The PHQ-4. *Psychosomatics* **2009**, *50*, 613–621.
31. Forbes, D.; Alkemade, N.; Mitchell, D.; Elhai, J.D.; McHugh, T.; Bates, G.; Novaco, R.W.; Bryant, R.; Lewis, V. Utility of the Dimensions of Anger Reactions-5 (DAR-5) scale as a brief anger measure. *Depress. Anxiety* **2014**, *31*, 166–173. [CrossRef]
32. Hughes, M.E.; Waite, L.J.; Hawkley, L.C.; Cacioppo, J.T. A Short Scale for Measuring Loneliness in Large Surveys: Results from two population-based studies. *Res. Ageing* **2004**, *26*, 655–672. [CrossRef] [PubMed]
33. Espie, C.A.; Kyle, S.D.; Hames, P.; Gardani, M.; Fleming, L.; Cape, J. Psychometric properties of the Sleep Condition Indicator and Insomnia Severity Index in the evaluation of insomnia disorder. *BMJ Open* **2014**, *4*, 004183. [CrossRef] [PubMed]
34. Espie, C.A.; Machado, P.F.; Carl, J.R.; Kyle, S.D.; Cape, J.; Siriwardena, A.N.; Luik, A.I. The sleep condition indicator: Reference values derived from a sample of 200,000 adults. *J. Sleep Res.* **2018**, *27*, e12643. [CrossRef] [PubMed]
35. Altena, E.; Micoulaud-Franchi, J.A.; Geoffroy, P.A.; Sanz-Arigita, E.; Bioulac, S.; Philip, P. The bidirectional relation between emotional reactivity and sleep: From disruption to recovery. *Behav. Neurosci.* **2016**, *130*, 336–350. [CrossRef] [PubMed]
36. Simon, E.B.; Oren, N.; Sharon, H.; Kirschner, A.; Goldway, N.; Okon–Singer, H.; Tauman, R.; Deweese, M.M.; Keil, A.; Hendler, T. Losing neutrality: The neural basis of impaired emotional control without sleep. *J. Neurosci.* **2015**, *35*, 13194–13205. [CrossRef] [PubMed]
37. Luo, M.; Guo, L.; Yu, M.; Jiang, W.; Wang, H. The psychological and mental impact of coronavirus disease 2019 (COVID19) on medical staff and general public—A systematic review and meta-analysis. *Psychiatry Res.* **2020**, *291*, 113190. [CrossRef]
38. Nickell, L.A.; Crighton, E.J.; Tracy, C.S.; Al-Enazy, H.; Bolaji, Y.; Hanjrah, S.; Hussain, A.; Makhlouf, S.; Upshur, R.E.G. Psychosocial effects of SARS on hospital staff: Survey of a large tertiary care institution. *CMAJ* **2004**, *170*, 793–798. [CrossRef]
39. Lee, S.M.; Kang, W.S.; Cho, A.R.; Kim, T.; Park, J.K. Psychological impact of the 2015 MERS outbreak on hospital workers and quarantined hemodialysis patients. *Compr. Psychiatr.* **2018**, *87*, 123–127. [CrossRef]
40. Su, T.P.; Lien, T.C.; Yang, C.Y.; Su, Y.L.; Wang, J.H.; Tsai, S.L.; Yin, J.C. Prevalence of psychiatric morbidity and psychological adaptation of the nurses in a structured SARS caring unit during outbreak: A prospective and periodic assessment study in Taiwan. *J. Psychiatr. Res.* **2007**, *41*, 119–130. [CrossRef] [PubMed]
41. Wang, C.; Pan, R.; Wan, X.; Tan, Y.; Xu, L.; Ho, C.S.; Ho, R.C. Immediate psychological responses and associated factors during the initial stage of the 2019 coronavirus disease (COVID-19) epidemic among the general population in China. *Int. J. Environ. Res. Public Health* **2020**, *17*, 1729. [CrossRef] [PubMed]
42. Qiu, D.; Yu, Y.; Li, R.Q.; Li, Y.L.; Xiao, S.Y. Prevalence of sleep disturbances in Chinese healthcare professionals: A systematic review and meta-analysis. *Sleep Med.* **2020**, *67*, 258–266. [CrossRef] [PubMed]
43. Pappa, S.; Sakkas, N.; Sakka, E. A year in review: Sleep dysfunction and psychological distress in healthcare workers during the COVID-19 pandemic. *Sleep Med.* **2022**, *91*, 237–245. [CrossRef] [PubMed]
44. Th'ng, F.; Rao, K.A.; Ge, L.; Mao, D.; Neo, H.N.; Molina, J.A.; Seow, E. A one-year longitudinal study: Changes in depression and anxiety in frontline emergency department healthcare workers in the COVID-19 pandemic. *Int. J. Environ. Res. Public Health* **2021**, *18*, 11228. [CrossRef] [PubMed]
45. Sasaki, N.; Asaoka, H.; Kuroda, R.; Tsuno, K.; Imamura, K.; Kawakami, N. Sustained poor mental health among healthcare workers in COVID-19 pandemic: A longitudinal analysis of the four-wave panel survey over 8 months in Japan. *J. Occup. Health* **2021**, *63*, 12227. [CrossRef] [PubMed]
46. Li, Y.; Qin, Q.; Sun, Q.; Sanford, L.D.; Vgontzas, A.V.; Tang, X. Sleep disturbances and psychological reactions during the COVID-19 outbreak in China. *J. Clin. Sleep Med.* **2020**, *16*, 1417–1418. [CrossRef] [PubMed]
47. Abdulah, D.M.; Musa, D.H. Sleep disturbances and Stress of Physicians during COVID-19 Outbreak. *Sleep Med. X* **2020**, *2*, 100017. [CrossRef] [PubMed]
48. Zhang, C.X.; Yang, L.; Liu, S.; Ma, S.; Wang, Y.; Cai, Z.; Du, H.; Li, R.; Kang, L.; Su, M.; et al. Survey of sleep disturbances and related social psychological factors among medical staff involved in the 2019 novel coronavirus disease outbreak. *Front. Psychiatry* **2020**, *1*, 306–312. [CrossRef]

49. Geoffroy, P.A.; Le Goanvic, V.; Sabbagh, O.; Richoux, C.; Weinstein, A.; Dufayet, G.; Lejoyeux, M. Psychological support system for hospital workers duringthe COVID-19 outbreak: Rapid design and implementation of the Covid-Psyhotline. *Front. Psychiatry* **2020**, *11*, 511. [CrossRef]
50. Htay, M.N.N.; Marz, R.R.; Al Rifai, A.; Kamberi, F.; El-Abasiri, R.A.; Nyamache, J.M.; Hlaing, H.A.; Hassanein, M.; Moe, S.; Suet, T.T.; et al. Immediate impact of COVID-19 on mental health and its associated factors among healthcare workers: A global perspective across 31 coutries. *J. Glob. Health* **2020**, *10*, 020381. [CrossRef]
51. Huang, Y.E.; Zhao, N. Generalized anxiety disorder, depressive symptoms and sleep quality during COVID-19 outbreak in China: A web-based crosssectional survey. *Psychiatry Res.* **2020**, *288*, 112954–112963. [CrossRef] [PubMed]
52. Patterson, P.D.; Weaver, M.D.; Frank, R.C.; Warner, C.W.; Martin-Gill, C.; Guyette, F.X.; Fairbanks, R.J.; Hubble, M.W.; Songer, T.J.; Callaway, C.W.; et al. Association between poor sleep, fatigue, and safety outcomes in emergency medical services providers. *Prehospital Emerg. Care* **2012**, *16*, 86–97. [CrossRef] [PubMed]
53. Diaz, F.; Cornelius, T.; Bramley, S.; Venner, H.; Shaw, K.; Dong, M.; Pham, P.; McMurry, C.L.; Cannone, D.E.; Sullivan, A.M.; et al. The association between sleep and psychological distress among New York City healthcare workers during the COVID-19 pandemic. *J. Affect. Disord.* **2022**, *298*, 618–624. [CrossRef] [PubMed]
54. McAlonan, G.M.; Lee, A.M.; Cheung, V.; Cheung, C.; Tsang, K.W.; Sham, P.C.; Chua, S.E.; Wong, J.G.W.S. Immediate and sustained psychological impact of an emerging infectious disease outbreak on health care workers. *Can. J. Psychiatry* **2007**, *52*, 241–247. [CrossRef]
55. Montemurro, N. The emotional impact of COVID-19: From medical staff to common people. *Brain Behav. Immun.* **2020**, *87*, 23–24. [CrossRef]
56. Alnofaiey, Y.H.; Alshehri, H.A.; Alosaimi, M.M.; Alswat, S.H.; Alswat, R.H.; Alhulayfi, R.M.; Alghamdi, M.A.; Alsubaieet, R.M. Sleep disturbances among physicians during COVID-19 pandemic. *BMC Res. Notes* **2020**, *13*, 493. [CrossRef] [PubMed]
57. Mo, Y.; Deng, L.; Zhang, L.; Lang, Q.; Liao, C.; Wang, N.; Liao, C.; Wang, N.; Qin, M.; Huang, H. Work stress among Chinese nurses to support Wuhan in fighting against COVID-19 epidemic. *J. Nurs. Manag.* **2020**, *28*, 1002–1009. [CrossRef]
58. Zhan, Y.; Liu, Y.; Liu, H.; Li, M.; Shen, Y.; Gui, L.; Zhang, J.; Luo, Z.; Tao, X.; Yu, J. Factors associated with insomnia among Chinese front-line nurses fighting against COVID-19 in Wuhan: A cross-sectional survey. *J. Nurs. Manag.* **2020**, *28*, 1525–1535. [CrossRef]
59. Jain, A.; Singariya, G.; Kamal, M.; Kumar, M.; Jain, A.; Solanki, R.K. COVID-19 pandemic: Psychological impact on anaesthesiologists. *Indian J. Anaesth.* **2020**, *64*, 774–783.
60. Wang, S.; Xie, L.; Xu, Y.; Yu, S.; Yao, B.; Xiang, D. Sleep disturbances among medical workers during the outbreak of COVID-2019. *Occup. Med.* **2020**, *70*, 364–369. [CrossRef] [PubMed]
61. Wang, W.; Song, W.; Xia, Z.; He, Y.; Tang, L.; Hou, J.; Lei, S. Sleep disturbance and psychological profiles of medical staff and non-medical staff during the early outbreak of COVID-19 in Hubei Province, China. *Front. Psychiatry* **2020**, *11*, 733. [CrossRef] [PubMed]
62. Rossi, R.; Socci, V.; Pacitti, F.; Mensi, S.; Di Marco, A.; Siracusano, A.; Siracusano, A.; Di Lorenzo, G. Mental health outcomes among healthcare workers and the general population during the COVID-19 in Italy. *Front. Psychol.* **2020**, *11*, 608986. [CrossRef] [PubMed]
63. Li, F.; Luo, S.; Mu, W.; Li, Y.; Ye, L.; Zheng, X.; Xu, B.; Ding, Y.; Ling, P.; Zhou, M.; et al. Effects of sources of social support and resilience on the mental health of different age groups during the COVID-19 pandemic. *BMC Psychiatry* **2021**, *21*, 16. [CrossRef] [PubMed]
64. Salari, N.; Khazaie, H.; Hosseinian-Far, A.; Ghasemi, H.; Mohammadi, M.; Shohaimi, S.; Daneshkhah, A.; Khaledi-Paveh, B.; Hosseinian-Far, M. The prevalence of sleep disturbances among physicians and nurses facing the COVID-19 patients: A systematic review and meta-analysis. *Global Health* **2020**, *16*, 92. [CrossRef] [PubMed]
65. Qi, J.; Xu, J.; Li, B.Z.; Huang, J.S.; Yang, Y.; Zhang, Z.T.; Yao, D.A.; Liu, Q.H.; Jia, M.; Gonget, D.K.; et al. The evaluation of sleep disturbances for Chinese frontline medical workers under the outbreak of COVID-19. *Sleep Med.* **2020**, *72*, 1–4. [CrossRef] [PubMed]
66. Herrero San Martin, A.; Parra Serrano, J.; Diaz Cambriles, T.; Arias Arias, E.V.; Muñoz Méndez, J.; Del Yerro Álvarez, M.J.; González Sánchez, M. Sleep characteristics in health workers exposed to the COVID-19 pandemic. *Sleep Med.* **2020**, *75*, 388–394. [CrossRef]
67. Zhao, X.; Zhang, T.; Li, B.; Yu, X.; Ma, Z.; Cao, L.; Gu, Q.; Dong, C.; Jin, Y.; Fan, J.; et al. Job-related factors associated with changes in sleep quality among healthcare workers screening for 2019 novel coronavirus infection: A longitudinal study. *Sleep Med.* **2020**, *75*, 21–26. [CrossRef] [PubMed]
68. Stewart, N.H.; Koza, A.; Dhaon, S.; Shoushtari, C.; Martinez, M.; Arora, V.M. Sleep Disturbances in Frontline Health Care Workers During the COVID-19 Pandemic: Social Media Survey Study. *J. Med. Internet Res.* **2021**, *2*, e27331. [CrossRef]
69. Di Filippo, P.; Attanasi, M.; Dodi, G.; Porreca, A.; Raso, M.; Di Pillo, S.; Chiarelli, F. Evaluation of sleep quality and anxiety in Italian pediatric healthcare workers during the first wave of COVID-19 pandemic. *Res. Notes* **2021**, *14*, 219. [CrossRef] [PubMed]
70. Lai, J.; Ma, S.; Wang, Y.; Cai, Z.; Hu, J.; Wei, N.; Wu, J.; Du, H.; Chen, T.; Li, R.; et al. Factors associated with mental health outcomes among health care workers exposed to Coronavirus disease 2019. *JAMA Netw. Open* **2020**, *3*, 203976. [CrossRef]

71. Alshekaili, M.; Hassan, W.; Al Said, N.; Sulaimani, F.; Jayapal, S.K.; Al-Mawali, A.; Chan, M.F.; Mahadevan, S.; Al-Adawi, S. Factors associated with mental health outcomes across healthcare settings in Oman during COVID-19: Frontline versus non-frontline healthcare workers. *BMJ Open* **2020**, *10*, 042030. [CrossRef]
72. Rossi, R.; Socci, V.; Pacitti, F.; Di Lorenzo, G.; Di Marco, A.; Siracusano, A.; Rossi, A. Mental health outcomes among frontline and second-line health care workers during the Coronavirus disease 2019 (COVID-19) pandemic in Italy. *JAMA Netw. Open* **2020**, *3*, 2010185. [CrossRef] [PubMed]
73. Zhuo, K.; Gao, C.; Wang, X.; Zhang, C.; Wang, Z. Stress and sleep: A survey based on wearable sleep trackers among medical and nursing staff in Wuhan during the COVID-19 pandemic. *Gen. Psychiatr.* **2020**, *33*, 100260. [CrossRef]
74. Hennein, R.; Mew, E.J.; Lowe, S.R. Socio-ecological predictors of mental health outcomes among healthcare workers during the COVID-19 pandemic in the United States. *PLoS ONE* **2021**, *16*, e0246602. [CrossRef] [PubMed]
75. The Lancet. COVID-19: Protecting health-care workers. *Lancet* **2020**, *395*, 922. [CrossRef]
76. Altena, E.; Baglioni, C.; Espie, C.A.; Ellis, J.; Gavriloff, D.; Holzinger, B.; Schlarb, A.; Frase, L.; Jernelöv, S.; Riemann, D. Dealing with sleep problems during home confinement due to theCOVID-19 outbreak: Practical recommendations from a task force of the European CBT-I Academy. *J. Sleep Res.* **2020**, *29*, 13052. [CrossRef] [PubMed]
77. West, C.; Dyrbye, L.; Shanafelt, T. Physician burnout: Contribution, consequences and solutions. *J. Intern. Med.* **2018**, *283*, 516–529. [CrossRef] [PubMed]
78. Meira e Cruz, M.; Miyazawa, M.; Gozal, D. Putative contributions of circadian clock and sleep in the context of SARS-CoV-2 infection. *Eur. Respir. J.* **2020**, *55*, 2001023. [CrossRef]

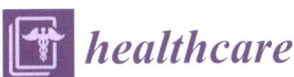

Article

Obstructive Sleep Apnea Syndrome Comorbidity Phenotypes in Primary Health Care Patients in Northern Greece

Panagiota K. Ntenta [1], Georgios D. Vavougios [1], Sotirios G. Zarogiannis [1,2,*] and Konstantinos I. Gourgoulianis [1]

[1] Department of Respiratory Medicine, Faculty of Medicine, School of Health Sciences, University of Thessaly, 41500 Larissa, Greece; yiotantenta@gmail.com (P.K.N.); gvavougyios@uth.gr (G.D.V.); kgourg@uth.gr (K.I.G.)
[2] Department of Physiology, Faculty of Medicine, School of Health Sciences, University of Thessaly, 41500 Larissa, Greece
* Correspondence: szarog@med.uth.gr

Abstract: Background: Obstructive sleep apnea syndrome (OSAS) is a significant public health issue. In the general population, the prevalence varies from 10% to 50%. We aimed to phenotype comorbidities in OSAS patients referred to the primary health care (PHC) system. Methods: We enrolled 1496 patients referred to the PHC system for any respiratory- or sleep-related issue from November 2015 to September 2017. Some patients underwent polysomnography (PSG) evaluation in order to establish OSAS diagnosis. The final study population comprised 136 patients, and the Charlson comorbidity index was assessed. Categorical principal component analysis and TwoStep clustering was used to identify distinct clusters in the study population. Results: The analysis revealed three clusters: the first with moderate OSAS, obesity and a high ESS score without significant comorbidities; the second with severe OSAS, severe obesity with comorbidities and the highest ESS score; and the third with severe OSAS and obesity without comorbidities but with a high ESS score. The clusters differed in age ($p < 0.005$), apnea–hypopnea index, oxygen desaturation index, arousal index and respiratory and desaturation arousal index ($p < 0.001$). Conclusions: Predictive comorbidity models may aid the early diagnosis of patients at risk in the context of PHC and pave the way for personalized treatment.

Keywords: comorbidities; Greece; OSAS; phenotyping; primary health care

1. Introduction

Obstructive sleep apnea syndrome (OSAS) is a disease characterized by recurrent episodes of partial or complete collapse of the upper airway. It occurs during sleep despite the documented ongoing effort to breath. This leads to a partial reduction in airflow, followed by arousal, with an abrupt reduction in blood oxygen saturation (hypopneas). A complete cessation of airflow lasting at least 10 s during sleep is defined as apnea. This pattern can occur many times during the night [1].

OSAS prevalence is estimated to be approximately 5–10% in the general population, regardless of race and ethnicity, with certain subgroups of the population bearing higher risk [2]. An estimated 10% of middle-aged men and 3% of middle-aged women suffer from moderate/severe disease [3].

Early OSAS diagnosis can make a significant contribution to reducing comorbidity, healthcare costs, mortality rates and facilitating the reference for medical services. Still, few studies have investigated the early detection of OSAS in patients attending primary health care (PHC) services either due to snoring and/or sleep interruption and daytime sleepiness. Predictive comorbidity models enrich our knowledge about OSAS heterogeneity and aid in the early diagnosis of patients at risk, facilitating better individualized treatment approaches for patients. Some years ago, we were the first to employ, categorical principal component analysis (CATPCA) in combination with cluster analysis in an OSAS population in order to detect comorbidity phenotypes [4]. Our scope was to identify the interplay between OSAS and its comorbidities, an approach that had served well in phenotyping in other areas and that also gained popularity after our study in the OSAS field [5–11].

The aim of the current study was to evaluate our previously published CATPCA and TwoStep cluster (TSC) predictive comorbidity phenotyping model in OSAS patients who underwent polysomnography (PSG) after referral from the Greek PHC services.

2. Materials and Methods

2.1. Study Population

We performed an epidemiological observational study to investigate the relationship between OSAS, concomitant diseases and the characteristics of the studied PHC population. We screened 1496 patients referred to the PHC system in the northern part of Greece for any respiratory or sleep problem from November 2015 to September 2017. The study population consisted of adults, 18 to 65 years of age, who had previously undergone a full standard PSG in the Sleep Unit of the "AGIOS PAVLOS" General Hospital. Patients previously diagnosed with respiratory failure were excluded from our study. We designed a database that included patient demographics and anthropometric and socio-economic data, along with behavioral characteristics, clinical history, and Epworth Sleepiness Scale and Berlin Questionnaire results, and all parameters were included in the patients' overnight PSGs in the laboratory. From the initially screened population, 136 patients were included in the final analysis. The study was conducted according to the guidelines of the Declaration of Helsinki and approved by the Institutional Review Board of the 4th HEALTH REGION–MACEDONIA & THRACE (21990/5 July 2016).

2.2. OSAS Definition Severity and Diagnosis

A common measurement of sleep apnea is the apnea–hypopnea index (AHI), which is the number of apneas and hypopneas that occur per hour of sleep, and it is used to grade the degree of OSAS severity [12]. In our study, the determination of AHI was achieved after a full-night PSG in the laboratory. According to the American Academy of Sleep Medicine (AASM), there are four types of OSAS [13,14]:

1. Normal (AHI < 5);
2. Mild (AHI $\geq$ 5–14);
3. Moderate (AHI $\geq$ 15–29);
4. Severe OSAS (AHI $\geq$ 30).

2.3. Polysomnography (PSG)

PSG is considered the "gold-standard" for sleep disorder diagnosis and requires an overnight stay in a sleep laboratory. Laboratory-based full-night PSG was performed in the studied population and included the monitoring of sleep state through the use of electroencephalography (EEG), electrooculography (EOG), electromyography (EMG), electrocardiography (ECG), oral thermistor, sound probe around the neck for snoring measurement, pulse oximetry-determined changes in blood oxygen levels and body position, and the respiratory effort was measured with the use of abdominal and thoracic belts. Arousals were measured as sudden shifts in brain wave activity. Apnea was defined as a pause in respiration nasal airflow using pressure transducers for at least 10 s. Apneas were further classified as obstructive, central or mixed based on whether the effort to breath was present during the event. Hypopnea was defined as a reduction in ventilation of at least 30% from the baseline in airflow reduction for >10 s. This results in a decreased arterial saturation associated with at least 4% oxygen desaturation due to partial airway obstruction [15].

2.4. Questionnaires

In addition to PSG, screening tools, such as questionnaires, indicate the risk of patients for OSAS. They are simple, cost effective and validated tools recommended for the initial screening of OSAS [15]. The Epworth Sleepiness Scale (ESS) consists of eight different situations, and the questionnaire asks the subject to rate the probability of falling asleep in specific situations. Patients with scores ≥ 11 and experiencing involuntary sleepiness during activities that require more active attention, such as talking or driving, are suggested to have excessive daytime sleepiness [14,16]. The Berlin Questionnaire (BQ) has three parts. The survey items address the presence and frequency of snoring behavior, daytime sleepiness or fatigue and history of obesity or hypertension [15].

2.5. Comorbidity Assessment

Comorbidity assessment is an important component of health services research and an inevitable clinical prognostic factor. Comorbidity may impact treatment, prognosis and quality of care assessment. In our study, the severity of comorbidity was determined based on the adjusted Charlson comorbidity index (CCI) score. The CCI score was calculated for the studied population based on an algorithm formatted as a Microsoft Excel Macro, which provides a rapid method for calculating the CCI score. The CCI score was developed by Hall et al. in 1987 and predicts the one-year mortality for a patient who may have a range of comorbid conditions (index consists of 19 medical conditions). Each condition is assigned a score of 1, 2, 3, or 6, with total scores ranging from 0 to 37. Comorbidity, in our study, was defined in terms of the absence or presence of one or more conditions included in and scored by the CCI criteria [17].

2.6. Statistical Analysis

The statistical analysis was performed using the IBM SPSS Statistics 21.0 software package. Data normality was assessed by the Kolmogorov–Smirnov test. Data are presented as mean $\pm$ standard deviation (SD) for data with normal distribution, and as median with interquartile ranges in parenthesis for skewed data. Independent samples *t* test or Mann–Whitney U test was used where appropriate. Categorical variables are expressed as percentages, and the chi-square or Fischer's exact test was used. Differences between clusters were tested by one-way ANOVA analysis with post-hoc Bonferroni correction. $p < 0.05$ is considered significant.

2.7. Categorical Principal Component Analysis (CATPCA)

CATPCA is a variant of the principal component analysis (PCA). This method is the nonlinear equivalent of the standard PCA and reduces the observed set of variables into a smaller set of uncorrelated variables called principal components, which represent most of the information found in the original variables. The most important advantages of nonlinear over linear PCA are that it incorporates multivariate variables and that it can handle and discover nonlinear relationships between variables [18]. The method is most useful when many variables prohibit an effective interpretation of the relationships between objects. It reduces the dimensionality of a set of variables while accounting for as much of the variation as possible, and this optimal scaling allows better performance. By reducing the dimensionality, the clustering process is facilitated. Categorical variables are optimally quantified in the specified dimensionality. As a result, nonlinear relationships between variables can be modeled. CATPCA maximizes the correlations of the object scores with each of the quantified variables for the number of components (dimensions) specified to be used as clustering variables. This method was used on the components of the CCI.

2.8. TwoStep Clustering

Subsequently, components extracted from the CATPCA were used as clustering variables along with the AHI. For this, the SPSS TwoStep cluster (TSC) method was used. TSC is a scalable cluster analysis algorithm designed to handle very large mixed datasets and to reveal data groups (clusters) within a dataset that would not otherwise be apparent. TSC integrates a hierarchical and partitioning clustering algorithm, adding attributes to cluster objects. This method defines the relationships among items and improves the weaknesses of applying a single clustering algorithm. Clusters are categories of items with many features in common.

The TSC method is divided into the following two steps: Step 1: the pre-cluster step identifies regions with dense intercorrelations in the input variables and produces primary sub-clusters [19]. Step 2: these initial sub-clusters resulting from the first step are merged into the final clusters using the hierarchical agglomerative clustering method. Determining the optimal number of clusters in a data set is a fundamental issue in partitioning clustering; the TwoStep algorithm automatically incorporates the Bayesian information criterion (BIC) and the change in the distance measurement by also calculating the log likelihood ratio distance [20].

Finally, a post-hoc test provided by the TSC method is the average silhouette coefficient, which is a measure that indicates how similar an object is to its own cluster (cohesion) compared to other clusters (separation). The silhouette ranges from −1 (indicating a very poor model) to +1 (indicating that the object is well matched to its own cluster and poorly matched to neighboring clusters). An average silhouette greater than 0.5 indicates a reasonable partitioning of data [21]. In our study, the optimal cutoff was set at >0.85 when comparing the differentiation between clusters.

3. Results

3.1. Participant Characteristics

Among the 288 participants, 115 patients were diagnosed with other sleeping breathing disorders, 28 declined to undergo PSG, and 9 recordings were technically unacceptable. Thus, a total of 136 patients were included in our study. In Table 1, the demographics and the respiratory and sleep apnea characteristics of the study participants are shown.

Table 1. Sample demographics, questionnaires, and PSG results.

	All Sample	Gender		p Value
	$n = 136$	Females	Males	
Age (years)	48 (38, 57.75)	50 (36.8%) 45 (36, 54)	86 (63.2%) 45 (36, 54)	$p < 0.001$
Weight (kgr)	91.50 (84, 105)	88.27 ± 20.32	96.5 (86, 11.3)	$p = 0.026$
Height (cm)	172 ± 9.99	163.5 ± 7.70	176.8 ± 7.33	$p < 0.001$
Body Mass Index (BMI)	32.37 (28.10, 34.08)	32.73 ± 7.59	31.60 (28.03, 33.63)	$p = 0.204$
Low Epworth Sleepiness Scale (ESS)	68 (50%) 8 (6, 9)	29 (58%) 9 (7, 9)	39 (45.3%) 8 (6, 9)	$p = 0.214$
High ESS	68 (50%) 13 (11.25, 15.75)	21 (42%) 13 (12, 14.5)	47 (54.7%) 13 (11, 16)	$p = 0.846$
Low-Risk Berlin Questionnaire (BQ)	30 (22%)	8 (16%)	22 (25.6%)	
High-Risk BQ	106 (78%)	42 (84%)	64 (74.4%)	
Apnea Hypopnea Index (AHI) Mild	20 (14.7%) 11.70 (10.30, 13.38)	8 (16%) 10.70 (9.20, 13.85)	12 (13.9%) 11.70 (11.40, 13.38)	$p = 0.333$
Moderate AHI	34 (25%) 21.50 (19.85, 25.45)	14 (28%) 20.70 (18.68, 25.55)	20 (23.3%) 22.40 (20.03, 25.53)	$p = 0.660$
Severe AHI	74 (54.4%) 60.40 (41.33, 81.53)	23 (46%) 60.20 (38.30, 70.10)	51 (59.3%) 63.20 (44.70, 86.60)	$p = 0.382$
AHI	31.75 (18.43, 63)	26.55 (14.43, 52.43)	34.95 (20.70, 71.25)	$p = 0.024$
Obstructive Apnea Index (OAI)	7.6 (1.93, 25.33)	4.25 (0.98, 11.38)	10.30 (3.08, 40.43)	$p = 0.001$

Table 1. Cont.

	All Sample	Gender		p Value
	n = 136	Females	Males	
Oxygen Desaturation Index (ODI)	24.40 (12.40, 54.53)	19.40 (10.98, 42.43)	27.85 (14.25, 60.98)	$p = 0.036$
Respiratory Arousal Index (RAI)	7.10 (0.5, 28.43)	14.85 (3.55, 30)	4.40 (0.2, 23.85)	$p = 0.016$
Desaturation Arousal Index (DAI)	0.9 (0.3, 2.55)	1 (0.4, 2.33)	0.65 (0.2, 3.1)	$p = 0.336$
Arousal Index (AI)	18.75 (8.33, 36.78)	21.40 (11.15, 34.95)	14.75 (5.98, 45.75)	$p = 0.228$
Charlson Comorbidity Index (CCI)	1 (0, 1)	1 (0, 1)	0 (0,1)	$p = 0.024$

Data are presented as mean ± SD for normally distributed data (height) or median (interquartile ranges) for skewed data (remaining data). Normally distributed data were analyzed by Student t-test and skewed data with Mann–Whitney U test.

3.2. Cluster Analysis

CATPCA produced three components (Table 2 represents Cronbach's alpha value) that were used with AHI staging as clustering variables in the TSC technique. Applying this method, three distinct clusters were identified from the analysis.

Table 2. Cronbach's alpha value.

Dimension	Cronbach's Alpha	Variance Accounted for Total (Eigenvalue)	Dimension	Cronbach's Alpha
1	0.729	1.946	1	0.729
2	−0.015	0.990	2	−0.015
Total	0.989	2.936	Total	0.989

Clusters can correspond to phenotypes. The first phenotype corresponds to moderate OSAS, obesity and a high ESS score without significant comorbidities; the second to severe OSAS, severe obesity with comorbidities and the highest ESS score; and the third to severe OSAS and obesity without comorbidities but with a high ESS score. The clusters differed significantly in age ($p < 0.005$), apnea–hypopnea index (AHI), oxygen desaturation index (ODI), arousal index (AI) and respiratory and desaturation arousal index ($p < 0.001$) (Tables 3–5).

Table 3. Correlation-transformed variables.

	AHI	ODI	CCI (0–37)
AHI	1.000	0.934	0.047
ODI	0.934	1.000	0.100
CCI (0–37)	0.047	0.100	1.000
Dimension	1	2	3
Eigenvalue	1.946	0.990	0.064

Table 4. One-way analysis of variance (ANOVA) descriptives.

	Cluster 1	Cluster 2	Cluster 3	p-value
	n = 67 (49.3%)	n = 25 (18.4%)	n = 44 (32.4%)	
Males	37 (27.2%)	16 (11.76%)	33 (24.26%)	
Females	30 (22.05%)	9 (6.61%)	11 (8.08%)	
Age (males) Age (females)	44.11 ± 9.74 49.43 ± 12.54 $p = 0.017$	48.94 ± 12.55 57.00 ± 7.87 $p = 0.96$	42.91 ± 11.15 55.64 ± 8.29 $p = 0.001$	

Table 4. Cont.

	Cluster 1	Cluster 2	Cluster 3	p-value
	n = 67 (49.3%)	n = 25 (18.4%)	n = 44 (32.4%)	
BMI (males)	29.43 ± 4.76	33.42 ± 3.75	34.14 ± 6.04	
BMI (females)	30.71 ± 7.57	37.49 ± 6.80	35.77 ± 6.03	
	$p = 0.25$	$p = 0.18$	$p = 0.46$	
ESS (0–24)	10.09 ± 4.13	11.60 ± 3.99	11.23 ± 3.19	$p = 0.146$
AHI	20.08 ± 10.29	44.85 ± 31.08	73.42 ± 20.46	$p = 0.001$
ODI	14.50 ± 8.73	40.47 ± 31.31	61.46 ± 22.01	$p = 0.001$
AI	14.99 ± 10.60	32.69 ± 28.26	42.70 ± 31.58	$p = 0.001$
RAI	7.49 ± 9.01	25.42 ± 29.13	32.36 ± 32.22	$p = 0.001$
DAI	1.02 ± 1.31	1.85 ± 2.47	3.08 ± 3.69	$p = 0.001$
SAI	0.64 ± 1.01	0.81 ± 1.10	0.52 ± 1.04	$p = 0.541$

Data are presented as mean ± standard deviation (SD). ESS = Epworth Sleeping Scale; AHI = apnea index + hypopnea index/h; ODI = Oxygen Desaturation Index; AI = Arousal Index; RAI = Respiratory Arousal Index; DAI = Desaturation Arousal Index; SAI = Snore Arousal Index.

Table 5. CCI (0–37) TwoStep Cluster Number crosstabulation.

			TwoStep Cluster Number			Total
			1	2	3	
CCI (0–37)	0	Count	40 a	0 b	23 a	63
		Residual	9.0	−11.6	2.6	
		Std. Residual	1.6	−3.4	0.6	
		Adjusted Residual	3.1	−5.1	1.0	
	1	Count	27 a	0 b	21 a	48
		Residual	3.4	−8.8	5.5	
		Std. Residual	0.7	−3.0	1.4	
		Adjusted Residual	1.2	−4.1	2.1	
	2	Count	0 a	14 b	0 a	14
		Residual	−6.9	11.4	−4.5	
		Std. Residual	−2.6	7.1	−2.1	
		Adjusted Residual	−3.9	8.3	−2.7	
	3	Count	0 a	8 b	0 a	8
		Residual	−3.9	6.5	−2.6	
		Std. Residual	−2.0	5.4	−1.6	
		Adjusted Residual	−2.9	6.1	−2.0	
	4	Count	0 a	2 a	0 a	2
		Residual	−1.0	1.6	−6	
		Std. Residual	−1.0	2.7	−8	
		Adjusted Residual	−1.4	3.0	−1.0	
	8	Count	0 a	1 a	0 a	1
		Residual	−5	8	−3	
		Std. Residual	−7	1.9	−6	
		Adjusted Residual	−1.0	2.1	−7	
Total		Count	67	25	44	136

Each subscript letter denotes a subset of TwoStep Cluster Number categories, whose column proportions do not differ significantly from each other at the 0.05 level.

Total Cronbach's alpha and total variance explained based on cumulative eigenvalue were determined for each scaled model in comparison to the previous model. The objective of this evaluation was to maintain internal consistency among comorbidity features, while aiming prospectively for an increase in variance explained by the scaled model.

4. Discussion

Although OSAS public awareness and its associated health consequences have increased, the prevalence of OSAS continues to rise, and a significant part of the affected population remains undiagnosed. Several studies have shown that a phenotyping approach is important in early detection and provides more adapted treatment to the patient's needs. The identification of subgroups based on comorbidities and symptoms is crucial to understand OSAS causality and to develop management strategies customized for each subgroup. Such approaches have not been validated in the context of a community-based population [22]. Our study aimed to apply an OSAS comorbidity phenotyping approach previously developed by our group in a sample of the primary health care population [4].

This study placed emphasis on the standardized definition of comorbidity and OSAS severity based on AHI. TSC revealed three distinct clusters referred to as moderate-to-severe OSAS in our study population. Comorbidity scores were segregated into the severe OSAS cluster without comorbidities and severe OSAS with comorbidities. Our results are in line with those of the study by Vavougios et al. [4], although we found three distinct clusters out of six, which was maybe due to the lower number of patients. Specifically, Vavougios et al. found six distinct clusters, where one corresponded to healthy subjects, one corresponded to mild OSAS without comorbidities, two corresponded to moderate OSAS with and without comorbidities and, finally, two corresponded to severe OSAS with and without comorbidities [4]. In both studies, clinical changes in age, BMI, ODI, AHI and AI were found to be associated with a higher risk of belonging to a more serious phenotype. Despite the strong association between OSAS and obesity, studies have shown that an important number of OSAS patients have a BMI within the normal range [23]. However, this relationship is reinforced by studies concluding that patients with a higher BMI experience frequent ODI periods, resulting in a higher AI and decreased sleep efficiency [24]. Moreover, a 10% increase in weight gain was associated with a huge probability of developing OSAS, and a 10% weight loss predicted a 26% decrease in AHI [25]. Furthermore, as others have noted, both the current study and the study by Vavougios et al. discovered a nonlinear relationship between comorbidity and OSAS severity [26]. This recurrent finding indicates that moderate-to-severe OSAS patients can be furthermore stratified by resiliency against comorbidities [27], albeit studies determining the trajectory of exposure to moderate or severe untreated OSAS are understandably lacking.

There are important differences between the current study and the study by Vavougios et al. that need to be addressed. The current study was a PHC population-based study, as opposed to a study involving OSAS patients recruited from a sleep clinic, where participants reported sleep-related disturbances without a diagnosis of OSAS or other sleeping breathing disorder. Furthermore, in the current study, there were different clinical features and criteria included in the analysis [4].

Few studies have formally characterized the distinct combinations of symptoms and comorbidities in OSAS patients. To our knowledge, the first study that applied cluster analysis and that identified distinct subgroups of OSAS patients was performed by Ye et al. (ISAC study), which only placed emphasis on patients with moderate-to-severe OSAS (AHI $\geq$ 15 events/h) who were referred to a sleep clinic [28], whereas we also included patients with mild OSAS in a community-based study. The ISAC study was relatively consistent in the severity of the disease and the presence of symptoms, including comorbidities, as they distinguished them in their study population. In contrast to our study, the use of a predetermined definition of comorbidity, such as CCI, is considered a major difference, because CCI excludes hypertension, and cardiovascular disease (CVD) has several different aspects [28]. Recently, Pien GW et al. studied the follow-up data from the ISAC cohort to assess the differences in symptom responses after 2 years of CPAP treatment among the defined clusters. More specifically, they examined the relationship between OSAS clusters and successful CPAP treatment, and they concluded that the clusters with more severe OSAS were more likely to respond to treatment [29]. Keenan et al. (SAGIC study) studied OSAS patients who were middle aged and obese and had predominantly severe OSAS. After using cluster analysis, they found five clusters, where three of them were similar to those of the ISAC study and the remaining two were less symptomatic [30].

The study by Saaresanta et al. studied a huge population in 18 countries who were referred to sleep centers. Four clinical phenotypes were reported based on daytime symptoms; insomnia; and comorbidities, including CVD and anatomical and phycological features. The results are in line with the findings of the ISAC study [31].

A recent clustering study studied a large French population of moderate-to-severe OSAS patients with the same inclusion criteria as in the SAGIC study. They assessed demographics, lifestyle factors, OSAS severity, comorbidities and environmental risk factors. They identified six clusters parallel to those of the SAGIC study, but the absence of insomnia-related symptoms was the key difference. However, the major difference with our study was that OSAS severity measurements (AHI/ODI) were not considered to define subgroups [32].

A smaller study in Italy (198 OSAS patients) identified three clusters in a sample referred to a sleep clinic that were similar to those of our study, and the differences between the clusters were a consequence of OSAS severity, BMI and ESS [33]. The first community-based study was the Wisconsin Sleep Cohort Study, with participants randomly selected from a working population. The study showed a high prevalence of SDB, using PSG in adults [34]. Moreover, a huge study from the Australian PHC system (BEACH) analyzed all adults for OSAS or snoring from 2000 to 2014; however, the data did not reveal if patients were formally tested for OSAS or which path they followed in doing so (direct referral for testing or only after seeing a specialist) [35]. Recently, two Spanish studies, PASHOS and GESAP, studied a program of the PHC system and a sleep unit for OSAS management. Although the protocol that both studies followed was similar to ours, PSG was not used as the standard test for OSAS diagnosis, and the upper age range was much larger in both studies than in our study [36,37].

5. Conclusions

The main strength of our study was that we studied a partnership of a PHC system and a sleep clinic to establish OSAS diagnosis and to evaluate the resulting OSAS clusters in the initial population. A potential limitation of our study was that it involved a small sample size, and our population was predominantly male. However, the design of our study was closely associated with clinical practice, and our findings indicate that PHC can be incorporated into the clinical management of OSAS patients in a similar way to that used for other chronic diseases. Our study also corroborated a nonlinear relationship between comorbidity and OSAS severity, indicating that moderate-to-severe OSAS patients can be further stratified by resiliency against comorbidities.

Author Contributions: Conceptualization, G.D.V., S.G.Z. and K.I.G.; methodology, G.D.V.; software, G.D.V.; validation, S.G.Z.; formal analysis, P.K.N.; investigation, P.K.N.; resources, P.K.N. and K.I.G.; data curation, P.K.N. and G.D.V.; writing—original draft preparation, P.K.N. and S.G.Z.; writing—review and editing, G.D.V. and K.I.G.; visualization, P.K.N.; supervision, S.G.Z.; project administration, P.K.N.; funding acquisition, P.K.N. All authors have read and agreed to the published version of the manuscript.

Funding: This research received no external funding. Panagiota Ntenta received a PhD fellowship from the Postgraduate Master Course in Primary Health Care of the Faculties of Medicine and Nursing of the School of Health Sciences of the University of Thessaly.

Institutional Review Board Statement: The study was conducted according to the guidelines of the Declaration of Helsinki and approved by the Institutional Review Board of the 4th Y.PE.–MACEDONIA & THRACE (21990/5 July 2016).

Informed Consent Statement: Informed consent was obtained from all subjects involved in the study.

Data Availability Statement: Data are available on reasonable request from the corresponding author.

Acknowledgments: The authors would like to thank Konstantina Tzereme for excellent administrative support.

Conflicts of Interest: The authors declare no conflict of interest.

References

1. Marin, J.M.; Carrizo, S.J.; Vicente, E.; Agusti, A.G.N. Long term cardiovascular outcome in men with OSASS with or without treatment with CPAP: An observational study. *Lancet* **2005**, *365*, 1046–1053. [CrossRef]
2. Punjabi, N.M. The Epidemiology of Adult of Adult Obstructive Sleep Apnea. *Proc. Am. Thorac. Soc.* **2008**, *5*, 136–143. [CrossRef] [PubMed]
3. Peppard, E.R.; Young, T.; Barnet, H.J.; Palta, M.; Hagen, E.W.; Jla, K.M. Increased Prevalence of Sleep-Disorders Breathing in Adults. *Am. J. Epidemiol.* **2013**, *177*, 1006–1014. [CrossRef] [PubMed]
4. Vavougios, D.G.; Natsios, G.; Pastaka, C.; Zarogiannis, S.G.; Gourgoulianis, K.I. Phenotypes of comorbidity in OSAS patients: Combining categorical principal component analysis with cluster analysis. *J. Sleep Res.* **2016**, *25*, 31–38. [CrossRef] [PubMed]
5. Benassi, M.; Garofalo, S.; Ambrosini, F.; Sant'angelo, R.P.; Raggini, R.; De Paoli, G.; Ravani, C.; Giovagnoli, S.; Orsoni, M.; Piraccini, G. Using Two-Step Cluster Analysis and Latent Class Cluster Analysis to Classify the Cognitive Heterogeneity of Cross-Diagnostic Psychiatric Inpatients. *Front. Psychol.* **2020**, *11*, 1085. [CrossRef]
6. Kent, P.; Jensen, R.K.; Kongsted, A. A comparison of three clustering methods for finding subgroups in MRI, SMS or clinical data: SPSS TwoStep Cluster analysis, Latent Gold and SNOB. *BMC Med. Res. Methodol.* **2014**, *14*, 113. [CrossRef] [PubMed]
7. Costa, D.; Rodrigues, A.M.; Cruz, E.B.; Canhão, H.; Branco, J.; Nunes, C. Driving factors for the utilisation of healthcare services by people with osteoarthritis in Portugal: Results from a nationwide population-based study. *BMC Health Serv. Res.* **2021**, *21*, 1022. [CrossRef]
8. Mihaicuta, S.; Udrescu, M.; Topirceanu, A.; Udrescu, L. Network science meets respiratory medicine for OSAS phenotyping and severity prediction. *PeerJ* **2017**, *5*, e3289. [CrossRef]
9. Ma, E.Y.; Kim, J.W.; Lee, Y.; Cho, S.W.; Kim, H.; Kim, J.K. Combined unsupervised-supervised machine learning for phenotyping complex diseases with its application to obstructive sleep apnea. *Sci. Rep.* **2021**, *11*, 4457. [CrossRef]
10. Van Overstraeten, C.; Andreozzi, F.; Youssef, S.B.; Bold, I.; Carlier, S.; Gruwez, A.; Bruyneel, A.V.; Bruyneel, M. Obstructive Sleep Apnea Syndrome Phenotyping by Cluster Analysis: Typical Sleepy, Obese Middle-aged Men with Desaturating Events are A Minority of Patients in A Multi-ethnic Cohort of 33% Women. *Curr. Med. Sci.* **2021**, *41*, 729–736. [CrossRef]
11. Topîrceanu, A.; Udrescu, L.; Udrescu, M.; Mihaicuta, S. Gender Phenotyping of Patients with Obstructive Sleep Apnea Syndrome Using a Network Science Approach. *J. Clin. Med.* **2020**, *9*, 4025. [CrossRef]
12. Olson, E.J.; Moore, W.R.; Morgenthaler, T.I.; Gay, P.C.; Staats, B.A. Obstructive sleep apnoea hypopnoea syndrome. *Mayo Clin. Proc.* **2003**, *78*, 1545–1552. [CrossRef]
13. American Academy of Sleep Medicine (AASM). Available online: https://www.aasm.org (accessed on 5 May 2020).
14. Epstein, L.J.; Kristo, D.; Strollo, P.J., Jr.; Friedman, N.; Malhotra, A.; Patil, S.P.; Ramar, K.; Rogers, R.; Schwab, R.J.; Weaver, E.M. Clinical guideline for the evaluation, management, and long-term care of obstructive sleep apnea in adults. *J. Clin. Sleep Med.* **2009**, *15*, 263–276.
15. Netzer, N.C.; Stoohs, R.A.; Netzer, C.M.; Clark, K.; Strohl, K.P. Using the Berlin Questionnaire to identify patients at risk for the sleep apnea syndrome. *Ann. Intern. Med.* **1999**, *5*, 485–491. [CrossRef]
16. Johns, M.W. A new method for measuring daytime sleepiness: The Epworth sleepiness scale. *Sleep* **1991**, *14*, 540–545. [CrossRef]
17. Hall, W.H.; Ramachandran, R.; Narayan, S.; Jani, A.B.; Vijayakumar, S. An electronic application for rapidly calculating Charlson comorbidity score. *BMC Cancer* **2004**, *4*, 94. [CrossRef]
18. Meulman, J.J.; Heiser, W.J.; SPSS. *SPSS Categories 13.0*; SPSS: Chicago, IL, USA, 2004.
19. Theodoridis, S.; Koutroumbas, K. *Pattern Recognition*, 4th ed.; Academic Press: New York, NY, USA, 2008.
20. Fraley, C.; Raftery, A.E. How many clusters? Which clustering method? Answers via model-based cluster analysis. *Comput. J.* **1998**, *4*, 578–588. [CrossRef]
21. Kaufman, L.; Rousseeuw, P.J. Partitioning around Medoids (Program PAM). In *Finding Groups in Data: An Introduction to Cluster Analysis*; Kaufman, L., Rousseeuw, P.J., Eds.; John Wiley & Sons, Inc.: Hoboken, NJ, USA, 1990; pp. 68–125.
22. Carberry, J.C.; Amatoury, J.; Eckert, D.J. Personalized management approach for OSA. *Chest* **2018**, *153*, 744–755. [CrossRef]
23. Gray, L.E.; McKenzie, K.D.; Eckert, J.D. Obstructive Sleep Apnea without Obesity Is Common and Difficult to Treat: Evidence for a Distinct Pathophysiological Phenotype. *J. Clin. Sleep Med.* **2017**, *13*, 81–88. [CrossRef]
24. Özdilekcan, Ç.; Özdemir, T.; Türkkanı, H.M.; Sur, H.Y.; Katoue, M.G. The Association of Body Mass Index Values with Severity and Phenotype of Sleep-Disordered Breathing. *Tuberk Toraks* **2019**, *67*, 265–271. [CrossRef]
25. Peepard, P.E.; Young, T.; Palta, M.; Depmsey, J.; Skatrud, J. Longitudinal study of moderate weight change and sleep-disordered breathing. *JAMA* **2000**, *284*, 3015–3021. [CrossRef]
26. Zinchuk, A.V.; Gentry, M.J.; Concato, J.; Yaggi, H.K. Phenotypes in obstructive sleep apnea: A definition, examples and evolution of approaches. *Sleep Med. Rev.* **2017**, *35*, 113–123. [CrossRef]

27. Gagnadoux, F.; Le Vaillant, M.; Paris, A.; Pigeanne, T.; Leclair-Visonneau, L.; Bizieux-Thaminy, A.; Alizon, C.; Humeau, M.P.; Nguyen, X.L.; Rouault, B.; et al. Relationship between OSA clinical phenotypes and CPAP treatment outcomes. *Chest* **2016**, *149*, 288–290. [CrossRef]
28. Ye, L.; Pien, G.; Ratcliffe, S.J.; Björnsdottir, E.; Arnardottir, E.S.; Pack, A.I.; Benediktsdottir, B.; Gislason, T. The different clinical faces of obstructive sleep apnoea: A cluster analysis. *Eur. Respir. J.* **2014**, *44*, 1600–1617. [CrossRef]
29. Pien, G.W.; Ye, L.; Keenan, T.B.; Maislin, G.; Bjornsdottir, E.; Arnardottir, E.S.; Benediktsdottir, B.; Gislason, T.; Pack, A.I. Changing faces of Obstructive Sleep Anea: Treatment Effects by Cluster designation in the Icelandic Sleep Apnea Cohort. *Sleep* **2018**, *41*, 1–13. [CrossRef]
30. Keenan, T.B.; Kim, J.; Singh, B.; Bittencourt, L.; Chen, N.-H.; Cistulli, A.P.; Magalang, U.J.; McArdle, N.; Mindel, J.W.; Benediktsdottir, B.; et al. Recognizable clinical subtypes of obstructive sleep apnea across international sleep centers: A cluster analysis. *SLEEP J.* **2018**, *41*, 1–14. [CrossRef]
31. Saaresanta, T.; Hedner, J.; Bonsignore, R.M.; Riha, R.L.; McNicholas, W.T.; Penzel, T.; Anttalainen, U.; Kvamme, J.A.; Pretl, M.; Sliwinski, P.; et al. Clinical Phenotypes and Comorbidity in European Sleep Apnoea Patients. *PLoS ONE* **2016**, *11*, e0163439.
32. Bailley, S.; Destors, M.; Grillet, Y.; Richard, P.; Stach, B.; Vivodtzev, I.; Timsit, J.-F.; Lévy, P.; Tamisier, R.; Pépin, J.-L.; et al. Obstructive Sleep Apnea: A Cluster Analysis at Time of Diagnosis. *PLoS ONE* **2016**, *11*, e0157318. [CrossRef]
33. Lacedonia, D.; Capragnano, E.G.; Sabato, R.; Storto, M.M.L.; Palmiotti, G.A.; Capozzi, V.; Barbaro, M.P.F.; Gallo, C. Characterization of obstructive sleep apnea-hypopnea syndrome (OSA) population by means of cluster analysis. *J. Sleep Res.* **2016**, *25*, 724–730. [CrossRef]
34. Young, T.; Palta, M.; Dempsey, J.; Skatrud, J.; Weber, S.; Badr, S. The occurrence of sleep-disordered breathing among middle-aged adults. *N. Engl. J. Med.* **1993**, *328*, 1230–1235. [CrossRef]
35. Nathan, E.C.; Harrison, M.C.; Yee, J.B.; Grunstein, R.R.; Wong, K.K.H.; Britt, H.V.C.; Marshall, N.S. Management of Snoring and Sleep Apnea in Australian Primary Care: The BEACH Study (2000–2014). *J. Clin. Sleep Med.* **2016**, *12*, 1167–1173.
36. Mayos, M.; Penacoba, P.; Ptro Pijoan, N.M.; Santiveri, C.; Flor, X.; Juvanteny, J.; Sampol, G.; Lioberes, P.; Aoiz, J.I.; Bayo, J.; et al. Coordinated program between primary care and sleep unit for the management of obstructive sleep apnea. *NPJ Prim. Care Respir. Med.* **2019**, *29*, 39. [CrossRef] [PubMed]
37. Tarraubella, N.; Battle, J.; Nadal, N.; Castro-Grattoni, A.L.; Gomez, S.; Sanchez-de-la-Torre, M.; Barbe, F. GESAP trial rationale and methodology: Management of patients with suspected obstructive sleep apnea in primary care units compared to sleep units. *NPJ Prim. Care Respir. Med.* **2017**, *27*, 8. [CrossRef]

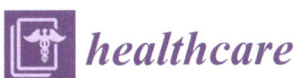

Article

Poor Diet, Long Sleep, and Lack of Physical Activity Are Associated with Inflammation among Non-Demented Community-Dwelling Elderly

Maria Basta [1,2,*], Christina Belogianni [1], Mary Yannakoulia [3], Ioannis Zaganas [4], Symeon Panagiotakis [5], Panagiotis Simos [1] and Alexandros N. Vgontzas [1,2]

- [1] Department of Psychiatry, University Hospital of Heraklion, 71500 Heraklion, Greece; belogianni.christina@gmail.com (C.B.); akis.simos@gmail.com (P.S.); avgontzas@psu.edu (A.N.V.)
- [2] Sleep Research and Treatment Center, Department of Psychiatry, Penn State University, State College, PA 16802, USA
- [3] Department of Nutrition and Dietetics, School of Health Science and Education, Harokopio University of Athens, 17671 Athens, Greece; mary.yannakoulia@gmail.com
- [4] Department of Neurology, University Hospital of Heraklion, 71500 Heraklion, Greece; johnzag@yahoo.com
- [5] Department of Internal Medicine, University Hospital of Heraklion, 71500 Heraklion, Greece; simeongpan@hotmail.com
- * Correspondence: mpasta@uoc.gr; Tel.: +30-2810392402; Fax: +30-2810392859

Abstract: Inflammation in elderly is associated with physical and cognitive morbidity and mortality. We aimed to explore the association of modifiable lifestyle parameters with inflammation among non-demented, community-dwelling elderly. A sub-sample of 117 patients with mild cognitive impairment (MCI, $n = 63$) and cognitively non-impaired controls (CNI, $n = 54$) were recruited from a large, population-based cohort in Crete, Greece, of 3140 elders (>60 years old). All participants underwent assessment of medical history/physical examination, extensive neuropsychiatric/neuropsychological evaluation, diet, three-day 24-h actigraphy, subjective sleep, physical activity, and measurement of IL-6 and TNFα plasma levels. Associations between inflammatory markers and diet, objective sleep duration, subjective sleep quality, and lack of physical activity were assessed using multivariate models. Regression analyses in the total group revealed significant associations between TNF-α and low vegetable consumption ($p = 0.003$), and marginally with objective long nighttime sleep duration ($p = 0.04$). In addition, IL-6 was associated with low vegetable consumption ($p = 0.001$) and lack of physical activity ($p = 0.001$). Poor diet and lack of physical activity appear to be modifiable risk factors of inflammation, whereas long sleep appears to be a marker of increased inflammatory response in elderly. Our findings may have clinical implications given the association of inflammatory response with morbidity, including cognitive decline, and mortality in elderly.

Keywords: inflammatory markers; elderly; objective sleep; diet; physical activity

1. Introduction

In the elderly, several molecular and cellular changes of the innate and acquired immunity have been described as potential contributors to biological aging [1]. Among others, dysregulation of the immune system, known as inflammaging, is characterized by low-grade but constant elevations of pro-inflammatory markers, such as interleukin (IL)-1, IL-6, IL-8, IL-13, C-reactive protein (CRP), interferon a (IFNa) and interferon b (IFNb), and tumor necrosis factor-alpha (TNFα). High levels of pro-inflammatory markers are evident in the majority of elderly, even among those without risk factors or clinically active diseases [2]. Pro-inflammatory responses, cellular senescence and immune senescence [3,4] are important components in the disorders of aging, including cardiovascular disease, cancer, chronic kidney disease, dementia, and depression, and other age-related conditions, such as functional decline, sarcopenia, frailty and mortality [2]. In light of these observations, there is a growing trend to approach overall mortality and morbidity, through the study of how various modifiable factors, such as diet, sleep and physical exercise, can affect the inflammatory load and consequently impact overall quality of life [5].

In older populations, research examining the relation of dietary parameters and inflammatory markers is rather scarce and has not produced consistent results so far. Observational and intervention studies, performed in either community-dwelling or hospitalized older individuals, concluded that sufficient evidence exists only regarding the protective role of n-3 polyunsaturated fatty acid intake [6,7]. In relation to diet overall, two studies in older adults from Italy and Scotland found that closer adherence to a Mediterranean diet, a plant-based dietary pattern, is related to decreases in inflammation-related markers over time (three or six years, respectively) [8,9]. However, little is known about the associations between inflammatory markers and specific food groups (i.e., vegetables, red meat, dairy, legumes, etc.) in older adults, including elderly with mild cognitive impairment (MCI), information that may be easily addressed in daily clinical practice.

Other studies have focused on possible links between sleep and inflammation in older adults. Sleep architecture changes significantly as we age [10,11], and health decline contributes to increasing sleep problems among the elderly, such as insomnia, sleep apnea, circadian rhythm sleep–wake disorders, and poor sleep quality and quantity [10,12]. Research so far indicates a U-shape association between objective sleep measurements and increased inflammatory markers among cognitively non-impaired elderly (CNI) [13–16], while others found no significant association between them [17,18].

Finally, in relation to physical activity, there is solid evidence reporting that physical activity based on amount and intensity of leisure time activities are related to lower concentrations of inflammatory markers in blood in older population groups [19–26]. Notably, this association has not been systematically studied using simple questions such as frequency of daily continuous brisk walking, reflecting a common and accessible for elderly form of physical activity with evidence for health benefits based on the UK Chief Medical Officer's guidelines [27].

In terms of exercise, higher levels based on rather strenuous exercise programs have a beneficial effect on inflammation levels in healthy elderly [22]. Longitudinal studies investigating associations between inflammatory markers and exercise in patients with MCI are very few. A recent pilot study demonstrated that 12 weeks of aerobic training in 30 CNI and 30 patients with MCI significantly decreased inflammatory markers in both groups [28]. Moreover, a recent meta-analysis has linked lifestyle interventions, including exercise, with significant reductions in IL-6 and TNFα levels in patients with MCI and dementia [29].

MCI is an early stage of impairment in memory and/or other cognitive functions (such as language, executive, or visuoconstruction capacity) in individuals who maintain the ability to independently perform most activities of daily living and sustain a normal level of function [30–32]. On the other hand, the prevalence of MCI is high (about 15–20% in elderly above 60 years), with a significant annual rate in which MCI progresses to dementia varying between 8 and 15% per year [31]. Based on that, MCI is an important condition to identify and treat. Therefore, identifying possible modifiable factors that may delay or reverse the progression of MCI to dementia is very important.

To our knowledge, there is no study evaluating the joint contribution of all three parameters of lifestyle, i.e., diet, sleep, and physical activity, as described above in relation to inflammation markers in older non-demented adults, including patients with MCI. To fill this gap in the literature, the aim of the present study was to examine in a comprehensive way the association between inflammation and diet based on food groups, subjective and objective sleep and mild physical activity based on daily continuous, brisk walking, in a sample of community-dwelling older adults. A secondary objective was to explore if the purported role of each of the three lifestyle parameters is modified by the presence of age-related cognitive impairment as indicated by diagnosis of MCI. Based on our previous work and existing literature, we hypothesized that objective sleep, diet, and physical activity will independently relate to inflammation levels, both in cognitively non-impaired elderly, as well as among persons with MCI.

2. Materials and Methods

2.1. Study Design

The present sample consisted of participants of the Cretan Aging Cohort, a cross-sectional study of community-dwelling elders, recruited from the rural and urban areas in the district of Heraklion, Crete, Greece, between March 2013 and June 2015. The primary aim of this study was to investigate the prevalence of and risk factors associated with cognitive decline [33]. The Cretan Aging Cohort study was conducted in two phases. The study was conducted according to the guidelines laid down in the Declaration of Helsinki and all procedures involving human subjects/patients were approved by the Bioethics Committee of the University Hospital of Heraklion, Crete (Protocol Number: 13541, 20 November 2010). Written informed consent was obtained from all subjects.

Phase I: Eligible participants were those aged > 60 years who visited selected primary health care facilities in areas of the Heraklion district for any reason. Consenting individuals (n = 3200) completed an interview with a specially trained nurse, who used a structured questionnaire to document sociodemographic information, anthropometric measurements, physical and mental health issues, and medication use. Cognitive function was evaluated using the Greek version of the Mini Mental State Examination (MMSE) test [34], applying a universal cut-off of 23/24 points (because the majority of participants had ≤6 years of formal education) for referral of patients for further evaluation. Based on this cut-off, participants were divided into two groups: those with MMSE <24, considered to be at risk for cognitive impairment, and the not-at-risk group with MMSE ≥24 [33]. After excluding participants with crucial missing data (MMSE score, age), the final study sample consisted of 3140 people (57.0% women) aged 73.7 ± 7.8 (60–100) years, who had completed an average of 5.8 ± 3.3 (0–18) years of formal education and lived mostly in rural areas.

Phase II: Participants who scored < 24 points on the MMSE (n = 636) were referred for an extensive neuropsychological and neuropsychiatric evaluation in phase 2 of the study. The 344 consenting subjects were similar with the 636 originally refereed subjects in terms of age, gender, and body mass index (BMI). Certified neurologists, psychiatrists and internists completed an extensive questionnaire based on the one used in the Hellenic Longitudinal Investigation of Aging and Dietstudy [35]. Trained neuropsychologists performed a test battery evaluating a variety of cognitive domains. Apart from medical and family history, daily activities, dietary patterns and sleep characteristics were assessed as well (for a detailed description of all tests and scales used, see [33]). Diagnosis of any type of MCI was based on modified Petersen criteria (IWG-1) [36] and on a consensus decision between two or more clinicians who took into account results from the comprehensive neuropsychiatric and neuropsychological evaluation. Diagnosis of MCI further required that cognitive deficits could not be accounted for by clinically significant mood or anxiety disorder.

To be included in the MCI group participants had to have age- and education-adjusted z scores <−1.5 on indices derived from at least two tests within a given cognitive domain (episodic memory, language, attention/executive) and demonstrate intact levels of everyday functionality according to a comprehensive, informant scale of instrumental activities of daily living [37] adapted for the Greek population from Lawton and Brody (1969). Using the non-cognitively impaired pool of subjects who scored >24 on the MMSE (n = 2504), a control group of 181 participants was created after stratifying for residence, gender, and age. Of those, 161 agreed to participate in phase 2 of the study (see Figure 1). In phase II, among 505 participants examined, 231 were diagnosed as MCI, 128 with dementia, and 146 were CNI [33].

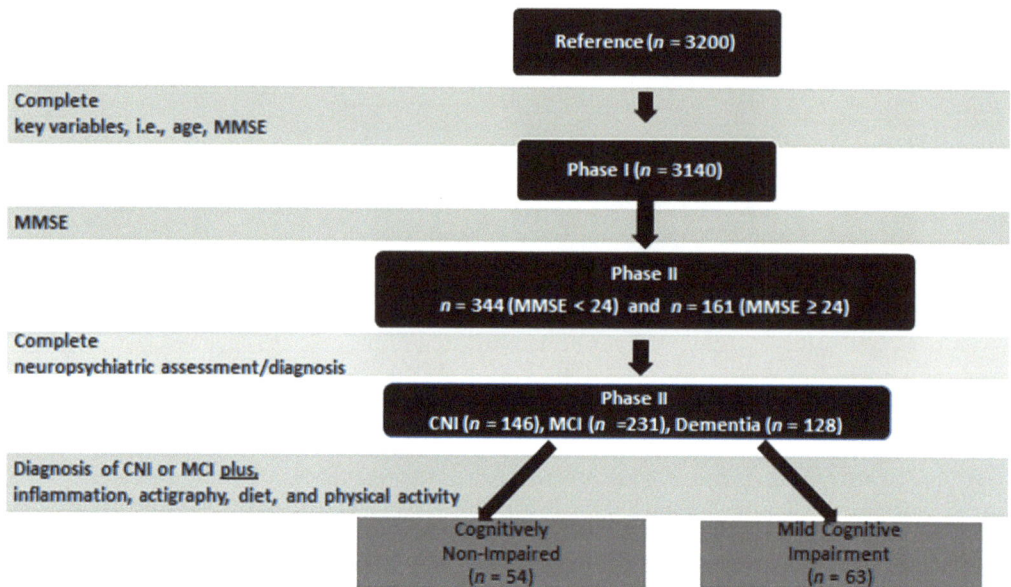

Figure 1. Study flowchart. Abbreviations; MMSE: Mini Mental State Examination, CNI: cognitively non-impaired, MCI: mild cognitive impairment.

2.2. Participants

The current analyses were performed on a sub-sample of participants from Phase II in whom we obtained complete data of objective (actigraphy) and subjective sleep, measurements of inflammatory markers (TNF-α and IL-6 plasma level), as well as dietary and physical activity habits based on valid questionnaires. The final sample included non-cognitively impaired participants (CNI) ($n = 54$), and participants with a diagnosis of MCI ($n = 63$) (Figure 1). Given that all participants in this cohort were community-dwelling members of primary care health units, elderly people with severe terminal medical illnesses or severe movement impairment were not included in this cohort.

2.3. Measurements

2.3.1. Inflammatory Markers

Blood samples were collected from each participant between 10:00 am and 12:00 pm, transferred to EDTA-containing tubes (three per participant) and refrigerated until centrifugation (within 3 h) for plasma isolation. Afterwards, the plasma samples were kept in deep freeze (-80 °C). Plasma TFN-α and IL-6 were measured by ELISA technique (Human TNF-alpha Quantikine HS ELISA and Human IL-6 Quantikine HS ELISA kits respectively, R&D Systems Europe, Abington, UK). For the TNF-α measurement, the inter-assay coefficient of variation was 12.74%, the intra-assay coefficient of variation was 19.04, and the lower detection limit was 0.209 pg/mL. For the IL-6 determination, the inter-assay coefficients of variation were 13.09%, the intra-assay coefficients of variation were 11.04, and the lower detection limit was 0.133 pg/mL.

2.3.2. Diet

Habitual diet was assessed using a validated semi-quantitative food frequency questionnaire [38]. It comprises 69 questions on the consumption of foods or combination of foods, including dairy products, cereals, fruits, vegetables, meat, fish, legumes, added fats, alcoholic beverages, stimulants and sweets. Using a 6-point scale ("never/rarely", "1–3 times/month", "1–2 times/week", "3–6 times/week", "1 time/day", "≥ 2 times/day"), participants were asked to indicate the absolute frequency of consuming a certain amount of food, expressed in g, millilitres, or in other common measures, such as slice, tablespoon or cup, depending on the food. Responses to the food frequency questionnaire were converted to daily intakes of specific food items and were extrapolated into macronutrient intakes. Energy intake was calculated by summing energy intake from macronutrients and alcohol, assuming 4 kcal/g for carbohydrates and proteins, 9 kcal/g for lipids, and 7 kcal/g for alcohol. Responses were also grouped into major groups (expressed as servings/day). Adherence to the Mediterranean dietary pattern was evaluated using the MedDietScore, an 11-item composite score calculated for each participant from the FFQ-based food consumption [39]. The score is based on the weekly consumption of 11 food groups (non-refined cereals, fruits, vegetables, legumes, potatoes, fish, meat and meat products, poultry, full fat dairy, olive oil use and alcohol). A score 0–5 is given for each food group. The potential range of MedDietScore is between 0 and 55, with higher values indicating greater adherence to the Mediterranean diet.

2.3.3. Sleep Measurements

Subjective Sleep: Subjective sleep and presence of any sleep disorder were evaluated using 20 sleep-related questions from a standardized questionnaire, used in the Penn State Cohort and described in detail elsewhere [40]. In the current analysis, subjective sleep variables examined were non-refreshing sleep, excessive daytime sleepiness (EDS), sleep apnea symptoms and insomnia symptoms qualified in terms of severity on a scale of 0–4 (0 = none, 1 = mild, 2 = moderate, 3 = severe). Non-refreshing sleep was evaluated by a positive response ("often" or "always") to the following question "Do you feel groggy and un-refreshed after you wake up in the morning". Excessive Daytime Sleepiness (EDS) was evaluated by a positive response ("often" or "always") to one or both of the questions: "Do you feel groggy or sleepy most of the day but manage to stay awake", and/or "Do you have irresistible sleep attacks". The presence of symptoms consistent with sleep apnea was indicated by a positive response on one or both of the following questions: "Do you know/Have you been told that you stop breathing or breath irregularly during sleep, occasionally, often or always?" and "Do you know/Have you been told that you snore during sleep to a moderate/severe degree?". Finally, the presence of "insomnia symptoms" was established on a "yes" answer to the questions: "Do you have difficulty falling asleep", "Do you have difficulty staying asleep" or "Do you wake up in the morning earlier than desired" often or always.

Objective Sleep: Objective measurement of sleep in a free-living environment was documented for three consecutive 24-h periods during weekdays using an actigraph (Actigraph, GT3XP model, Pensacola, FL, USA) placed on the non-dominant arm of the participant. The actigraphic data were examined together with sleep diaries in which the actigraph was removed and "bedtime"/"out of bedtime" times were reported daily. Night was defined based on the questions "What time did you go to bed" and "What time did you get out of bed" answered by the participant in the sleep diary. Naps, defined as daytime sleep for more than 20 min, were based on the actigraphy and the sleep diary provided by the participant [41,42]. Actigraphy data including among other night sleep efficiency (SE), night sleep onset latency (SOL), night total sleep time (TST), night time in bed (TMB), night wake time after sleep onset (WASO), number of awakenings during the night, night average duration of awakenings, 24-h (nighttime and daytime) sleep time (24-hTST), and 24-h (nighttime and daytime) time in bed (24-h TMB) were analyzed using the ActLife 6 software (Actlife v6.9.5 LLC, Pensacola, FL, USA). Periods without actigraphic activity which, based on the sleep diaries, were not identified as sleep were considered as artifacts and were removed from the analysis. Sleep parameters were averaged over three consecutive 24-h. Participants with actigraphy recorded over fewer than three days or average night TST ≤ 3 h were excluded from the analysis. The start time of the 24-h period was set at 11:00 am on the day that the actigraph was applied on the participant's hand by our staff. Objective sleep parameters were analyzed as continuous variables in all group comparisons. From the objectively recorded sleep time data, we regrouped the entire study sample into two ordinal groups. Initially, the total group was divided in quartiles. Our previous findings based on the same cohort have shown that long but not short sleep duration is associated with cognitive impairment both among CNI and MCI participants. Based on that, we divided the sample to the top 25% of persons above the median percent sleep time (long sleep duration group), and the 75% of persons in the bottom half (normal sleep duration group). We then rounded the cut-off points to meaningful numbers and thus created the following two sleep duration groups: the long sleep duration group consisted of those who slept ≥ 7.5 h (coded as 1), and the normal sleep duration group of those who slept <7.5 h (coded as 0) [43].

Finally, short sleep duration was defined as total night <360 min, corresponding to the lower quartile of the distribution of night total sleep time (TST) in the total sample of the present study.

2.3.4. Physical Activity

Regular physical activity was based on participant responses to a single question "How many days did you walk for more than 10 min in a row in a brisk manner during the last week". Since we aimed to evaluate the role of mild physical activity, lack of physical activity was defined if participants had less than three days of 10 min of brisk walking in a row during the last week, given that adults engaging in less than 30 min of activity per week are considered as significantly inactive [44]. Lack of activity was coded with a value of 1 and presence of activity with 0.

2.3.5. Other Variables

Demographic variables such as gender, and age, and body mass index (BMI) were also assessed. Additionally, prescription of any type of psychotropic medication (including benzodiazepines) was recorded. Finally, a diagnosis of late-life depression was based on the Phase II clinical interview by a team of a certified psychiatrist, a neurologist and a geriatrician, score on self-report psychiatric symptom scales, and the thorough neuropsychological evaluation.

2.4. Statistical Analysis

In preliminary univariate analyses we assessed diagnostic group differences on demographic variables, sleep, and lifestyle habits and proinflammatory cytokines. Group differences on continuous variables (total sleep time, sleep efficiency, sleep latency, wake time after sleep onset, cytokine levels, dietary intake) were assessed through ANOVAs and on categorical variables (subjective sleep indices, physical activity) using chi-square tests. In these analyses age, gender, BMI, use of psychotropic medications, sleep apnea symptoms, and diagnosis of depression served as covariates.

The main objective of the study involved assessing the joint contribution of demographic, sleep (objective and subjective), and lifestyle variables on IL-6 or TNF-a levels in a sample of elders varying considerably in cognitive status. Variable selection for multivariate models was based on partial correlations, computed in the total sample, between each independent variable and IL-6 or TNF-a levels, controlling for MCI diagnosis (coded as 0 for the NCI group and 1 for the MCI group). Variables of interest were entered in the multivariate models if their corresponding partial correlation with IL-6 or TNF-a had a p-value < 0.1. These multiple linear regression models included IL-6 or TNF-a as the dependent variable and age, gender, BMI, and MCI diagnosis as confounders. Both models (the first with IL-6 and the second with TNF-a as the dependent variable) were recomputed, stratified by clinical group (with age, gender, and BMI as confounders). The effects of interest in these analyses were (i) R^2 change (evaluated at study-wise $p < 0.05/6 = 0.008$), and (ii) the regression coefficients for each independent variable entered in the second step of each model (following all covariates), which were evaluated at family-wise $p < 0.05/3 = 0.017$ for the model predicting TNF-a and at $p < 0.05/2 = 0.025$. A priori power estimation (using

G*Power 3.1 [45]) indicated that the sample size was adequate to detect a minimum change in $R^2 = 0.095$ (corresponding to a small effect size) to ensure power of 80% at $p = 0.05$.

3. Results

3.1. Sample Demographics, Clinical and Preclinical Variables

The final sample included 117 participants (63.7% women; Table 1) aged 74.5 years (SD = 7.4), who had attained an average of 5.1 (SD = 3.1) years of formal education. The sample average MMSE score was 24.9 points (SD = 3.6) and comprised 54 cognitively non-impaired (CNI) and 63 persons diagnosed with MCI (Figure 1). Table 2 shows inflammatory markers, diet, subjective and objective sleep variables, and physical activity in the total sample (corresponding values by clinical group are presented in the Supplementary Tables S1 and S2). In univariate analyses, the two clinical groups were comparable on levels of IL-6/TNF-a, sleep parameters, frequency of mild activity ($p > 0.1$) and the majority of dietary variables with some exceptions (descriptives by clinical group and corresponding effect sizes are presented in Table 3). Specifically, CNI participants reported greater adherence to the Mediterranean diet, greater daily energy intake, and greater consumption of red meat, non-refined and refined cereals, and sweets, compared to MCI participants.

Table 1. Demographic and clinical parameters of the total sample and by diagnostic group.

	Total Group I (n = 117)		CNI (n = 54)		MCI (n = 63)		p	Cohen's d
	Mean	SD	Mean	SD	Mean	SD		
Age (years)	74.0	7.4	72.3	7.6	75.6	7.0	0.005	0.45
Education (years)	5.1	3.1	5.4	2.7	4.8	3.5	0.3	0.19
Gender (%)								
Men	36.3	-	40.7		28.6		0.3	0.18
Women	63.7	-	59.3		71.4			
MMSE	24.9	3.6	27.0	2.8	22.9	2.8	<0.001	1.19
GDS	3.5	3.4	2.7	3.4	4.5	3.3	0.008	0.50
HADS-Anxiety	2.8	3.3	2.6	3.4	3.4	3.3	0.3	0.25
Depression (%)	27.4	-	11.1	-	39.7	-	0.001	0.65
Psychotropic medication (%)	31.9	-	24.2	-	44.2	-	0.011	0.53
Benzodiazepine use (%)	8.8	-	9.7	-	8.2	-	0.9	0.11
BMI	30.0	4.8	30.5	4.9	29.3	4.5	0.06	0.26

MMSE: Mini Mental State Examination; GDS: Geriatric Depression Scale; HADS: Hospital Anxiety and Depression Scale. BMI: body mass index, CNI: cognitively non-impaired, MCI: mild cognitive impairment. Note: Corresponding values for the combined, total sample of CNI and MCI participants in the Cretan Aging cohort (n = 377, Mean age = 75.4, SD = 7.3) are as follows. MMSE: Mean = 24.5, SD = 3.5; GDS: Mean = 3.7, SD = 3.5; HADS-Anxiety: Mean = 3.0, SD = 3.4; BMI: Mean = 30.1, SD = 4.7. Total CNI group; MMSE: Mean = 26.4 (SD = 3.1); GDS: Mean = 3.1 (SD = 3.2); HADS-Anxiety: Mean = 2.9 (SD = 3.6); BMI: Mean = 30.5 (4.7). Total MCI group; MMSE: Mean = 22.3 (SD = 2.6); GDS: Mean = 4.3 (SD = 3.5); HADS-Anxiety: Mean = 3.3 (3.2); BMI: Mean = 29.9 (SD = 4.6).

Table 2. Inflammatory markers, sleep, diet, and physical activity levels of the entire sample (n = 117).

	Mean	SD		Mean	SD
IL-6 (pg/mL)	1.28	0.9	Energy	2228.1	536.20
TNF-α (pg/mL)	1.12	0.6	MDS	34.7	4.6
Night TST (min)	411.2	70.9	Servings per day of:		
24-h TST (min)	448.7	84.2	Vegetables	2.54	1.28
Night TST > 450 min (%)	21.0	-	Red meat	1.27	0.84
Night TST < 360 min (%)	26.1	-	Dairy	1.06	0.80
Night TMB (min)	503.2	78.8	Legumes	0.65	0.45
24-h TMB (min)	560.4	107.5	Non-refined cereal	0.91	0.94
Night Sleep Efficiency	83.0	8.8	Refined cereal	2.56	1.20
Night WASO	77.0	42.3	Potatoes	0.38	0.24
Night Sleep latency	13.0	12.0	Fruit	2.83	1.95
Number of Awakenings	15.9	6.1	Fish	0.83	0.66

Table 2. Cont.

	Mean	SD		Mean	SD
Sleep duration (min)	394.0	115.9	Poultry	0.52	0.37
Non-refreshing sleep (%)	12.9	-	Eggs	0.19	0.19
Leg movement (%)	1.7	-	Sweets	0.44	0.45
EDS (%)	2.6	-	Alcoholic beverages	0.54	0.97
Sleep Apnea symptoms (%)	17.2	-			
Insomnia-type symptoms (%)	32.5	-			
Physical activity (%)	64.0	-			

Note: Consumption of major food categories is in servings/day. TST: total sleep time, TMB: time in bed, WASO: wake time after sleep onset, EDS: excessive daytime sleepiness, Energy: total energy intake (kcal/day), MDS: Mediterranean diet score. IL-6 normal levels < 2 pg/mL [46], TNFα normal levels < 3.1 pg/mL [47].

Table 3. Inflammatory Markers, diet, sleep, and physical activity by diagnostic group.

	CNI (n = 54)	MCI (n = 63)	p	Cohen's d		CNI (n = 54)	MCI (n = 63)	p	Cohen's d
IL-6 (pg/mL)	1.36 (1.0)	1.21 (0.7)	0.7	0.17	Energy Intake	2455.8 (472.2)	2017.9 (508.7)	0.2	0.89
TNF-α (pg/mL)	1.07 (0.6)	1.16 (0.6)	0.1	0.16	MDS	35.9 (4.3)	33.6 (4.6)	0.016	0.49
Night TST (min)	408.9 (77.8)	414.5 (64.6)	0.4	0.09					
Night TST > 450 min (%)	16.1	25.0	0.2	0.24	Servings per day of:				
Night TST < 360 min (%)	25.8	27.3	0.9	0.02	Vegetables	2.72 (1.30)	2.41 (1.22)	0.7	0.24
24-h TST (min)	438.0 (92.9)	457.8 (75.3)	0.2	0.24	Red meat	1.47 (0.95)	1.12 (0.68)	0.002	0.55
Night TMB (min)	493.4 (88.1)	511.6 (68.3)	0.14	0.25	Dairy products	1.08 (0.80)	1.05 (0.82)	0.5	0.04
24-h TMB (min)	539.8 (117.9)	578.0 (95.9)	0.1	0.36	Legumes	0.64 (0.40)	0.66 (0.49)	0.8	0.05
Night Sleep Efficiency	82.9 (8.0)	81.2 (9.3)	0.3	0.22	Non-refined cereals	1.14 (1.08)	0.73 (0.78)	0.3	0.44
Night WASO	71.1 (41.3)	82.0 (43.2)	0.3	0.25	Refined cereals	2.65 (1.16)	2.48 (1.24)	0.2	0.13
Night Sleep latency	11.2 (7.0)	14.5 (14.7)	0.1	0.28	Potatoes	0.38 (0.23)	0.40 (0.25)	0.3	0.08
Number of Awakenings	15.4 (6.5)	16.3 (5.8)	0.9	0.15	Fruit	3.14 (1.77)	2.57 (2.07)	0.2	0.34
Sleep duration (min)	412.3 (123.1)	378.0 (106.6)	0.5	0.29	Fish	0.89 (0.74)	0.78 (0.58)	0.5	0.17
Non-refreshing sleep (%)	11.1	14.5	0.5	0.16	Poultry	0.51 (0.36)	0.53 (0.39)	0.7	0.06
Leg movement (%)	1.9	1.6	0.9	0.02	Eggs	0.24 (0.22)	0.15 (0.14)	0.017	0.47
EDS (%)	1.6	3.7	0.6	0.16	Sweets	0.54 (0.48)	0.35 (0.41)	0.006	0.43
Sleep Apnea symptoms (%)	16.7	17.7	0.9	0.04	Alcoholic beverages	0.74 (1.21)	0.38 (0.69)	0.1	0.39
Insomnia-type symptoms (%)	27.8	36.5	0.3	0.23					
Physical activity (%)	62.0	65.6	0.9	0.03					

Notes: Consumption of major food categories is in servings/day. Unless otherwise indicated, values are means (SD), CNI: cognitively non-impaired, MCI: mild cognitive impairment, TST: total sleep time, TMB: time in bed, WASO: wake time after sleep onset, EDS: excessive daytime sleepiness, Energy: total energy intake (kcal/day), MDS: Mediterranean diet score.

3.2. Associations of Inflammatory Markers with Sleep, Diet and Physical Activity

Univariate analyses: As shown in Table 4, in the entire sample, higher TNF-α levels were significantly associated with age (r = 0.230, p = 0.017), nighttime TST over 450 min (r = 0.202, p = 0.03), less frequent consumption of vegetables (r = −0.407, p < 0.001) and red meat (r = −0.190, p = 0.03). These correlations were adjusted for MCI diagnosis, which was weakly associated with inflammatory markers (Spearman r < 0.13). Moreover, higher levels of IL-6 were significantly associated with lack of mild physical activity (r = −0.303, p = 0.002) and less frequent consumption of vegetables (r = −0.393, p < 0.001). Correlations of inflammatory markers with all other variables (including depression diagnosis) were also very small (Spearman r < 0.15).

A similar pattern of associations between pro-inflammatory markers and food groups/physical activity was observed within each group, although the association between TNF-a and red meat consumption failed to reach significance, probably due to reduced statistical power (p > 0.4).

Multivariate analyses: According to the results of the univariate analyses, the following variables of interest were included in the model accounting for TNF-a levels: long nighttime TST, consumption of vegetables, and consumption of red meat. Entered together in the second step of the model (following age, gender, BMI, and MCI diagnosis which were entered as confounders in the first step), these variables resulted in significant model improvement (change in R^2 = 0.168, p < 0.001). As shown in Table 5, high TNF-α levels were significantly associated with lower vegetable consumption (p = 0.001) and marginally with night TST of more than 450 min (p = 0.04). In the analyses stratified by MCI diagnosis, consumption of vegetables remained significant in both groups (p < 0.016), although long nighttime TST failed to reach significance (p > 0.2).

Table 4. Partial correlations of demographic, clinical, sleep, and lifestyle parameters with proinflammatory cytokine levels in the entire sample.

	TNF-α	IL-6
Age	0.230 †[1]	0.157
Gender (male)	0.157	0.147
Depression Diagnosis	−0.164	−0.081
Physical activity	−0.070	−0.303 †[5]
Night TST > 450 min	0.202 *[2]	0.079
Insomnia Symptoms	−0.131	−0.043
Consumption of vegetables	−0.407 †[3]	−0.393 †[6]
Consumption of red meat	−0.190 *[4]	−0.140
Consumption of dairy	0.142	0.059
Consumption of legumes	−0.049	−0.134

Note: Pearson or Spearman r values controlling for Mild Cognitive Impairment diagnosis. Variables are listed if the zero-order correlations with either IL-6 or TNF-a were associated with $p < 0.1$. TST: total sleep time. * $p < 0.05$, † $p < 0.01$, [1] CNI: r = 0.192, p = 0.2; MCI: r = 0.245, p = 0.06, [2] CNI: r = 0.288, p = 0.04; MCI: r = 0.069, p = 0.5, [3] CNI: r = −0.418, p < 0.001; MCI: r = −0.328, p = 0.01, [4] CNI: r = −0.144, p = 0.3; MCI: r = −0.100, p = 0.4, [5] CNI: r = −0.318, p = 0.02; MCI: r = −0.298, p = 0.02, [6] CNI: r = −0.402, p = 0.002; MCI: r = −0.369, p = 0.003.

Table 5. Associations of TNF-α with modifiable lifestyle habits using Multiple Linear Regression analysis in the entire sample.

	B	95% CI	p Value
Night TST > 450 min	0.230	(0.010 to 0.449)	0.04 [1]
Consumption of vegetables	−0.203	(−0.289 to −0.117)	**0.001** [2]
Consumption of red meat	−0.102	(−0.077 to 0.282)	0.3
Constant	0.595	(−0.741 to 1.931)	0.4

TST: total sleep time; variables were included in the final models if they correlated with TNF-a at $p < 0.1$. Confounders: age, gender, BMI, Mild Cognitive Impairment diagnosis. Change in $R^2 = 0.174$, $p < 0.001$. Unstandardized regression coefficients are reported throughout, in bold if significant at Bonferroni-adjusted $p < 0.017$. [1] CNI: B = 0.287, p = 0.2; MCI: B = 0.130, p = 0.2, [2] CNI: B = −0.240, p = 0.002; MCI: B = −0.152, p = 0.016.

The following variables of interest were entered in the model accounting for IL-6 levels in the total sample: physical activity and consumption of vegetables jointly accounted for 24.2% of variance beyond that explained by step 1 confounders (age, gender, BMI, MCI diagnosis; change in $R^2 = 0.246$, $p < 0.001$). As shown in Table 6, higher levels of IL-6 were significantly associated with lack of physical activity ($p = 0.001$) and less frequent consumption of vegetables ($p = 0.001$). In the analyses stratified by MCI diagnosis, consumption of vegetables remained significant in both groups ($p < 0.009$), while lack of physical activity failed to reach significance ($p = 0.06$). Post-hoc power estimation indicated that the present sample size ensured adequate power (80%) to reveal a statistically significant independent contribution of physical activity to IL-6 levels (at $p < 0.05$), modest power (56–63%) to reveal statistically significant contribution of vegetable and meat consumption to TNF-a levels, and much lower power (26–36%) regarding the contribution of long nighttime TST and vegetable consumption to TNF-a and IL-6 levels, respectively.

Table 6. Associations of IL-6 with modifiable lifestyle habits using Multiple Linear Regression analysis in the entire sample.

	B	95% CI	p Value
Physical activity	−0.538	(−0.847 to −0.230)	**0.001** [1]
Consumption of vegetables	−0.300	(−0.428 to −0.172)	**0.001** [2]
Constant	1.887	(−1.169 to 3.943)	0.07

Variables were included in the final models if they correlated with IL-6 at $p < 0.1$. Confounders: age, gender, BMI, Mild Cognitive Impairment diagnosis. Change in $R^2 = 0.242$, $p < 0.001$. Unstandardized regression coefficients are reported throughout, in bold if significant at Bonferroni-adjusted $p < 0.025$. [1] CNI: B = −0.739, p = 0.06; MCI: B = −0.315, p = 0.09, [2] CNI: B = −0.303, p = 0.008; MCI: B = −0.222, p = 0.009.

4. Discussion

The main findings of this study are that the plasma levels of pro-inflammatory cytokines, i.e., TNF-α and IL-6, among community-dwelling elderly with and without mild cognitive impairment are independently and significantly associated with decreased consumption of vegetables, objective long sleep duration and self-reported lack of physical activity. It appears that poor diet and lack of physical activity may be predisposing factors related with inflammation in elderly, whereas long sleep duration seems to be a marker of increased inflammation in this population.

The first key finding of this study is that a diet low in vegetables correlates with high levels of both TNF-α and IL-6. This correlation was significant in the entire elderly group, as well as both in the cognitively non-impaired and the MCI patients' subgroups, separately. Previous literature has examined associations between Mediterranean diet and inflammation in various age groups, however few studies have reported associations between inflammatory markers and specific food groups in elderly populations. Specifically, some studies in young-middle-aged or wide age range cohorts reported associations between inflammatory markers such as CRP, IL-6, IL-1β and TNFα, TNFαR2 and vegetables /or vegetables and fruit combined [48–52]. However, none of these studies were focused on the elderly. One previous study in healthy, elderly men failed to find associations between vegetables consumption and CRP [20]. This study showed that in non-demented elderly, IL-6 and TNFα were significantly associated with low consumption of vegetables. Our finding may be explained by the special characteristics and environment of our sample, i.e., rural population, residing in a region in the Mediterranean Sea with mild sunny climate, and local produce of a large variety of vegetables and fruit, which were easily accessible, cheap and part of daily diet consumed in rather high amounts. It is known that the Cretan cuisine makes wide use of a large variety of greens and vegetables; based on previous research, Cretans consume up to three times more vegetables compared to other Europeans [53,54]. Moreover, based on previous literature, vegetables intake in Crete is high compared to other cohorts of older adults in western countries [55–57], but also in Greece [58].

Furthermore, to our knowledge, this is the first study to report an association between pro-inflammatory cytokines, IL-6 and TNFα and low vegetable consumption in elderly with mild cognitive impairment. Previous literature reports elevation of pro-inflammatory cytokines, IL-6 and TNFα in patients with degenerative dementias [59–61], while other studies have shown that adherence to Mediterranean diet, rich in specific food groups including vegetables, may be beneficial to cognitive function [62,63]. Future interventional studies in larger samples, focusing on the elderly with or without MCI, are needed to validate and expand our findings.

The second significant finding is that long objective total sleep time (TST) > 450 min is associated with higher levels of TNF-α in non-demented community-dwelling elderly. This effect reached significance after correcting for multiple comparisons in the subgroup of persons with MCI and approached significance in the analyses on the total sample. Although a recent meta-analysis including both objective and subjective sleep measurements in a wide age-range of adults [64] also reported an association between long sleep and inflammation, to our knowledge, only one previous original study reported this association in elderly men without cognitive impairment [65]. Our study confirms and expands previous findings on the association between long-sleep and higher inflammatory levels in elderly populations.

A study based on objective actigraphic sleep found a U-shape association between sleep duration and all-cause mortality among elderly [66]. Several studies have reported associations between long sleep duration and cardiovascular disease, coronary heart disease, cognitive decline, and all-cause mortality in this age group [43,67–70]. It appears that objective long sleep is a result/marker of increased inflammation in elderly subjects [65]. In contrast, and at the other end of the spectrum, short sleep duration, either habitual or as a result of experimental sleep deprivation, appears to induce higher levels of inflammatory markers both in elderly [14] and younger populations [71–75]; a condition that is reversed by lengthening sleep duration [76,77]. The underlying mechanisms relating long sleep and increased inflammation involve the pro-inflammatory cytokines IL-1β and TNFα, which have a significant role in the regulation of sleep both in animals and humans [78,79]. In addition, elevated cytokine levels are associated with excessive sleep and daytime sleepiness. Previous literature has demonstrated that exogenous administration of IL-1β and IL-6 to patients can induce somnolence and/or increased sleep [79]. Furthermore, in patients with excessive daytime sleepiness disorders, such as sleep apnea and narcolepsy, peripheral levels of IL-6 and TNFα are elevated and appear to mediate sleepiness and fatigue [80]; indeed, in a pilot study, Etanercept, a TFNα antagonist, significantly and markedly reduced daytime sleepiness in patients with sleep apnea [81].

Finally, we found that lack of physical activity is correlated with increased IL-6 levels. Many studies in the past have shown the inverse association of physical activity/exercise and inflammation in elderly populations [20–24,26,82–84]. In some of these studies physical activity based on self-reported amount and intensity of leisure activities or exercise programs appeared to be strenuous [20–24,84], whereas others used objective measures of physical activity such as step count, hand grip and accelerometry, and the chair stand test among others [24,26,82,83]. Furthermore, this study including MCI patients further confirms and expands earlier findings involving determinants of proinflammatory cytokines among these patients, i.e., associations between exercise and IL-6 and TNFα among patients with MCI with co-morbid insulin resistance, and significant decrease of inflammatory markers, such as IL-6, TNFα and CRP, in MCI patients after a 12-week exercise program [28]. This study showed that even mild self-reported activity assessed with a single question easily administered in a primary care setting, i.e., walking for a minimum of 10 min in a row in a brisk manner on three or more days per week, may have a significant impact on systemic inflammation in both cognitively intact and MCI elderly.

4.1. Strengths and Limitations

The main strength of the current study is the inclusion of multiple, modifiable lifestyle factors such as diet, sleep, and physical activity as potential correlates with underlying inflammation in elderly. Furthermore, our study has included a fairly large sample living in an area with unique dietetic habits such as large consumption of fresh vegetables. In addition, our outcome variables are easily measurable and applicable in a primary care setting such as single questions or actigraphy. Finally, the associations between diet, physical activity and inflammation were significant in the entire group and remained significant or borderline significant in both subgroups, i.e., cognitively intact or patients with MCI.

However, some limitations should also be acknowledged. In our study, actigraphy was performed for three consecutive 24-h periods, compared to 1–2 weeks of actigraphy recordings which is the recommended duration. Additionally, we used only self-reported symptoms of apnea to screen for obstructive sleep apnea (OSA), a condition highly prevalent among the elderly [85]. Similarly, EDS and subjective sleep duration were based on participants' self-reports. Additionally, in our model we did not include other factors potentially associated with inflammation, such as medication use and medical co-morbidities. Moreover, physical activity was based on self-report. However, the fact that vegetables are significantly related with both inflammatory markers examined in the regression models supports their independent role in inflammation in our sample. Finally, because of the cross-sectional nature of this study, causality between inflammation and lifestyle variables such as diet, sleep and physical activity cannot be examined.

4.2. Implications

Inflammatory response is associated with morbidity, including cognitive decline and mortality in elderly. Our study extends the existing literature by linking in a comprehensive way poor vegetable consumption, long sleep duration, and lack of physical activity with higher levels of inflammation among non-demented community-dwelling elderly. We propose that adopting a diet rich in vegetables and a physically active lifestyle, by lowering inflammation, could help reduce mortality and morbidity, including cognitive decline among elderly. Furthermore, given that long sleep seems to relate with inflammation levels, as well as cognition and disease severity among elders with cognitive decline [42,43,86], we and others have previously reported that treatment with sedative/sleep-prolonging psychotropic medication in this population should be given with caution [42,43,86,87]. These simple practical recommendations could be easily applied in a primary care setting.

Supplementary Materials: The following are available online at https://www.mdpi.com/article/10.3390/healthcare10010143/s1, Table S1: Zero order and partial correlations of variables of interest with levels of IL-6, Table S2: Zero order and partial correlations of variables of interest with levels of TNF-a.

Author Contributions: M.B.: contributed to the design of the study, collection of data, data analysis, interpretation of results and writing of the manuscript; C.B.: contributed to literature search and writing of the manuscript; M.Y.: contributed to data analysis, interpretation of results and preparation of the manuscript; I.Z.: contributed to the design of the study, collection of data, inflammatory markers measurement and writing of the manuscript; P.S.: contributed to the design of the study, data analysis, interpretation of results and preparation of the manuscript; S.P.: participated in data collection and preparation of the manuscript; A.N.V.: participated in the design and overall supervision of the study, interpretation of results and preparation of the manuscript. All authors have read and agreed to the published version of the manuscript.

Funding: This study was supported by a grant from the National Strategic Reference Framework (ESPA) 2007–2013, Program: THALES, University of Crete, entitled: "A multi-disciplinary network for the study of Alzheimer's Disease" (Grant No. MIS 377299). No other financial support is associated with the current research for any of the authors. The content of the manuscript is solely the responsibility of the authors.

Institutional Review Board Statement: The study was conducted according to the guidelines laid down in the Declaration of Helsinki and all procedures involving human subjects/patients were approved by the Bioethics Committee of the University Hospital of Heraklion, Crete (Protocol Number: 13541, (20 November 2010).

Informed Consent Statement: Written informed consent was obtained from all subjects involved in the study.

Data Availability Statement: The data presented in this study are available on request from the corresponding author.

Acknowledgments: We thank study coordinator Cynthia Manasaki for her continuing support. We also thank all primary care physicians from the primary health care facilities and all the individuals who participated in this study.

Conflicts of Interest: None of the authors have any other conflict of interest to declare.

References

1. Irwin, M.; Opp, M. Sleep Health: Reciprocal Regulation of Sleep and Innate Immunity. *Neuropsychopharmacology* 2017, 42, 129–155. Available online: https://pubmed.ncbi.nlm.nih.gov/27510422/ (accessed on 6 March 2021). [CrossRef]
2. Ferrucci, L.; Fabbri, E. Inflammageing: Chronic Inflammation in Ageing, Cardiovascular Disease, and Frailty. *Nat. Rev. Cardiol.* 2018, 15, 505–522. Available online: https://www.nature.com/articles/s41569-018-0064-2 (accessed on 7 March 2021). [CrossRef]
3. Franceschi, C.; Campisi, J. Chronic Inflammation (Inflammaging) and Its Potential Contribution to Age-Associated Diseases. *J. Gerontol. Ser. A Biol. Sci. Med. Sci.* 2014, 69 (Suppl. 1), S4–S9. Available online: http://www.ncbi.nlm.nih.gov/pubmed/24833586 (accessed on 3 August 2019). [CrossRef]
4. Kennedy, B.K.; Berger, S.L.; Brunet, A.; Campisi, J.; Cuervo, A.M.; Epel, E.S.; Franceschi, C.; Lithgow, G.J.; Morimoto, R.I.; Pessin, J.E.; et al. Geroscience: Linking aging to chronic disease. *Cell* 2014, 159, 709–713. [CrossRef] [PubMed]
5. Ngandu, T.; Lehtisalo, J.; Solomon, A.; Levälahti, E.; Ahtiluoto, S.; Antikainen, R.; Bäckman, L.; Hänninen, T.; Jula, A.; Laatikainen, T.; et al. A 2 Year Multidomain Intervention of Diet, Exercise, Cognitive Training, and Vascular Risk Monitoring versus Control to Prevent Cognitive Decline in at-Risk Elderly People (FINGER): A Randomised Controlled Trial. *Lancet* 2015, 385, 2255–2263. Available online: https://pubmed.ncbi.nlm.nih.gov/25771249/ (accessed on 6 March 2021). [CrossRef]

6. Ticinesi, A.; Meschi, T.; Lauretani, F.; Felis, G.; Franchi, F.; Pedrolli, C.; Barichella, M.; Benati, G.; Di Nuzzo, S.; Ceda, G.P.; et al. Nutrition and Inflammation in Older Individuals: Focus on Vitamin, D, n-3 Polyunsaturated Fatty Acids and Whey Proteins. *Nutrients* **2016**, *8*, 186. Available online: https://pubmed.ncbi.nlm.nih.gov/27043616/ (accessed on 7 March 2021). [CrossRef]
7. Custodero, C.; Mankowski, R.T.; Lee, S.A.; Chen, Z.; Wu, S.; Manini, T.M.; Echeverri, J.; Sabbà, C.; Beavers, D.P.; Cauley, J.A.; et al. Evidence-Based Nutritional and Pharmacological Interventions Targeting Chronic Low-Grade Inflammation in Middle-Age and Older Adults: A Systematic Review and Meta-Analysis. *Ageing Res. Rev.* **2018**, *46*, 42–59. Available online: https://pubmed.ncbi.nlm.nih.gov/29803716/ (accessed on 7 March 2021). [CrossRef]
8. Milaneschi, Y.; Bandinelli, S.; Penninx, B.W.; Vogelzangs, N.; Corsi, A.M.; Lauretani, F.; Kisialiou, A.; Vazzana, R.; Terracciano, A.; Guralnik, J.M.; et al. Depressive Symptoms and Inflammation Increase in a Prospective Study of Older Adults: A Protective Effect of a Healthy (Mediterranean-Style) Diet. *Mol. Psychiatry* **2011**, *16*, 589–590. Available online: https://jhu.pure.elsevier.com/en/publications/depressive-symptoms-and-inflammation-increase-in-a-prospective-st-4 (accessed on 7 March 2021). [CrossRef]
9. Luciano, M.; Mõttus, R.; Starr, J.M.; McNeill, G.; Jia, X.; Craig, L.C.A.; Deary, I.L. Depressive Symptoms and Diet: Their Effects on Prospective Inflammation Levels in the Elderly. *Brain Behav. Immun.* **2012**, *26*, 717–720. Available online: https://abdn.pure.elsevier.com/en/publications/depressive-symptoms-and-diet-their-effects-on-prospective-inflamm (accessed on 7 March 2021). [CrossRef] [PubMed]
10. Ancoli-Israel, S.; Poceta, J.S.; Stepnowsky, C.; Martin, J.; Gehrman, P. Identification and Treatment of Sleep Problems in the Elderly. *Sleep Med. Rev.* **1997**, *1*, 3–17. Available online: http://www.ncbi.nlm.nih.gov/pubmed/15310520 (accessed on 3 August 2019). [CrossRef]
11. Martin, J.; Shochat, T.; Ancoli-Israel, S. Assessment and Treatment of Sleep Disturbances in Older Adults. *Clin. Psychol. Rev.* **2000**, *20*, 783–805. Available online: http://www.ncbi.nlm.nih.gov/pubmed/10983268 (accessed on 3 August 2019). [CrossRef]
12. Loiselle, M.M.; Means, M.K.; Edinger, J.D. Sleep Disturbances in Aging. *Adv. Cell Aging Gerontol.* **2005**, *17*, 33–59. Available online: https://www.sciencedirect.com/science/article/abs/pii/S1566312404170028 (accessed on 3 August 2019).
13. Vgontzas, A.N.; Zoumakis, M.; Bixler, E.O.; Lin, H.-M.; Prolo, P.; Vela-Bueno, A.; Kales, A.; Chrousos, G.P. Impaired Nighttime Sleep in Healthy Old *Versus* Young Adults Is Associated with Elevated Plasma Interleukin-6 and Cortisol Levels: Physiologic and Therapeutic Implications. *J. Clin. Endocrinol. Metab.* **2003**, *88*, 2087–2095. Available online: https://academic.oup.com/jcem/article-lookup/doi/10.1210/jc.2002-021176 (accessed on 12 August 2019). [CrossRef] [PubMed]
14. Von Känel, R.; Dimsdale, J.E.; Ancoli-Israel, S.; Mills, P.J.; Patterson, T.L.; McKibbin, C.L.; Ms, C.A.; Grant, I. Poor Sleep Is Associated with Higher Plasma Proinflammatory Cytokine Interleukin-6 and Procoagulant Marker Fibrin D-Dimer in Older Caregivers of People with Alzheimer's Disease. *J. Am. Geriatr. Soc.* **2006**, *54*, 431–437. Available online: http://doi.wiley.com/10.1111/j.1532-5415.2005.00642.x (accessed on 12 August 2019). [CrossRef] [PubMed]
15. Vgontzas, A.N.; Zoumakis, M.; Papanicolaou, D.A.; Bixler, E.O.; Prolo, P.; Lin, H.-M.; Vela-Bueno, A.; Kales, A.; Chrousos, G.P.; Vgontzas, A.N.; et al. Chronic Insomnia Is Associated with a Shift of Interleukin-6 and Tumor Necrosis Factor Secretion from Nighttime to Daytime. *Metabolism* **2002**, *51*, 887–892. Available online: http://www.ncbi.nlm.nih.gov/pubmed/12077736 (accessed on 26 July 2019). [CrossRef] [PubMed]
16. Burgos, I.; Richter, L.; Klein, T.; Fiebich, B.; Feige, B.; Lieb, K.; Voderholzer, U.; Riemann, D. Increased Nocturnal Interleukin-6 Excretion in Patients with Primary Insomnia: A Pilot Study. *Brain Behav. Immun.* **2006**, *20*, 246–253. Available online: https://www.sciencedirect.com/science/article/pii/S0889159105001108?via%3Dihub (accessed on 12 August 2019). [CrossRef]
17. Taheri, S.; Austin, D.; Lin, L.; Nieto, F.J.; Young, T.; Mignot, E. Correlates of Serum C-Reactive Protein (CRP)—No Association with Sleep Duration or Sleep Disordered Breathing. *Sleep* **2007**, *30*, 991–996. Available online: http://www.ncbi.nlm.nih.gov/pubmed/17702268 (accessed on 12 August 2019). [CrossRef] [PubMed]
18. Matthews, K.A.; Zheng, H.; Kravitz, H.M.; Sowers, M.; Bromberger, J.T.; Buysse, D.J.; Owens, J.F.; Sanders, M.; Hall, M. Are Inflammatory and Coagulation Biomarkers Related to Sleep Characteristics in Mid-Life Women?: Study of Women's Health across the Nation Sleep Study. *Sleep* **2010**, *33*, 1649–1655. Available online: http://www.ncbi.nlm.nih.gov/pubmed/21120127 (accessed on 12 August 2019). [CrossRef] [PubMed]
19. Abramson, J.L.; Vaccarino, V. Relationship between Physical Activity and Inflammation among Apparently Healthy Middle-Aged and Older US Adults. *Arch. Intern. Med.* **2002**, *162*, 1286–1292. Available online: https://pubmed.ncbi.nlm.nih.gov/12038947/ (accessed on 7 March 2019). [CrossRef]
20. Wannamethee, S.G.; Lowe, G.D.O.; Whincup, P.H.; Rumley, A.; Walker, M.; Lennon, L. Physical Activity and Hemostatic and Inflammatory Variables in Elderly Men. *Circulation* **2002**, *105*, 1785–1790. Available online: https://pubmed.ncbi.nlm.nih.gov/11956120/ (accessed on 7 March 2019). [CrossRef]
21. Reuben, D.B.; Judd-Hamilton, L.; Harris, T.B.; Seeman, T.E. The Associations between Physical Activity and Inflammatory Markers in High-Functioning Older Persons: MacArthur Studies of Successful Aging. *J. Am. Geriatr. Soc.* **2003**, *51*, 1125–1130. Available online: http://doi.wiley.com/10.1046/j.1532-5415.2003.51380.x (accessed on 18 April 2019). [CrossRef] [PubMed]
22. Colbert, L.H.; Visser, M.; Simonsick, E.M.; Tracy, R.P.; Newman, A.B.; Kritchevsky, S.B.; Pahor, M.; Taaffe, D.; Brach, J.; Rubin, S.; et al. Physical Activity, Exercise, and Inflammatory Markers in Older Adults: Findings from the Health, Aging and Body Composition Study. *J. Am. Geriatr. Soc.* **2004**, *52*, 1098–1104. Available online: https://pubmed.ncbi.nlm.nih.gov/15209647/ (accessed on 7 March 2019). [CrossRef] [PubMed]
23. Jankord, R.; Jemiolo, B. Influence of physical activity on serum IL-6 and IL-10 levels in healthy older men. *Med. Sci. Sports Exerc.* **2004**, *36*, 960–964. [CrossRef]

24. Elosua, R.; Bartali, B.; Ordovas, J.M.; Corsi, A.M.; Lauretani, F.; Ferrucci, L. Association Between Physical Activity, Physical Performance, and Inflammatory Biomarkers in an Elderly Population: The InCHIANTI Study. *J. Gerontol. Ser. A Biol. Sci. Med. Sci.* 2005, *60*, 760–767. Available online: https://academic.oup.com/biomedgerontology/article-abstract/60/6/760/590349 (accessed on 18 April 2019). [CrossRef]
25. Nicklas, B.J.; Beavers, D.P.; Mihalko, S.L.; Miller, G.D.; Loeser, R.F.; Messier, S.P. Relationship of Objectively-Measured Habitual Physical Activity to Chronic Inflammation and Fatigue in Middle-Aged and Older Adults. *J. Gerontol. Ser. A Biol. Sci. Med. Sci.* 2016, *71*, 1437–1443. Available online: https://pubmed.ncbi.nlm.nih.gov/27382039/ (accessed on 7 March 2019). [CrossRef]
26. Draganidis, D.; Jamurtas, A.; Stampoulis, T.; Laschou, V.; Deli, C.; Georgakouli, K.; Papanikolaou, K.; Chatzinikolaou, A.; Michalopoulou, M.; Papadopoulos, C.; et al. Disparate Habitual Physical Activity and Dietary Intake Profiles of Elderly Men with Low and Elevated Systemic Inflammation. *Nutrients* 2018, *10*, 566. Available online: http://www.mdpi.com/2072-6643/10/5/566 (accessed on 7 March 2019). [CrossRef] [PubMed]
27. Public Health England, 10 Minutes Brisk Walking Each Day in Mid-Life for Health Benefits and towards Achieving Physical Activity Recom-Mendations. Evidence Summary. Available online: https://assets.publishing.service.gov.uk/government/uploads/system/uploads/attachment_data/file/639030/Health_benefits_of_10_mins_brisk_walking_evidence_summary.pdf (accessed on 7 March 2019).
28. Alghadir, A.H.; Gabr, S.A.; Al-Momani, M.; Al-Momani, F. Moderate Aerobic Training Modulates Cytokines and Cortisol Profiles in Older Adults with Cognitive Abilities. *Cytokine* 2021, *138*, 155373. Available online: https://pubmed.ncbi.nlm.nih.gov/33248912/ (accessed on 7 March 2019). [CrossRef]
29. Stigger, F.S.; Zago Marcolino, M.A.; Portela, K.M.; Della Méa Plentz, R. Effects of Exercise on Inflammatory, Oxidative, and Neurotrophic Biomarkers on Cognitively Impaired Individuals Diagnosed with Dementia or Mild Cognitive Impairment: A Systematic Review and Meta-Analysis. *J. Gerontol. Ser. A Biol. Sci. Med. Sci.* 2019, *74*, 616–624. Available online: https://pubmed.ncbi.nlm.nih.gov/30084942/ (accessed on 7 March 2019). [CrossRef]
30. Petersen, R. Mild Cognitive Impairment. *N. Engl. J. Med.* 2011, *364*, 2227–2234. [CrossRef]
31. Petersen, R. Mild Cognitive Impairment. *Continuum Lifelong Learn. Neurol.* 2016, *22*, 404–418. [CrossRef]
32. Roberts, R.; Knopman, D. Classification and Epidemiology of MCI. *Clin. Geriart. Med.* 2013, *29*, 753–772. [CrossRef]
33. Zaganas, I.V.; Simos, P.; Basta, M.; Kapetanaki, S.; Panagiotakis, S.; Koutentaki, I.; Fountoulakis, N.; Bertsias, A.; Duijker, G.; Tziraki, C.; et al. The Cretan Aging Cohort: Cohort Description and Burden of Dementia and Mild Cognitive Impairment. *Am. J. Alzheimer's Dis. Other Dement.®* 2019, *34*, 23–33. Available online: http://www.ncbi.nlm.nih.gov/pubmed/30259758 (accessed on 11 September 2019). [CrossRef] [PubMed]
34. Fountoulakis, K.N.; Tsolaki, M.; Chantzi, H.; Kazis, A. Mini Mental State Examination (MMSE): A Validation Study in Greece. *Am. J. Alzheimer's Dis. Other Dement.®* 2000, *15*, 342–345. Available online: http://aja.sagepub.com/cgi/doi/10.1177/153331750001500604 (accessed on 11 September 2019). [CrossRef]
35. Dardiotis, E.; Kosmidis, M.H.; Yannakoulia, M.; Hadjigeorgiou, G.M.; Scarmeas, N. The Hellenic Longitudinal Investigation of Aging and Diet (HELIAD): Rationale, Study Design, and Cohort Description. *Neuroepidemiology* 2014, *43*, 9–14. Available online: https://www.karger.com/Article/FullText/362723 (accessed on 11 September 2019). [CrossRef]
36. Winblad, B.; Palmer, K.; Kivipelto, M.; Jelic, V.; Fratiglioni, L.; Wahlund, L.-O.; Nordberg, A.; Bäckman, L.; Albert, M.; Almkvist, O.; et al. Mild Cognitive Impairment—Beyond Controversies, towards a Consensus: Report of the International Working Group on Mild Cognitive Impairment. *J. Intern. Med.* 2004, *256*, 240–246. Available online: http://doi.wiley.com/10.1111/j.1365-2796.2004.01380.x (accessed on 22 March 2021). [CrossRef]
37. Simos, P.; Papastefanakis, E.; Panou, T.; Kasselimis, D. *The Greek Memory Scale*; Laboratory of Applied Psychology, University of Crete: Rethymno, Greece, 2011.
38. Bountziouka, V.; Bathrellou, E.; Giotopoulou, A.; Katsagoni, C.; Bonou, M.; Vallianou, N.; Barbetseas, J.; Avgerinos, P.C.; Panagiotakos, D.B. Development, Repeatability and Validity Regarding Energy and Macronutrient Intake of a Semi-Quantitative Food Frequency Questionnaire: Methodological Considerations. *Nutr. Metab. Cardiovasc. Dis.* 2012, *22*, 659–667. Available online: https://pubmed.ncbi.nlm.nih.gov/21269818/ (accessed on 7 March 2021). [CrossRef]
39. Panagiotakos, D.B.; Pitsavos, C.; Stefanadis, C. Dietary Patterns: A Mediterranean Diet Score and Its Relation to Clinical and Biological Markers of Cardiovascular Disease Risk. *Nutr. Metab. Cardiovasc. Dis.* 2006, *16*, 559–568. Available online: https://pubmed.ncbi.nlm.nih.gov/17126772/ (accessed on 7 March 2021). [CrossRef]
40. Vgontzas, A.N.; Liao, D.; Pejovic, S.; Calhoun, S.; Karataraki, M.; Basta, M.; Fernández-Mendoza, J.; Bixler, E.O. Insomnia with short sleep duration and mortality: The Penn State cohort. *Sleep* 2010, *33*, 1159–1164. [CrossRef]
41. Mednick, S.C.; Ehrman, M. *Take a Nap! Change Your Life*, 1st ed.; Workman Publishing: New York, NY, USA, 2006; ISBN 978-0-7611-4290-4.
42. Basta, M.; Koutentaki, E.; Vgontzas, A.N.; Zaganas, I.; Vogiatzi, E.; Gouna, G.; Bourbouli, M.; Panagiotakis, S.; Kapetanaki, S.; Fernandez-Mendoza, J.; et al. Objective daytime napping is associated with disease severity and inflammation in patients with mild to moderate dementia. *J. Alzheimer's Dis.* 2020, *74*, 803–815. [CrossRef]
43. Basta, M.; Simos, P.; Vgontzas, A.; Koutentaki, E.; Tziraki, S.; Zaganas, I.; Panagiotakis, S.; Kapetanaki, S.; Fountoulakis, N.; Lionis, C. Associations between sleep duration and cognitive impairment in mild cognitive impairment. *J. Sleep Res.* 2019, *28*, e12864. [CrossRef]

44. Department of Health. Start Active Stay Active. 2011. Available online: https://www.gov.uk/government/publications/start-active-stay-active-a-report-on-physical-activity-from-the-four-home-countries-chief-medical-officers (accessed on 7 March 2019).
45. Faul, F.; Erdfelder, E.; Buchner, A.; Lang, A.G. Statistical Power Analyses Using G*Power 3.1: Tests for Correlation and Regression Analyses. *Behav. Res. Methods* **2009**, *41*, 1149–1160. Available online: https://pubmed.ncbi.nlm.nih.gov/19897823/ (accessed on 9 April 2021). [CrossRef]
46. Puzianowska-Kuźnicka, M.; Owczarz, M.; Wieczorowska-Tobis, K.; Nadrowski, P.; Chudek, J.; Slusarczyk, P.; Skalska, A.; Jonas, M.; Franek, E.; Mossakowska, M. Interleukin-6 and C-reactive protein, successful aging, and mortality: The PolSenior study. *Immun. Ageing* **2016**, *13*, 21. [CrossRef]
47. Charlton, R.A.; Lamar, M.; Zhang, A.; Ren, X.; Ajilore, O.; Pandey, G.N.; Kumar, A. Associations between pro-inflammatory cytokines, learning, and memory in late-life depression and healthy aging. *Int. J. Geriatr. Psychiatry* **2018**, *33*, 104–112. [CrossRef] [PubMed]
48. Root, M.M.; Mcginn, M.C.; Nieman, D.C.; Henson, D.A.; Heinz, S.A.; Shanely, R.A.; Knab, A.M.; Jin, F. Combined Fruit and Vegetable Intake Is Correlated with Improved Inflammatory and Oxidant Status from a Cross-Sectional Study in a Community Setting. *Nutrients* **2012**, *4*, 29–41. Available online: https://pubmed.ncbi.nlm.nih.gov/22347616/ (accessed on 7 March 2021). [CrossRef]
49. Piccand, E.; Vollenweider, P.; Guessous, I.; Marques-Vidal, P. Association between Dietary Intake and Inflammatory Markers: Results from the CoLaus Study. *Public Health Nutr.* **2019**, *22*, 498–505. Available online: https://pubmed.ncbi.nlm.nih.gov/30333073/ (accessed on 11 March 2021). [CrossRef]
50. Jiang, Y.; Wu, S.H.; Shu, X.O.; Xiang, Y.B.; Ji, B.T.; Milne, G.L.; Cai, Q.; Zhang, X.; Gao, Y.; Zheng, W.; et al. Cruciferous Vegetable Intake Is Inversely Correlated with Circulating Levels of Proinflammatory Markers in Women. *J. Acad. Nutr. Diet.* **2014**, *114*, 700–708.e2. Available online: https://pubmed.ncbi.nlm.nih.gov/24630682/ (accessed on 7 March 2021). [CrossRef]
51. Hildreth, K.L.; Van Pelt, R.E.; Moreau, K.L.; Grigsby, J.; Hoth, K.F.; Pelak, V.; Anderson, C.A.; Parnes, B.; Kittelson, J.; Wolfe, P.; et al. Effects of Pioglitazone or Exercise in Older Adults with Mild Cognitive Impairment and Insulin Resistance: A Pilot Study. *Dement. Geriatr. Cogn. Dis. Extra* **2015**, *5*, 51–63. Available online: https://pubmed.ncbi.nlm.nih.gov/25852732/ (accessed on 7 March 2021). [CrossRef]
52. Tabung, F.K.; Smith-Warner, S.A.; Chavarro, J.E.; Wu, K.; Fuchs, C.S.; Hu, F.B.; Chan, A.T.; Willett, W.C.; Giovannucci, E.L. Development and validation of an empirical dietary inflammatory index. *J. Nutr.* **2016**, *146*, 1560–1570. [CrossRef]
53. Willett, W.C.; Sacks, F.; Trichopoulou, A.; Drescher, G.; Ferro-Luzzi, A.; Helsing, E.; Trichopoulos, D. Mediterranean Diet Pyramid: A Cultural Model for Healthy Eating. *Am. J. Clin. Nutr.* **1995**, *61*, 1402S–1406S. Available online: https://pubmed.ncbi.nlm.nih.gov/7754995/ (accessed on 7 March 2021). [CrossRef]
54. Bertsias, G.; Linardakis, M.; Mammas, I.; Kafatos, A. Fruit and vegetables consumption in relation to health and diet of medical students in Crete, Greece. *Int. J. Vitam. Nutr. Res.* **2005**, *75*, 107–117. [CrossRef] [PubMed]
55. Rehm, C.D.; Peñalvo, J.L.; Afshin, A.; Mozaffarian, D. Dietary Intake among US Adults, 1999–2012. *JAMA* **2016**, *315*, 2542–2553. [CrossRef]
56. Hoy, M.K.; Goldman, J.D.; Sebastian, R.S. Fruit and vegetable intake of US adults estimated by two methods: What We Eat in America, National Health and Nutrition Examination Survey 2009–2012. *Public Health Nutr.* **2016**, *19*, 2508–2512. [CrossRef] [PubMed]
57. Nicklett, E.J.; Kadell, A.R. Fruit and vegetable intake among older adults: A scoping review. *Maturitas* **2013**, *75*, 305–312. [CrossRef]
58. Anastasiou, C.A.; Yannakoulia, M.; Kosmidis, M.H.; Dardiotis, E.; Hadjigeorgiou, G.M.; Sakka, P.; Arampatzi, X.; Bougea, A.; Labropoulos, I.; Scarmeas, N. Mediterranean diet and cognitive health: Initial results from the Hellenic Longitudinal Investigation of Ageing and Diet. *PLoS ONE* **2017**, *12*, e0182048. [CrossRef] [PubMed]
59. Yang, L.; Lu, R.; Jiang, L.; Liu, Z.; Peng, Y. Expression and Genetic Analysis of Tumor Necrosis Factor-α (TNF-α) G-308A Polymorphism in Sporadic Alzheimer's Disease in a Southern China Population. *Brain Res.* **2009**, *1247*, 178–181. Available online: https://pubmed.ncbi.nlm.nih.gov/18992723/ (accessed on 7 March 2021). [CrossRef]
60. Bagyinszky, E.; Van Giau, V.; Shim, K.; Suk, K.; An, S.S.A.; Kim, S.Y. Role of Inflammatory Molecules in the Alzheimer's Disease Progression and Diagnosis. *J. Neurol. Sci.* **2017**, *376*, 242–254. Available online: https://pubmed.ncbi.nlm.nih.gov/28431620/ (accessed on 7 March 2021). [CrossRef] [PubMed]
61. Kaplin, A.; Carroll, K.A.L.; Cheng, J.; Allie, R.; Lyketsos, C.G.; Calabresi, P.; Kaplin, A. IL-6 Release by LPS-Stimulated Peripheral Blood Mononuclear Cells as a Potential Biomarker in Alzheimer's Disease. *Int. Psychogeriatr.* **2009**, *21*, 413–414. Available online: https://www.ncbi.nlm.nih.gov/pmc/articles/pmid/19040786/?tool=EBI (accessed on 7 March 2021). [CrossRef] [PubMed]
62. Weiner, M.W.; Veitch, D.P.; Aisen, P.S.; Beckett, L.A.; Cairns, N.J.; Green, R.C.; Harvey, D.; Jack, C.R.; Jagust, W.; Liu, E.; et al. The Alzheimer's Disease Neuroimaging Initiative: A Review of Papers Published since Its Inception. *Alzheimer's Dement.* **2013**, *9*, e111–e194. Available online: http://www.ncbi.nlm.nih.gov/pmc/articles/PMC4108198/ (accessed on 7 March 2019). [CrossRef]
63. Morris, M.C.; Tangney, C.C.; Wang, Y.; Sacks, F.M.; Bennett, D.A.; Aggarwal, N.T. MIND Diet Associated with Reduced Incidence of Alzheimer's Disease. *Alzheimer's Dement.* **2015**, *11*, 1007–1014. Available online: http://www.ncbi.nlm.nih.gov/pubmed/25681666 (accessed on 8 October 2019). [CrossRef]
64. Irwin, M.R.; Olmstead, R.; Carroll, J.E. Sleep disturbance, sleep duration, and inflammation: A systematic review and meta-analysis of cohort studies and experimental sleep deprivation. *Biol. Psychiatry* **2016**, *80*, 40–52. [CrossRef]
65. Smagula, S.F.; Harrison, S.; Cauley, J.A.; Ancoli-Israel, S.; Cawthon, P.M.; Cummings, S.; Stone, K.L. Determinants of Change in Objectively Assessed Sleep Duration among Older Men. *Am. J. Epidemiol.* **2017**, *185*, 933–940. [CrossRef]

66. Kripke, D.F.; Langer, R.D.; Elliott, J.A.; Klauber, M.R.; Rex, K.M. Mortality Related to Actigraphic Long and Short Sleep. *Sleep Med.* **2011**, *12*, 28–33. Available online: https://pubmed.ncbi.nlm.nih.gov/20870457/ (accessed on 7 March 2021). [CrossRef]
67. Irwin, M.R.; Vitiello, M.V. Implications of sleep disturbance and inflammation for Alzheimer's disease dementia. *Lancet Neurol.* **2019**, *18*, 296–306. [CrossRef]
68. Spira, A.P.; Stone, K.L.; Redline, S.; Ensrud, K.E.; Ancoli-Israel, S.; Cauley, J.A.; Yaffe, K. Actigraphic Sleep Duration and Fragmentation in Older Women: Associations with Performance across Cognitive Domains. *Sleep* **2017**, *40*, zsx073. [CrossRef]
69. Jike, M.; Itani, O.; Watanabe, N.; Buysse, D.J.; Kaneita, Y. Long sleep duration and health outcomes: A systematic review, meta-analysis and meta-regression. *Sleep Med. Rev.* **2018**, *39*, 25–36. [CrossRef]
70. Azevedo Da Silva, M.; Singh-Manoux, A.; Shipley, M.J.; Vahtera, J.; Brunner, E.J.; Ferrie, J.E.; Kivimäki, M.; Nabi, H. Sleep duration and sleep disturbances partly explain the association between depressive symptoms and cardiovascular mortality: The Whitehall II cohort study. *J. Sleep Res.* **2014**, *23*, 94–97. [CrossRef]
71. Patel, S.R.; Zhu, X.; Storfer-Isser, A.; Mehra, R.; Jenny, N.S.; Tracy, R.; Redline, S. Sleep duration and biomarkers of inflammation. *Sleep* **2009**, *32*, 200–204. [CrossRef] [PubMed]
72. Irwin, M.R. Why Sleep Is Important for Health: A Psychoneuroimmunology Perspective. *Annu. Rev. Psychol.* **2015**, *66*, 143–172. Available online: http://www.ncbi.nlm.nih.gov/pubmed/25061767 (accessed on 3 August 2019). [CrossRef]
73. Taveras, E.M.; Rifas-Shiman, S.L.; Rich-Edwards, J.W.; Mantzoros, C.S. Maternal Short Sleep Duration Is Associated with Increased Levels of Inflammatory Markers at 3 Years Postpartum. *Metabolism* **2011**, *60*, 982–986. Available online: http://www.ncbi.nlm.nih.gov/pubmed/21040938 (accessed on 23 October 2019). [CrossRef]
74. Miller, M.A.; Kandala, N.-B.; Kivimaki, M.; Kumari, M.; Brunner, E.J.; Lowe, G.D.O.; Marmot, M.G.; Cappuccio, F.P. Gender Differences in the Cross-Sectional Relationships between Sleep Duration and Markers of Inflammation: Whitehall II Study. *Sleep* **2009**, *32*, 857–864. Available online: http://www.ncbi.nlm.nih.gov/pubmed/19639748 (accessed on 7 October 2019).
75. Vgontzas, A.N.; Zoumakis, E.; Bixler, E.O.; Lin, H.-M.; Follett, H.; Kales, A.; Chrousos, G.P. Adverse Effects of Modest Sleep Restriction on Sleepiness, Performance, and Inflammatory Cytokines. *J. Clin. Endocrinol. Metab.* **2004**, *89*, 2119–2126. Available online: https://academic.oup.com/jcem/article-lookup/doi/10.1210/jc.2003-031562 (accessed on 26 July 2019). [CrossRef]
76. Vgontzas, A.N.; Pejovic, S.; Zoumakis, E.; Lin, H.M.; Bixler, E.O.; Basta, M.; Fang, J.; Sarrigiannidis, A.; Chrousos, G.P. Daytime Napping after a Night of Sleep Loss Decreases Sleepiness, Improves Performance, and Causes Beneficial Changes in Cortisol and Interleukin-6 Secretion. *Am. J. Physiol. Metab.* **2007**, *292*, E253–E261. Available online: http://www.physiology.org/doi/10.1152/ajpendo.00651.2005 (accessed on 16 July 2019). [CrossRef]
77. Pejovic, S.; Basta, M.; Vgontzas, A.N.; Kritikou, I.; Shaffer, M.L.; Tsaoussoglou, M.; Stiffler, D.; Stefanakis, Z.; Bixler, O.E.; Chrousos, G.P. Effects of Recovery Sleep after One Work Week of Mild Sleep Restriction on Interleukin-6 and Cortisol Secretion and Daytime Sleepiness and Performance. *Am. J. Physiol. Metab.* **2013**, *305*, E890–E896. Available online: https://www.physiology.org/doi/10.1152/ajpendo.00301.2013 (accessed on 7 March 2021). [CrossRef]
78. Opp, M.R.; Kapas, L.; Toth, L.A. Cytokine involvement in the regulation of sleep. *Proc. Soc. Exp. Biol. Med.* **1992**, *201*, 16–27. [CrossRef]
79. Moldofsky, H.; Lue, F.A.; Eisen, J.; Keystone, E.; Gorczynski, R.M. The relationship of interleukin-1 and immune functions to sleep in humans. *Psychosom. Med.* **1986**, *48*, 309–318. [CrossRef] [PubMed]
80. Vgontzas, A.N.; Papanicolaou, D.A.; Bixler, E.O.; Kales, A.; Tyson, K.; Chrousos, G.P. Elevation of plasma cytokines in disorders of excessive daytime sleepiness: Role of sleep disturbance and obesity. *J. Clin. Endocrinol. Metab.* **1997**, *82*, 1313–1316. [CrossRef]
81. Vgontzas, A.N.; Zoumakis, E.; Lin, H.M.; Bixler, E.O.; Trakada, G.; Chrousos, G.P. Marked decrease in sleepiness in patients with sleep apnea by etanercept, a tumor necrosis factor-alpha antagonist. *J. Clin. Endocrinol. Metab.* **2004**, *89*, 4409–4413. [CrossRef]
82. Moy, M.L.; Teylan, M.; Weston, N.A.; Gagnon, D.R.; Danilack, V.A.; Garshick, E. Daily Step Count Is Associated with Plasma c-Reactive Protein and il-6 in a us Cohort with COPD. *Chest* **2014**, *145*, 542–550. Available online: https://pubmed.ncbi.nlm.nih.gov/24091482/ (accessed on 7 March 2021). [CrossRef] [PubMed]
83. Wåhlin-Larsson, B.; Carnac, G.; Kadi, F. The Influence of Systemic Inflammation on Skeletal Muscle in Physically Active Elderly Women. *Age* **2014**, *36*, 9718. Available online: https://pubmed.ncbi.nlm.nih.gov/25311555/ (accessed on 7 March 2021). [CrossRef]
84. Fischer, C.P.; Berntsen, A.; Perstrup, L.B.; Eskildsen, P.; Pedersen, B.K. Plasma Levels of Interleukin-6 and C-Reactive Protein Are Associated with Physical Inactivity Independent of Obesity. *Scand. J. Med. Sci. Sport* **2007**, *17*, 580–587. Available online: https://pubmed.ncbi.nlm.nih.gov/17076827/ (accessed on 7 March 2021). [CrossRef] [PubMed]
85. Bixler, E.O.; Vgontzas, A.N.; Ten Have, T.; Tyson, K.; Kales, A. Effects of Age on Sleep Apnea in Men. *Am. J. Respir. Crit. Care Med.* **1998**, *157*, 144–148. Available online: http://www.atsjournals.org/doi/abs/10.1164/ajrccm.157.1.9706079 (accessed on 8 October 2019). [CrossRef] [PubMed]
86. Basta, M.; Zaganas, I.; Simos, P.; Koutentaki, E.; Dimovasili, C.; Mathioudakis, L.; Bourbouli, M.; Panagiotakis, S.; Kapetanaki, S.; Vgontzas, A. Apolipoprotein E $\epsilon 4$ (APOE $\epsilon 4$) Allele is Associated with Long Sleep Duration among Elderly with Cognitive Impairment. *J. Alzheimer's Dis.* **2021**, *79*, 763–771. [CrossRef] [PubMed]
87. Moga, D.C.; Taipale, H.; Tolppanen, A.M.; Tanskanen, A.; Tiihonen, J.; Hartikainen, S.; Wu, Q.; Jicha, G.A.; Gnjidic, D. A Comparison of Sex Differences in Psychotropic Medication Use in Older People with Alzheimer's Disease in the US and Finland. *Drugs Aging* **2017**, *34*, 55–65. Available online: https://europepmc.org/articles/PMC5253689 (accessed on 7 March 2021). [CrossRef] [PubMed]

MDPI AG
Grosspeteranlage 5
4052 Basel
Switzerland
Tel.: +41 61 683 77 34

Healthcare Editorial Office
E-mail: healthcare@mdpi.com
www.mdpi.com/journal/healthcare

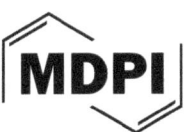

Disclaimer/Publisher's Note: The title and front matter of this reprint are at the discretion of the Guest Editor. The publisher is not responsible for their content or any associated concerns. The statements, opinions and data contained in all individual articles are solely those of the individual Editor and contributors and not of MDPI. MDPI disclaims responsibility for any injury to people or property resulting from any ideas, methods, instructions or products referred to in the content.

www.ingramcontent.com/pod-product-compliance
Lightning Source LLC
LaVergne TN
LVHW070001100526
838202LV00019B/2603